Breaching Safe Nursing Practice

T0094294

Breaching Safe Nursing Practice

Case Studies of Failures, Omissions, Commissions and Crimes

Edited by Zane Robinson Wolf
and Denise Nagle Bailey

McFarland & Company, Inc., Publishers
Jefferson, North Carolina

This book has undergone peer review.

ISBN (print) 978-1-4766-8339-3
ISBN (ebook) 978-1-4766-4476-9

Library of Congress and British Library
cataloguing data are available

Library of Congress Control Number 2022026661

© 2022 Zane Robinson Wolf and Denise Nagle Bailey. All rights reserved

*No part of this book may be reproduced or transmitted in any form
or by any means, electronic or mechanical, including photocopying
or recording, or by any information storage and retrieval system,
without permission in writing from the publisher.*

Front cover photograph © 2022 Shutterstock

Printed in the United States of America

*McFarland & Company, Inc., Publishers
Box 611, Jefferson, North Carolina 28640
www.mcfarlandpub.com*

To the nurses in our family: Zana Wolf DeProspo,
Gwynneth Jarrell, Gale Robinson-Smith, and Elise Robinson
Pizzi; to my grandchildren, Ciara and Rory Dasher, Elizabeth
and Robinson Wolf, and Zane Leo DeProspo; to my husband,
Charles J. Wolf; and to my nursing students and colleagues.
—Zane Robinson Wolf

and

To my husband, G. Alan Bailey, and family for their
many years of collective support in my academic endeavors
and to all of my former nursing students, who are now
practicing in varied clinical settings.
—Denise Nagle Bailey

Acknowledgments

Dr. Bailey and I appreciate the contributions of our colleagues to this book. They were asked to examine difficult issues in nursing practice and delivered excellent chapters. We also benefited from the comments of reviews. The support of La Salle University's Connelly Library staff is a continued gift and contributed mightily to this work. Thanks also goes to Dr. Shirley Gordon, past president of the International Association for Human Caring, for granting permission to use a table published in the *International Journal for Human Caring*.

Reviewers

We appreciate the recommendations of the reviewers and Dré Person, assistant editor at McFarland. Their reviews helped us to improve the manuscript. Thank you for your critique.

Table of Contents

Introduction

Zane Robinson Wolf, PhD, RN, CNE,
FCPP, ANEF, FAAN, *and* Denise Nagle Bailey,
EdD, RN, MEd, MSN, CSN, FCPP

Health care professionals carry out actions that promote the safety of patients and employees whenever they provide health care services. Whether caring for patients in their homes or in acute care institutions and long-term care settings, teams of caregivers work to improve the well-being and health of patients and families who trust in their expertise and commitment to excellent care. The access that nurses and their colleagues have to patients and families is a sacred trust. Many health care providers live that trust. They are alone in caregiving situations with vulnerable patients and ethically carry out their work. Few harm patients.

Nurses might suspect that something is not right with their colleagues' nursing care or that of other health care providers. They might witness situations that threaten patient safety and may or may not act as protectors of the defenseless. Nurses may hesitate to share misgivings or suspicions with managers and administrators, perhaps fearing retribution in the form of ostracism at work or worse (Wolf, 2020). The same concerns apply to interactions between nurses. Bullying events can be public or private. Witnesses may or may not intervene. Some nurses resign positions to work at other institutions because of toxic providers.

Literature on threats to patient and nurse safety, security, happiness, and satisfaction with health care and with work environments is scattered throughout published works. Few have combined challenging, difficult nursing practice topics in one document. This book was conceived as a resource for nursing students and practicing nurses to highlight some aspects of the shadows and gray and dark sides of nursing practice. Chapters include examples and circumstances of gray or dark side nursing activities and challenges that threaten the welfare of patients and nursing staff.

The book addresses selected violations of professional nursing conduct and practices that take place in shadows or on the margins of clinical practice. A nursing practice violation is defined as an infraction or abuse of professional nursing standards; it is conduct that involves action or inaction in the delivery of patient care (Benner et al., 2010). A professional nursing violation is defined as unprofessional conduct that involves action or inaction at work that harms a nurse colleague. Examples are found in this book.

Since patients and nurse colleagues are harmed resulting from intentional acts or failure to act, examples of the dark side of nursing were selected to assist nurses in understanding these violations and deviations in professional nursing practice. We also chose examples of practices that are often used but seldom questioned, such as those in the gray zone. We hope that by reviewing strategies, based on empirical and theoretical literature and concepts incorporated in relevant theories, that instances of violations or accepted but seldom-questioned practice activities might be reduced or eliminated from professional nursing.

Ethical principles are examined in chapters of the book as is nurses' professional responsibility to care for vulnerable people. The book is based on these standards as the nurse-patient relationship unfolds; nurses' knowledge and capabilities are used as they act on behalf of patients (Benner et al., 2010). Nurses put patients first and advocate for them (Benner et al., 2010). References to caring theories are also found in the chapters of this book. This is not surprising, because many contributors are grounded in caring theories and science; these theories are framed by ethical principles.

Each chapter presents a critical incident showing the gray or dark side of nursing. Chapters are framed by peer-reviewed theoretical and empirical literature and strategies that might help to improve nursing care and address professional challenges. Authors use evidence-based interventions, activities, or strategies that assist nurses in analyzing and reducing such problems in nursing. The hope is to acknowledge the gray zones of practice, to prevent the dark side of nursing incidents, and to illustrate the complexities of caregiving situations. Recommendations are made, selected from professional literature, poetry, and film, and critical incidents are described, showing the gray or dark side of nursing and approaches to eliminate or address them.

Different types of references support the chapters in the book in the main reference section. Authors conducted a search of various databases to locate relevant citations. References from personal collections were also used. However, literature on some topics was not abundant.

Each chapter includes a table on strategies, such as actions and models, targeting the chapter's problem and highlighting specific research. Other references, chosen by authors (Author Selection), highlight their preferences from professional literature, poetry, films, etc., that match chapter topics. Answers to test questions for each chapter are found at the end of the book, before the index.

The chapters of the book were guided by the following structure:

Objectives	Author selections of professional
Critical Incident	literature, poetry, films, etc.,
Background	illustrating gray or dark side of
Literature	nursing topics
Strategies	References
Conclusion	Multiple-Choice Questions
Discussion Questions	

We hope by bringing examples of nursing in the shadows and the dark side forward that discussions may follow. Conversations that are inspired by chapters in this book could shed light on the issues examined and stimulate changes in nursing practice and health care settings.

The aims of this book are to:

1. identify threats to patient and nurse well-being that are antithetical to nurses' principles, common practices, caring work, and ethics,

2. sensitize nurses and other stakeholders to gray and dark side of nursing incidents and practices through case examples and empirical, theoretical, ethical, legal, and artistic literature and products,

3. examine concepts associated with strategies for eliminating the dark side of nursing incidents, and

4. pose evidence-based solutions for eliminating, mitigating, and addressing examples representing the gray or dark side of nursing.

In Chapter 1, "The Dark Side of Nursing," the presence of the dark and gray side of nursing practice is explored as is classic literature in which the opposite of good nursing practice was introduced by pioneers who learned about noncaring nursing practice from patients. Ethical practice and regulatory standards are explored. Research on practice violations is reviewed; few studies were located on state board data. Chapter 2, "Justifying Coercion in Patient Care," describes the practice of coercion to accomplish improved patient outcomes when clinical situations are difficult. Various types of coercion are explored. Nurses use coercive approaches to manage patients seen to be in danger. Chapter 3, "Lying to Patients for Therapeutic Ends," also reviews an assumed-to-be-helpful and practical strategy, lying to patients, that nurses and other professionals use to convince patients to change behavior and consequently progress to desired clinical outcomes. Types of lying are discussed, specifically compassionate lying. Placebos and health care errors are also explored.

Chapter 4, "Blurred Lines: Professional Boundary Violations," delves into professional boundary issues between nurses and patients, whereby boundaries gradually dissolve as boundary crossings transition to boundary violations. State boards of nursing complaints and resulting sanctions for practice violations are noted. Guidelines for dealing with boundary violations are discussed. Chapter 5, "'Difficult' Patients," explores the challenges of carrying out a therapeutic nurse-patient relationship when patients' care burden or patients' behavior result in nurse frustration and avoidance. The power gradient between nurses and patients is examined as is a recommendation for nurses to self-reflect on their practice.

Chapter 6, "Neglect and Negligence of Patients," notes that nurses and others fail to provide appropriate and timely care to patients, with the result of patient suffering, even death. Examples of patient neglect and nurse negligence are described. Vulnerable groups of patients are at risk for harmful outcomes; interventions are framed by providers' obligation to provide safe care. Definitions of neglect and negligence are compared. In Chapter 7, "Physical Abuse of Patients," examples of physical abuse of patients are provided, including abuse of older persons, application of restraints and use of seclusion for psychiatric patients, and abuse of maternity patients. Cultural and social status implications are explored, and a recommendation is made that nursing assistants receive education on conflict resolution and interventions for caring for residents with dementia.

Chapter 8, "Bullying by Nurses," situates bullying in health care using historical antecedents. Terminology on bullying types is contrasted with incivility and discrimination. Bullying across health care and educational settings is explored. In Chapter 9, "Relational Incompetence: The Witnessing Nurse," relational incompetence, or the intentional act of not intervening when witnessing a peer's incompetence, is examined. The ethical roots of nursing practice focus the chapter on the obligation to report incompetence and explore the construct of competence in Roach's (2002) caring theory.

Reckless behavior is discussed in Chapter 10, "Reckless Nursing Care," in the context of the complexities of high-consequence health care delivery systems. It considers the patterns of providers that intentionally disregard professional standards and ethical codes of conduct. Threats to patient safety are framed by health care administrators' challenges to address behaviors and counsel and discipline nurses and others recognized as they typically and consistently bend the rules. The next step of submitting complaints to a state board of nursing is reviewed. Chapter 11, "Missed Nursing Care: A Covert Error of Omission," considers the daily threat to patient safety of missed nursing care, whether missed in part or whole or delayed. Examples include prescribed treatments and basic nursing care. The responsibility of registered nurses to delegate and supervise other health care workers is discussed, along with professional standards and nursing models, the Quality Caring Model©, and the Missed Nursing Care Model.

Chapter 12, "Shielding from Bad News," contemplates health care providers' responsibility of truth-telling about bad news in situations in which cancer, other difficult diagnoses, and death are in the foreground. The barriers restricting the sharing of weighty messages are countered by suggestions to plan communication episodes in consideration of patients' personal, family, and cultural orientations. So, too, is nurses' responsibility to share information following the initial episode of sharing of bad news.

Chapter 13, "Failure to Report Abuse and Whistleblowing," explains cases in which nurse defendants were tried for failure to report abuse and lapses of care. The need to change organizational cultures is noted, specifically in institutions appearing to condone disturbing employee conduct. The implications of whistleblowing are presented in cases involving nurse whistleblowers. Fear of retaliation resulting from reporting unsafe work environments could influence responses to unsafe care and create ethical dilemmas for nurses.

In Chapter 14, "Homicide and Nursing Staff," murder is examined as the worst example of nursing practice. Although the incidence of murder is very low, nonetheless it requires attention. Often nurse colleagues are naïve about its possibility. Charges against nurses lead to convictions and imprisonment or ruined reputations, in the case of those for whom acquittal decisions are published. Of note is that checklists on troublesome behavior have to be used carefully, because most evidence is circumstantial.

In Chapter 15, "Mistakes Versus Crimes," categories of behavioral concepts associated with health care errors are examined. The criminalization of mistakes is explored. Errors do not show intent; however, reckless nursing care and crimes do indicate intent. In contrast, the recognition and support of nurses and other health care providers who make errors and consequently suffer need to continue in health care institutions.

It is important to acknowledge the nursing pioneers who have considered the gray and dark sides of nursing practice. Two pioneers need to be thanked; they inspired us to go forward. We appreciate the work of Drs. Mary Corley and Suzanne Goren for their article on the dark side of nursing (Corley & Goren, 1998). We are also indebted to Dr. Beatrice Crofts Yorker Schumacher (2018) who is an expert on murder of patients in health care settings. Drs. Doris Riemen (1986) and Sigridur Halldorsdottir (1991) caught the attention of nurses fluent in caring science to consideration of patients' perspectives when uncaring nursing practice was received.

We thank the health care providers who continue to provide excellent care to patients and families and who strive daily for safety and excellent outcomes for those served and for those who serve them. They are our heroes, as seen in the caring work of colleagues throughout the COVID-19 pandemic. We hope that during clinical situations, where nurses and their colleagues are caring for patients, families, and each other, they remember to practice loving kindness for themselves and others each day.

REFERENCES

Benner, P., Leonard, V., Shulman, L.S., Day, L., & Sutphen, M. (2010). *Nurses: A Call for Radical Transformation*. Jossey Bass.

Corley, M.C., & Goren, S. (1998). The dark side of nursing: Impact of stigmatizing responses on patients. *Scholarly Inquiry for Nursing Practice: An International Journal, 12*(2), 99–119.

Halldorsdottir, S. (1991). Five basic modes of being with another. In D. Gaut, & M.M. Leininger (Eds.), *Caring: The compassionate healer* (pp. 37–49). National League for Nursing Press.

National Council of State Boards of Nursing, Benner, P.E., Scott, K., Sheets, V., Goettsche, V., & Patterson, L. (2010). Practice breakdown: Professional responsibility and patient advocacy. In P.E. Benner, K. Malloch, & V. Sheets, *Nursing pathways for patient safety* (pp. 138–149). Mosby Elsevier.

Riemen, D. (1986). Noncaring and caring in the clinical setting: Patient descriptions. *Topics in Clinical Nursing, 8* (2), 30–36.

Roach, M.S. (2002). *Caring, the human mode of being: A blueprint for the health professions* (2nd Rev. ed.). CHA Press.

Schumacher, B.C.Y. (2018, May 27). *Exhibit-163: Expert Report. To Mark Zigler, Toronto, Canada*. https://-Exhibit-163_Expert-Report-of-Professor-Beatrice-Crofts-Yorker.pdf.

Watson Caring Science Institute. (2010). *Core concepts of Jean Watson's theory of human caring/caring science*. https://www.scribd.com/document/245464310/Watsons-Theory-of-Human-Caring-Core-Concepts-and-Evolution-to-Caritas-Processes-Handout.

Wolf, Z.R. (2019). The dark side of nursing [Editorial]. *International Journal for Human Caring, 23*(1), 1–3.

CHAPTER 1

The Dark Side of Nursing

Zane Robinson Wolf, PhD, RN,
CNE, FCPP, ANEF, FAAN

Objectives

1. Define the dark side of nursing in the context of clinical nursing practice.
2. Describe ethical principles violated when patients receive bad nursing care.
3. Compare examples of good and bad nursing care.
4. Explain instances of the dark side of nursing in research.

Critical Incident

My first encounter with the dark side of nursing occurred in the critical care unit where I worked as a new nurse. One of the nursing staff recorded a value for a normal respiratory rate that did not coincide with a patient's definitive tachypnea. Another incident happened when my second daughter was born; I asked a nursing assistant in the newborn nursery to please give my baby to me so I could breastfeed her. She threatened me and cursed at me. The situation was witnessed by a registered nurse who did not intervene. The nursing assistant later came to my room and threatened me again. I left the hospital sooner than expected.

Ten years later, a registered nurse student shared with her class that a nurse coworker struck a patient in the emergency unit, an act followed by no administration-led consequences. Around that time, I was conducting research on medication errors. I discovered two studies in which nurses were suspected of killing critically ill patients. These efforts led to discovering Corley and Goren's (1998) seminal article on the dark side of nursing. They cited Jameton's (1992) definition of nursing's dark side as the absence of caring. Jameton's assertions about nursing ethics are consistent with the American Nurses Association (ANA, 2015) Code of Ethics. Nurses' caring ethics mandate that nurses:

> bring attention to human rights violations in all setting and contexts … with particular attention to preserving the human rights of vulnerable groups such as the poor, the homeless, the elderly, the mentally ill, prisoners, refugees, women, children, and socially stigmatized groups [ANA, 2015, p. 33].

Ethical principles govern nurse behavior; the most important is beneficence, to do good. The do no harm principle anchors the clinical practice of all health care providers.

Background

The persistence of dark side of nursing events might be explained by nursing's stressful work. This and other rationalizations are not enough, regardless of nurses' claim that patients' problematic behaviors evoke negative staff responses. Admittedly, health care providers are sometimes in danger from patients, family members, and friends; staff safety is paramount. However, nurses should never stigmatize, neglect, act angrily or hostilely, or otherwise harm patients despite reflex responses to their conspicuously difficult, threatening, or assaultive behavior. Furthermore, when nurses label patients *difficult,* they provide an opening in organizational cultures for nursing staff and other health care providers to deliver poor nursing care. Unless the label is eliminated, it follows patients until discharge (Price, 2013).

Dark Side of Nursing: Classics

In a thoughtful analysis of the moral situation of nursing practice, Jameton (1992) explored the distinguishing characteristics of the nursing profession, based on nurses' daily care of patients and their commitment to caring for patients. Connected with this assertion was his notice of the struggle between nurse caring and the more objective nature of institutionalized health care, including its technical and procedural aspects. He emphasized the importance of the information exchange during nurse-patient interactions, nurses' limited authority in health care settings, and nurses' decisions about the use and prioritization of resources for patient care based on the ethical principle of justice. In this case, justice was related to the allocation of the resource of nurses' work and the time needed to care for patients. Jameton (1992) emphasized that communication with patients and families and friends of patients is accompanied by complex ethical issues. He suggested that nurses' positions in organizations are further complicated; they serve as moral witnesses of care that they categorize as unethical or unwise, including procedures they themselves perform.

Jameton (1992) noted that the concept of caring is important in relation to nursing ethics, particularly because the professional labor of nurses incorporates task-oriented and emotive care, as seen in nurses' personal commitment to the welfare of patients. According to Jameton (1992), nursing involves a commitment to emotional labor. Although he observed that the status of nurses in relation to physicians and administrators may restrict nurses' perceived impact, Jameton (1992) recognized nursing's contributions to health care systems.

Toward the end of his analysis of nurses' work and ethical principles relevant to nursing practice, Jameton (1992) proposed that a main objective of nurses' emotional labor is control of patients, including assurances of safety and compliance with medical regimens. Connected to this suggestion is manipulation and control of patients by nurses to achieve these objectives. He invited a full examination of this example of the dark side of nursing.

Since Jameton's (1992) work, nursing literature on the dark side has proliferated, with many publications addressing bullying in nursing. Corley and Goren (1998) explored the dark side of nursing and listed several examples of nurses' behavior, including failure to provide care to meet patients' needs, rough physical handling, breaches of confidence, or patient manipulation. They framed dark side examples in the social-psychological concepts of marginalization, stigmatization, and stereotyping. They proposed that when patients' behavior is judged to be difficult by nurses or when they do not like patients or find them offensive, nursing care quality declines.

Nurses may distance themselves from patients identified as difficult (Corley & Goren, 1998). Distancing behaviors are revealed as nurses continue to provide physical care to stigmatized patients, but they withhold emotional care. In this and other dark side instances, patient outcomes can be negatively affected. Corley and Goren inferred that institutional leaders may support stereotyping implicitly; employee groups then stigmatize patients who threaten the social order of hospitals by their behavior. Nurses react by carrying out coercive behaviors when patient behavior is difficult to manage. When staff place patients in seclusion or use physical and chemical restraints, patients' well-being may not be the priority.

Corley and Goren (1998) suggested that staff might consistently view some patients negatively, such as suicidal, homeless, alcoholic, and substance abusing (Clarke et al., 2015) persons. Staff withdraw their support. As with societal expectations of the moral conduct of nurses, these vulnerable groups merit the best nursing care possible. Corley and Goren addressed the importance of nurses' relationships with patients and the need for nurses to do good and to do the right thing as framed by their moral sense and caring ethics. They recommended that leaders of health care institutions support ethical decision making by focusing on mission-based activities and the moral obligation to maintain ethical practices and eliminate the dark side behaviors of nurses and other staff.

Nurse leaders need to acknowledge publicly that dark side of nursing behaviors exist and foster change by influencing abandonment of stigmatizing assumptions (Corley & Goren, 1998). Team training is called for to develop organizational cultures oriented in ethically conscious behaviors. Such efforts can form creative strategies to eliminate patient avoidance and neglect. Nurse faculty members also must model students' ethical behaviors.

In contrast, love of self and others is the antidote to nursing's dark side. For example, an examination of *caritas*, giving altruistic love to humans, was proposed as the basis of caring and was oriented by philosophical and academic literature (Arman & Rehnsfeldt, 2006) and caring theories of Eriksson (2002). Caritas represented the ontological basis of compassion, relationships, and presence (Løgstrup, 1997). Whether or not unselfish love or caritas sounded unprofessional and threatening to nurses was explained by nurses' insecurity and fear about showing love in patient care. The authors proposed that nurses who practice love in professional practice are risk takers, perhaps going beyond earlier conceptualizations of the role of nurse. Of concern was the question raised that compassionate care, a visible sign of love in caring, was a health care resource and might be considered in the fair distribution of care. The authors proposed that acts of love were essential to reduce human suffering.

Roach (1990) suggested that caring expresses individuals' humanity and shapes human development and fulfillment. She noted the paradox of caring is that it is "more obvious by its absence than by its presence in human affairs" (p. 9). To describe the convergence of caring and ethics, Roach (1998) suggested that patients' suffering typifies a professional call for nurses to be in relationship with them. She reflected on the ontology or the meanings of the ethical life of nurses, such as human caring for nursing. Roach conceptualized caring as an essential human attribute. Her model's initial categories—compassion, competence, confidence, conscience, and commitment—incorporated specific activities, attitudes, values, and skills. The model has been used as a framework for understanding nursing's caring role. Caring as a total way of being involves acting, relating to, investing in, and engaging in others. For Roach, caring was a synonym for love.

Roach (1998) indicated that ethics, in the context of caring, governs behaviors that demonstrate relational responsibility and the moral call to be human. As nurses strive to do good, they respond to the suffering of others, the call to care. Roach remarked that Western inquiry has produced much scholarship on knowledge of the good and the means of achieving good. By these understandings, nurses and others are in touch with what it means to be human. As moral persons, nurses are challenged to acknowledge and engage in caring and to recognize it in daily life, in colleagues at work, and in all persons whom nurses serve.

Roach (1998) proposed that caring is the human mode of being; human beings are caring by their nature. If they are uncaring, they are less than human. Crimes against persons are evidence of less than human behavior. Her contentions partially explain dark side of nursing behaviors.

Caring and Noncaring: Conceptual Orientations

An early study (Riemen, 1993; 1986) on nurse-patient interactions was based on accounts of patients' ($N = 10$) descriptions of caring actions of nurses. Although patients were asked about caring nursing actions first, their responses focused on noncaring actions by nurses. The essential structure of caring and noncaring behaviors and attitudes of nurses was described. Noncaring attitudes and behaviors consisted of being in a hurry and efficient, doing a job, being rough and belittling patients, not responding when called, and treating patients as objects. One patient mentioned that a nurse "made me feel like a little kid" (Riemen, 1986, p. 32). A nurse "washed me as though I was a toy; I was not a human being to her" (p. 33). During a noncaring interaction, nurses devalued patients and were present physically but distant emotionally.

Adding to Riemen's (1996) essential concepts on noncaring, Halldorsdottir (1991; 1996; 2008) created a caring theory based on a synthesis of six qualitative studies in which nurses' encounters with patients were described as caring and uncaring. She observed that patients were vulnerable when they needed professional nursing services. Halldorsdottir (1991) induced the basic modes of being with another, presented in a caring/uncaring dimension or continuum. The life-giving or biogenic mode was the highest form of being. The nurse affirms the patient as a person and connects with them. The life-sustaining or bioactive mode occurs when the nurse validates the personhood of the patient, providing a supportive environment. The life-neutral or biopassive mode is evident when the nurse/caregiver does not influence the life of the other. The life-restraining or biostatic mode is uncaring. The patient perceives the nurse as indifferent, insensitive, and detached. The patient is discouraged and his or her life is negatively affected. The life-destroying or biocidic mode is the most negative, destructive, uncaring mode. The patient is depersonalized; the joy of life is destroyed, and the vulnerability of the patient is increased. Uncaring nurses were seen by patients as incompetent.

Halldorsdottir (1996) offered metaphors to represent caring and uncaring theory, the bridge and the wall. The bridge illustrates an open exchange of communication and connectedness that occurs during the caring relationship shared by nurses and patients. Respect and compassion are perceived by patients. Well-being and health are outcomes. The wall indicates negative or non-existent caring (Bailey, 2011) and negative or no communication between patient and nurse. The wall typifies indifference, disconnection, and incompetence. Halldorsdottir's caring and uncaring theory is the first to include the dialectic and the continuum and provides descriptions to illustrate each mode of being (Bailey, 2011). Dark side behaviors by nurses align with biopassive, biostatic (e.g., neglect, avoidance), and biocidic (e.g., psychological and physical abuse, murder) modes.

Good and Bad Nursing

Ethical nursing practice was studied to describe when a nurse does the right thing as framed by virtue ethics (Smith & Godfrey, 2002). In a qualitative descriptive study, initial comparisons were made on the ethics of care, emphasizing individuality, relationships, responsibility, justice, autonomy, and rights. To orient the study, Aristotelian perspectives on moral virtue as character linked character to conduct. Character was a standard for action. Registered nurses ($N = 53$) recorded answers to open-ended questions on who a good nurse is and how a good nurse goes about doing the right thing. Personal characteristics were what a good nurse brings to nursing; these attributes are demonstrated each day, including caring, compassion, and respect for self and others. Professional characteristics were illustrated in membership in the nursing profession, commitment to persons cared for, nursing's code of ethics, nurse practice acts, standards of care, personal philosophy and personal code of ethics, and role modeling for the profession.

Knowledge base was associated with competency, including personal facts, skills, and information gained by education and experience (Smith & Godfrey, 2002). Patient centeredness was often nurses' priority. Advocacy included empowering others and intervening on behalf of patients; critical thinking was accomplished through reflective analysis and making appropriate and/or right decisions, planning care, and evaluating outcomes. Finally, the performance of safe, competent nursing care was essential as the nurse uniquely expressed himself or herself to care for and about patients (pp. 305–307). One limitation was a bias toward positive responses. Assessing the subjective characteristics of applicants to nursing programs was stressed. The authors confirmed virtue ethics as lived or present in nursing.

Critical incident technique and hermeneutic analysis were used to explore the meaning of patients' experiences when a nurse *cares for* and *does not care for* patients (Karlsson et al., 2004). Patients ($N = 23$) at a medical/geriatric clinic who were formerly hospitalized wrote about one or more situations in which nurses cared for or did not care for them. The subcategories of the *to care for* category included to abandon your heart, to consider a wish, and the fact that somebody has been thinking of me. *Does not care for* subcategories consisted of to be of no importance, to be troublesome, and to have no thoughtfulness. To unburden your heart meant that nurses stayed at patients' sides, took time with them, and patients felt supported. To consider a wish meant that nurses saw need, complied with patients' wishes, and showed they cared about how patients felt. That somebody was thinking of them was noticed in nurses' small acts on behalf of patients; nurses asked how patients felt, helped patients to feel recognized and important, and were available when patients needed help. To be of no importance, the first of the *does not care for* category, showed that patients felt neglected by nurses, were not acknowledged, received incorrect information, and felt like a package. The subcategory, to be troublesome, indicated that patients felt of no importance or a bother to nurses and that their words and the delivery of words communicated this sentiment. To have no thoughtfulness was experienced by patients feeling disregarded by nurses and nurses not asking if they could make patients comfortable.

Fagerstöm (2006) conducted a hermeneutic study, part of a larger study, to understand nurses' (*N* = 13) workload and experiences in relation to different levels of nursing intensity. Eriksson's (2002) caritative caring theory framed the study: ethical caring is important for nurses wanting to be good nurses. Nurses experienced a chaotic work environment; they worried about making fatal errors. Multiple tasks complicated work intensity and threatened nurses' sense of control of patient care; tasks threatened relationships with patients, family members, and nurse colleagues. Nurses preferred a combination of high and low intensity patient care. Their inner demand was that nurses were able to satisfactorily meet patients' needs and patients' expectations of receiving good nursing care. Nurses preferred a combination of complex and meaningful caring situations. The root metaphor for the study was based on understanding caring situations. Nurses struggled between being a good nurse and not being a good nurse. They needed time to see and care for patients.

A focus group study with nursing students (*N* = 14) described the meaning of moral responsibility in nursing and how moral responsibility was expressed in the clinical context (Lindh et al., 2007). Moral responsibility, experiences with ethical problems, and ethical challenges in daily practice were themes orienting the study. Nurses' inherent values were shaped by home, educational program, and workplace. Moral responsibility in nursing practice represented the relational way nurses connected with others and the way responsibility showed in their lives every day. Nurses' inner compass and dialogue showed in personal reflections related to ideals, values, and knowledge. Helping others, humaneness, and benevolence were implicit and explicit. Students viewed good role models as competent and committed; less than good nurses lacked knowledge, respect, and sensitivity. The moral principles of autonomy, beneficence, and nonmaleficence shaped student knowledge.

According to students, patients' suffering called for sensitivity, understanding, and compassion (Lindh et al., 2007). Striving to do good in nursing practice was present in clinical responses to illness and suffering; striving was relational, implying doing good for others and self (acting in accordance with one's ideas and values). Nurses respected patients by being positive about their expressions of suffering and protecting them from harm, such as unprofessional treatment. Advocacy showed as nurses acted for patients whose power was diminished. The subjective nature of doing good for others was seen in nurses never being sure of its effect. Acting in accordance with nurses' own values could place patients at risk. A relational way of being, consistent with nurses' moral responsibility enacted in nursing practice, was also a burden due to the demands of clinical work.

A grounded theory study (Sutherland & Gilbert, 2008) described how nursing students managed the work of clinical practicums. Rules consisted of nursing program, individual faculty, hospital and unit, and staff regulations. The rules structured students' clinical experiences, how they navigated the practicum, and the strategies they used to complete the practicum. Good nurses permitted students to perform procedures. The good patient label was linked with students having several procedures to perform and by patients who kept them busy and supported smooth care planning processes. Students' stress was reduced by patients who helped them complete assessment data and having few or no medications to give. Bad patients limited students' completion of clinical work by being independent, having complex psychosocial problems, and needing complex medication regimes or complicated equipment. Patients were therefore objectified and judged by their contributions to students completing assignments; they were objects of care rather than subjects or persons experiencing an illness. Physical care predominated. Students' concern with their educational needs showed some self-absorption, that ideally would change with more exposure to patients.

Good and bad nurses were contrasted in a study on development of professional identity (Traynor & Buus, 2016). Students ($N = 49$) enrolled in a university baccalaureate nursing program participated in a focus group study exploring their development during clinical experiences. Students viewed nursing work as caring and an expression of innate attributes; they equated caring with good nursing. Good nurses performed patient care well, identified with patients, and supported students. Bad nurses were uncaring toward patients and students. Bad nurses lacked or had lost some necessary qualities when performing nursing care for patients. They were not compassionate and their "minds and hearts are not really for caring.... Sometimes, they forget that (compassion).... They ... are just burned out" (Traynor & Buus, p. 190). Students did not want to become bad nurses and criticized those that neglected patients. Students feared being corrupted by working too long in health care.

The experiences of a group of new graduate nurses who worked in mental health service settings were presented in a participatory action research study (Hazelton et al., 2011). Graduate nurses, members of three mentorship groups, participated in group discussions and were observed by research team members. They described the significance of the newcomer experience. Major themes indicated that newcomers: found it difficult to fit into work environments, observed neglectful and hostile treatment of patients, and were hindered from acquiring therapeutic skills. In addition to working through feeling they were not being accepted by the seasoned staff, new graduates judged uncaring staff as disinterested or aggressive when working with patients. They were troubled by staff indifference to vulnerable and distressed patients and saw that staff sometimes demonized patients with a diagnosis of borderline personality disorder or a history of child abuse.

In this study (Hazelton et al., 2011), the dark side of nursing involved veteran staff's lack of conviction that more effective interventions, guided by health policy initiatives, were worth implementing, and were a waste of time and resources. The difference between ideal care, based on high professional standards, versus what the new graduates described they witnessed was concerning. Caring values that supported patients' autonomy, dignity, and complexities were in little evidence. The researchers judged the dark side of mental health services as below the surface of physician and nurse roles in psychiatric settings. They projected that new graduate nurses would view their work either as a duty to care for patients or a duty to control them. If they followed the institutionalized models of care carried out by cynical and uncaring staff, newcomer nurses might remain in an organizational environment in which poor care persists.

A phenomenological-hermeneutic study was conducted on patients that received care from mental health nurses (Talseth et al., 1999). Patients ($N = 21$) were admitted to psychiatric institutions in Norway if they intended to kill themselves or had attempted suicide. Caregivers included physicians and nurses. Experiences with receiving care were described in interviews. Negative experiences outweighed positive ones in narratives. Confirming nursing care was represented by attending to patients' basic needs through physical contact. Nurses were considerate and asked patients how they were and cared for them; they spent time with patients, sat down, and talked with them. Being with patients was important, as was listening without prejudice; nurses were understanding and open to patients so that they felt safe. Nurses were calm and evidenced relaxed body language with good eye contact, so that patients felt welcome. As nurses communicated hope, patients understood that it would take time to work through their painful situations.

Lack of confirming patients (Talseth et al., 1999) stood for negative care: nurses overlooked patients' basic needs and had limited personal contact, so they did not see or spend time with patients, but instead performed tasks. Nurses left patients alone, so that patients were isolated in their rooms. They listened to patients with prejudice and did not recognize who patients were; nurses were not open to patients, showing disinterest in them. By implicitly denying patients' feelings, patients did not share suicidal thoughts and other feelings; patients felt empty and communicated their hopelessness. Patients needed to feel confirmed during interactions with nurses; nurses needed to demonstrate interest in them, see them as persons, and respect and listen to them.

In one part of a phenomenological study, Davis (2005) interviewed hospitalized patients and examined expectations of patients on good and bad nursing. She invited patients to share expectations of nurses for good nursing care and definitions of it. Being there and being with patients were defining characteristics of good nursing care. Nurses' presence with patients was important. Good nurses were calm, gentle, courteous, attentive, comforting, and available. Bad nurses were strident, brash, and abrupt. They lacked caring and kindness. Patients also expected nurses to be technically competent.

Legal and Professional Oversight of Nursing Practice

The goal of professional practice laws is protection of the public. Professional nursing laws and other guidelines, such as standards, policies, and procedures, govern nursing conduct. In Pennsylvania, the Professional Nursing Law (Act) (1951) defines the practice of professional nursing; the law provides structure to nursing practice and stipulates nursing diagnosis and treatment of human responses to health problems, both actual and potential. Nursing services are specified and include case finding, health teaching, health counseling, and supportive or restorative care to assure life and well-being of people needing nursing care. Carrying out prescribed medical regimens of physicians and dentists is also included. Nursing programs that educate students for the role of nurse are accredited by state boards of nursing. Professional nursing laws regulate and approve these programs (Pennsylvania Code, n.d.).

The right to use the title of nurse and the initials, RN, is explained in nurse practice laws (Professional Nursing Law [Act], 1951). Charges are filed when nurses violate norms of professional conduct as determined by evidence provided, state board of nursing decisions, and courts. Penalties are applied when nurses' conduct is interpreted as violations of the law.

The public's expectations of professional nurses' conduct are based on moral, legal, and professional standards. The title registered nurse implies that nurses have passed RN licensing examinations. Applicant eligibility for admission to examinations for professional nurse licensure requires endorsements by approved professional nursing education programs that applicants are of good moral character. Schools of nursing are therefore the first filter on the path to achieve registered nurse status and role.

Violations of professional nursing practice laws consist of various infractions. Misdemeanors and other civil or criminal penalties are covered by law (Professional Nursing Law [Act], 1951). Negligent and physically and mentally incompetent professional nursing practices are examples. Causes of incompetence may be attributed to drug or alcohol dependency (Orr, 1993).

Boards of nursing bear the responsibility of overseeing statutory law and determine nurses who are competent to practice professional nursing (Carruth & Booth, 1999; Professional Nursing Law [Act], 1951). State boards of nursing, according to professional nursing law, do not issue licenses to applicants convicted of felonies, except after 10 years post-conviction, have demonstrated personal rehabilitation since conviction, and other qualifications (Professional Nursing Law [Act], 1951). Further, violations of professional nursing laws can be stipulated by states and other entities, depending on local, state, and country regulations. A nursing board may refuse, suspend, or revoke licenses. A nurse must have the ability to practice with reasonable skill and safety when patient care is required; evidence or testimony of nurse behaviors may be requested by state boards of nursing.

Fraud and deceit commissions are violations of the professional nursing practice law (Professional Nursing Law [Act], 1951). Convictions, pleading guilty, pleas of nolo contendere, or guilty verdicts for felonies or crimes of moral turpitude are serious violations. In such cases, state boards of nursing control licensure often based on court decisions. Impaired professional programs are available and may assist nurses to demonstrate satisfactory progress in treatment so that licenses are reissued by boards of nursing.

The Pennsylvania Department of State publishes disciplinary actions each month for the Bureau of Professional and Occupational Affairs' professional licensing boards. Selected examples of infractions for three months (March, July, & November) in 2020 disciplinary actions for the Pennsylvania Board of Nursing include the following examples of infractions of registered nurses:

- license indefinitely suspended because of inability to practice nursing with reasonable skill and safety to patients and for violating a Board order
- suspension of practical and professional nursing licenses and certification to practice as a Certified Registered Nurse Practitioner suspended and ordered to complete remedial continuing education for violating the Board's regulations by engaging in conduct defined as sexual impropriety in the course of a professional relationship
- license revocation by the State Board of Nursing based on felony conviction
- indefinite suspended license because of violation of a Board order and addiction to hallucinogenic, narcotic or other drugs which tend to impair judgment or coordination
- indefinite suspension due to inability to practice professional nursing with reasonable skill and safety
- convicted of crimes of moral turpitude and committing fraud or deceit in the practice of nursing or in securing her admission to such practice
- licenses placed on probation for two years for having misappropriated Lasix from a patient or employer

- automatic license suspension based on being convicted of a misdemeanor under the Controlled Substance, Drug, Device and Cosmetic Act
- indefinite suspension for being convicted of a felony [Pennsylvania Department of State, 2020].

State boards of nursing execute their responsibility and commitment to public safety as guided by professional nursing laws. In addition to board efforts at the state level, National Council of State Boards of Nursing (NCSBN) leaders' concern with differentiating nursing errors from intentional, harmful acts (Benner et al., 2006) resulted in work on a database to record characteristics of nurses' errors. They engaged Benner and colleagues who identified elements of the database. The challenge was that state boards of nursing focused on individual nurse culpability as compared to a systems approach to understanding error causation and perhaps to differentiate error from malpractice.

Initially an expert panel was formed by the NCSBN (Benner et al., 2006). Deliberations emphasized the connection between systems analysis and clinician knowledge and judgment that provide situated problem saving on prevention of predictable errors. A national database was created to collect data on nursing practice breakdowns as reported to state boards of nursing. The goal was to present evidence on nursing errors.

The complexity of nurses' errors can include patient factors, nurse characteristics, working conditions, and other system elements. Documenting nursing error details on a national database might promote understanding of safety breaches, provide evidence that helps to prevent and remediate patient safety threats, and distinguish malpractice from mistake. Key information was identified from investigative cases of boards of nursing; a taxonomy was created, Taxonomy of Error, Root Cause Analysis and Practice Responsibility (TERCAP). The expert panel predicted that findings for TERCAP might help to prevent errors, especially repeatable errors, and differentiate "human errors from willful negligence and intentional misconduct" (Brennan et al., 2006, p. 54). The TERCAP instrument was shared by NCSBN with state boards of nursing in the United States (NCSBN, n.d.).

The Texas Board of Nursing (2016) adapted the NCSBN instrument; minor error incidents were documented in the TERCAP instrument and not reported to the board. State board of nursing reports submitted to the Texas pilot study excluded incidents that might endanger the public. Remediation for errors included nurse education and employing agency changes, such as policy revision and guideline development. A pilot update was presented (Texas Board of Nursing, 2016); 26 boards of nursing submitted cases to TERCAP. The pilot results included nursing errors, not professional nursing law violations. A Texas peer review system is available to foster objectivity and to support committee evaluations of nursing practice breakdowns; the process assists in the assessment of nurses' conduct on facility or state board reporting of conduct.

Literature

Literature on nursing practice violations has varied widely. A few studies addressed practice violations from a legal perspective. This literature highlighted a need to differentiate nursing practice breakdowns (Benner et al., 2006) from nursing practice violations. For example, nursing errors are considered preventable (and accidental), if the widely accepted definition of medication errors is applied (National Coordinating Council for Medication Error Reporting, n.d.). Nursing practice violations are intentional.

Nursing practice violations were described in a qualitative study (Collins & Mikos, 2008). In addition to identifying state board of nursing actions on professional nurse licenses, researchers recognized patterns in licensure disciplinary cases. They affirmed that professional misconduct violated social policy statements, codes of ethics, or professional standards, and that competencies and certifications of professional bodies also regulate practice. They presented nursing practice violations as five domains: employment, professional, licensure disciplinary, criminal, or civil actions. Concurrent actions in these different domains might be carried out during different investigations on the same complaint. Permanent public records from state board cases and judicial records were the data sources on complaints filed against nurses suspected of violations.

Collins and Mikos (2008) mentioned additional sources of data on provider infractions. Data banks are accessible to evaluate nurses' and various health care providers' status on practice violations. Examples are Nursys, an online verification source for endorsement of a nurse requesting to practice in another state (National Council of State Boards of Nursing, n.d.), and the National Practitioner Data Bank (United States Department of Health and Human Services Health Resources and Services Administration, n.d.).

Continuing to provide additional background information for their study, Collins and Mikos (2008) categorized types of sanctions against violators: reprimand/discipline; education; recovery program; fine/costs; money judgment; practice restriction; payer exclusion; suspension/termination/revocation; and incarceration. Criminal offenses are the most serious. The researchers analyzed practice act violations using composite cases. Nursing practice violators included impaireds, incompetents, criminals, rule benders, and good nurse having a bad day. Their initial taxonomy was unique. The researchers invited critique and testing of the taxonomic structure. They projected that the findings might benefit nurse attorneys and risk managers.

Another study used grounded theory methods to describe the transformation of professional identity of nurses accused of violating a nurse practice act (Hutchinson, 1992). The Department of Professional Regulation investigated allegations and the Florida Board of Nursing regulated the process of review. Thirty nurses were interviewed and described experiences and perceptions of being investigated for having violated the nurse practice act. Board meetings and document analysis were other data sources.

Nurses underwent a status passage when accused of such violations (Hutchinson, 1992). The initial threat in the form of a letter signaled the alleged violation of the nurse practice act, the basic social problem. The transformation of professional identity, the basic social process, incorporated several phases: being confronted, assuming a stance, going through it, living the consequences, and re-visioning. Nurses reviewed events, considered causation, evaluated work situations, and questioned their own professionalism. They admitted, partially admitted, or denied violations. They built a case in their defense and assembled resources.

An observational study was conducted on a randomly selected sample of nurse violators (*N* = 249) from 1991 to 1995 on cases that were closed files, concluded by the Louisiana State Board of Nursing. Most were female (81.9 percent), held associate degrees (41 percent), were disciplined by suspension (58 percent), and had less than 10 years' (30 percent) experience. Three had their licenses revoked. Men were disciplined dispropor-tionately more than women; middle aged ($M = 42.4$ years) nurses were more often disci-plined than others.

Nurses considered options as they went through the bureaucratic process (e.g., hearings, board orders, license relinquishment), depending on charges (Hutchinson, 1992). The board might dismiss, reprimand, fine, require continuing education courses and/or probation, suspend licenses, or revoke licenses. They lived through the conse-quences of allegations, the complaint process, and case reviews. Embarrassment, guilt, terror, degradation, and financial stress were expressed; they were uncertain about the future. Some changed jobs and blamed work situations for violations. Nurses saw the board of nursing experience as an important personal experience, having become more self-aware and self-protective. Some left nursing or changed employers; they were more cautious at work and tended to distance themselves from coworkers. They had a trans-formed professional identity and recognized nursing power anew and personal attri-butes needed to practice nursing. Since interpersonal conflicts and medication errors resulted in disciplinary actions, Hutchinson recommended that nurse administrators learn which violations of nurse practice acts need to be reported to state boards of nurs-ing and manage other problems internally.

Summary

Understanding dark side of nursing behaviors required searching and analyz-ing related literature. Selected empirical, qualitative sources were obtained in which good and bad nursing care was described. Evidence showed in the form of quotes from patients, nursing students, and nurses about care demonstrated by nurses. Other indica-tors of bad nursing care can be inferred through state board of nursing reports showing summaries of offenses and dispositions.

Although nursing is viewed as the most trusted profession in Gallup poll results, more attention is needed to examine dark side of nursing problems and to suggest some strategies to reduce and eliminate them. The following shows the most recent Gallup poll results:

> More than four in five Americans (84 percent) again rate the honesty and ethical standards of nurses as "very high" or "high," earning them the top spot among a diverse list of professions for the 17th consecutive year. At the same time, members of Congress are again held in the low-est esteem, as nearly 58 percent of Americans say they have "low" or "very low" ethical standards. Telemarketers join members of Congress as having a majority of low/very low ratings [Brenan, 2018, para. 1].

At the core of nursing behaviors are ethical principles held by members of the nurs-ing profession. Both moral and ethical principles guide nurses' and health care provid-ers' conduct and shape their care of patients, families, and communities. These and other standards of conduct, including laws, frame nursing care and clinical environments.

The complexity and stress of daily nursing care apparent in work situations might present a rationale for dark side of nursing behaviors. However, excuses are indefensible, for example, a rationale for neglect of patients given extraordinarily busy unit activi-ties. Excuses might comfort those nurses who are guilty because of missed nursing care, or actions not delivered during shifts. Often nurse staffing problems are cited as real restrictions to providing ideal nursing care.

Not surprising are the critical judgments of nursing students and new nurses who witness dark side of nursing behaviors in more seasoned nurses. The idea that moral and ethical standards, which are developed prior to admission to nursing programs, highlights nurse educators' duty to sort out candidates during programs of study prior to endorsing candidates for testing for professional nursing licensure.

Nurse-patient relationships contribute greatly to nursing care and the way patients perceived being cared for. Relationships with fellow nurses stand out, too. The culture of nursing is passed from role models to newcomers and influences the milieu of work environments.

The impact of nurse caring for patients is an antidote to the dark side of nursing. Patients expect good nursing care. However, experiencing less than good care or even harmful care adds to patients' suffering.

Conclusion

Although dark side of nursing examples have been described in literature and addressed by changes in health care systems, more exposure is needed (Wolf, 2012). Using the lens of research and theory, this book examines dark side of nursing exemplars. We hope that these discussions and strategies help nurses individually and collectively to decrease and eradicate dark side attitudes and behaviors.

Strategies

See Table 1 for strategies aimed at fostering communication and caring relationships.

Table 1. Strategies to Decrease and Eradicate Dark Side Attitudes and Behaviors

Strategies to Effect Change	Evidence-Based Citations
Develop caring relationships among nursing staff and with faculty and students by teaching from the heart; review of professional characteristics: ongoing assessment of caring behaviors in performance evaluation instruments in clinical settings and courses with clinical components	Vitali (2019)
Workshops to transform work environments that are hostile and neglectful: caritas themes and caritas coaches are integrated throughout the nursing organization to build caring literacy	Somerville & Lee (2019)
Exercises presented as staff meetings to help nurses open themselves to accepting patients' positive and negative feelings: exercises explore mutual vulnerability between nurses and patients and developing self-reflective practices	King & Barry (2019)

Conclusion

Nursing staff in clinical settings provide nursing care in situations that are very stressful. Focusing on strategies that remind staff about the benefits of nurse caring and explorations of the idea of mutual vulnerability of nurses, patients, and families might help to reduce the effects of the workplace. Many stressors also operate for nursing students and faculty. A refocus on caring behaviors could operate to build caring bridges between students and faculty.

Discussion Questions

1. What are the major differences in the definitions of nursing practice breakdowns, nursing practice violations, and professional nursing violations?

2. What ethical principles govern nursing care? Provide examples of unethical nursing care.

3. What are the distinctions between nursing errors (nursing practice breakdowns) and nursing practice violations in relation to root causes?

4. What are behaviors exhibited by nurses that patients perceive as caring and compassionate?

5. What are behaviors exhibited by nurses that patients perceive as noncaring?

AUTHOR SELECTIONS

Levitas, A. (Producer). (2019). *Lullaby* [Film]. Radiant Films International.
Motley Rice LLC. (2019). *See Me* [Poem]. Nursing Home Alert. http://www.nursinghomealert. com/share-this-poem.

REFERENCES

American Nurses Association. (2015). *Code of ethics for nurses with interpretive statements*. https://www. nursingworld.org/practice-policy/nursing-excellence/ethics/code-of-ethics-for-nurses/.
Arman, M., & Rehnsfeldt, A. (2006). The presence of love in ethical caring. *Nursing Forum, 41*(1), 4–12.
Bailey, D.N. (2011). Framing client care using Halldorsdottir's theory of caring and uncaring behaviors within nursing and healthcare. *International Journal for Human Caring, 15*(4), 54–64.
Benner, P., Malloch, K., Sheets, V., Bitz, K., Emrich, L., Thomas, M.B., Bowen, K., Scott, K., Patterson, L., Schwed, K., & Farrell, M. (2006). TERCAP: Creating a national database on nursing errors. *Harvard Health Policy Review, 7*(1), 48–63.
Brenan, M. (2018, December 20). Nurses again outpace other professions for honesty, ethics. Gallup Poll. https://news.gallup.com/poll/245597/nurses-again-outpace-professions-honesty-ethics.aspx.
Carruth, A.K. (1999). Disciplinary actions against nurses: Who is at risk? *Journal of Nursing Law, 6*(3), 55–62.
Clarke, D.E., Gonzales, M., Pereira, A., Bouce-Gaudreau, K., Waldman, C., & Demczuk, L. (2015). The impact of knowledge on attitudes of emergency department staff towards patients with substance related presentations: A quantitative systematic review protocol. *JBI Database of Systematic Reviews & Implementation Reports, 13*(10), 133–145.
Collins, S.E., & Mikos, C.A. (2008). Evolving taxonomy of nurse practice act violators. *Journal of Nursing Law, 12*(2), 85–91.
Corley, M.C., & Goren, S. (1998). The dark side of nursing: Impact of stigmatizing responses on patients. *Scholarly Inquiry for Nursing Practice, 2*(2), 99–122.
Davis, L. (2005). A phenomenological study of patient expectations concerning nursing care. *Holistic Nursing Practice, 19*(3), 126–133.
Eriksson, K. (2002). Caring science in new key. *Nursing Science Quarterly, 15*(1), 61–65.
Fagerström. L. (2006). The dialectic tension between 'being' and 'not being' a good nurse. *Nursing Ethics, 13*(6), 622–632. https://doi.org/10.1177/0969733006069697.
Halldorsdottir, S. (1991). Five basic modes of being with another. In D.A. Gaut & M. Leininger (Eds.), *Caring: The compassionate healer* (pp. 37–40). National League for Nursing.
Halldorsdottir, S. (1996). *Caring and uncaring encounters in nursing and health care: Developing a theory.*

[Doctoral dissertation No. 493. Department of Caring Sciences, Faculty of Health Sciences, Linköping University, S-581 85]. Linköping University Medical Dissertations.

Halldorsdottir, S. (2008). The dynamics of the nurse-patient relationship: Introduction of a synthesized theory from the patient's perspective. *Scandinavian Journal of Caring Sciences, 22*, 643–652. https://doi.org/10.1111/j.1471-6712.2007.00568.x.

Hazelton, M., Rossiter, R., Sinclair, E., & Morrell, P. (2011). Encounters with the 'dark side': New graduate nurses' experiences in a mental health service. *Health Sociology Review, 20*(2), 172–186.

Hutchinson, S.A. (1992). Nurses who violate the nurse practice act: Transformation of professional identity. *Journal of Nursing Scholarship, 24*(2), 133–139.

Jameton, A. (1992). Nursing ethics and the moral situation of the nurse. In E. Friedman (Ed.), *Choices and conflict* (pp. 101–109). American Hospital Publishing.

Karlsson, M., Bergbom, I., vonPost, I., & Berg-Nordenberg, L. (2004). Patient experiences when the nurse cares for and does not care for. *International Journal for Human Caring, 8*(3), 30–36.

King, B.M., & Barry, C.D. (2019). Mutual vulnerability: Creating healing environments that nurture wholeness and well-being. In W. Rosa, S. Horton-Deutsch, & J. Watson, *A handbook for caring science: Expanding the paradigm* (pp. 373–384). Springer Publishing.

Lindh, I-B., Severinsson, E., & Berg, A. (2007). Moral responsibility: A relational way of being. *Nursing Ethics, 14*(2), 130–140.

Løgstrup, K.E. (1997). *The ethical demand*. University of Notre Dame.

National Coordinating Council for Medication Error Reporting. (n.d.). *Medication error definition*. https://www.google.com/search?q=ncc+merp+medication+error+definition&rlz=1C1EJFA_enUS791US791&oq=ncc+merp+medication+error&aqs=chrome.1.69i59j0l3j69i60l2.9950j0j8&sourceid=chrome&ie=UTF-8.

National Council of State Boards of Nursing. (n.d.). Nursing Practice Breakdown: TERCAP Pilot. Summary. https://www.thefreelibrary.com/Nursing+Practice+Breakdown%3A+TERCAP+Pilot+Project+Summary.-a0562370973.

National Council of State Boards of Nursing. (n.d.). *Nursys*. https://www.nursys.com/.

Orr, R.L. (1993). A profile of disciplined nurses in Tennessee, 1990–1992. (Publication No. 109871788). [Dissertation, University of Tennessee]. University Microfilms.

Pennsylvania Code. (n.d.). Chapter 21. State Board of Nursing, Subchapter A. Registered Nurses. Approval of Schools of Nursing. https://www.pacode.com/secure/data/049/chapter21/chap21toc.html.

Pennsylvania Department of State. (2020). Disciplinary actions. https://www.dos.pa.gov/ProfessionalLicensing/VerifyaProfessional/DisciplinaryActions/Documents/2020/July-2020.pdf

Price, B. (2013). Countering the stereotype of the unpopular patient. Nursing Older People, 25(6), 27–35.

Professional Nursing Law Act, PA.P.L. 317, No. 69. (May 22, 1951). https://www.dos.pa.gov/ProfessionalLicensing/VerifyaProfessional/DisciplinaryActions/Documents/2018/March%202018.pdf.

Riemen, D.J. (1983). *The essential structure of a caring interaction: A phenomenological study*. (Publication No. 8401214). [Dissertation, Texas Women's University]. University Microfilms International.

Riemen, D.J. (1986). Noncaring and caring in the clinical setting: Patients' descriptions. *Topics in Clinical Nursing, 8*(2), 30–36.

Roach, M.S. (1990). A call to consciousness: Compassion in today's health world. In D.A. Gaut, & M. Leininger (Eds.), *Caring: The compassionate healer*. National League for Nursing.

Roach, M.S. (1998). Caring ontology: Ethics and the call of suffering. *International Journal for Human Caring, 2*(2), 30–34.

Smith, K.V., & Godfrey, N.S. (2002). Being a good nurse and doing the right thing: A qualitative study. *Nursing Ethics, 9*(3), 301–312.

Somerville, J., & Lee, S.M. (2019). A blueprint for caritas health "care." In W. Rosa, S. Horton-Deutsch, & J. Watson, *A handbook for caring science: Expanding the paradigm* (pp. 401–412). Springer Publishing.

Sutherland, L.L., & Gilbert, V. (2008). The good patient–bad patient: A consequence of following the rules of a clinical practicum. Chapter 5. *Annual Review of Nursing Education, 6*, 83–101.

Talseth, A-G., Lindsith, A., Jacobsson, L., & Norberg, A. (1999). The meaning of psychiatric in-patients' experiences of being cared for by mental health nurses. *Journal of Advanced Nursing, 29*(5), 1034–1041.

Texas Board of Nursing (2016, April). Texas TERCAP pilot project update. *Texas Board of Nursing Bulletin, 47*(2), 1, 4.

Thomas, M.B., McDermott, E., Danielle, G., & Benbow, D. (2020). Evaluation of nursing practice breakdown: A resource for peer review. *Journal of Nursing Regulation, 11*(1), 42–47. https://doi.org/10.1016/S2155-8256(20)30060-0.

Traynor, M., & Buus, N. (2016). Professional identity in nursing: UK students' explanation for poor standards of care. *Social Science & Medicine, 166*, 186–194.

United States Department of Health and Human Services Health Resources and Services Administration. (n.d.). *National Practitioner Data Bank*. https://www.npdb.hrsa.gov/.

Vitali, N. (2019). Teaching from the heart. In W. Rosa, S. Horton-Deutsch, & J. Watson, *A handbook for caring science: Expanding the paradigm* (pp. 225–241). Springer Publishing.

Wolf, Z.R. (2012). Nursing practice breakdowns: Good and bad nursing. *MEDSURG Nursing, 21*(1), 16–22, 36.

MULTIPLE-CHOICE QUESTIONS

1. **Which of the following examples illustrates the dark side of nursing practice?**
   A. Labeling patients as difficult
   B. Reflecting on personal biases
   C. Carrying out patient management strategies
   D. Asserting preferences for quiet situations

2. **Which of the following patients are often viewed negatively by nursing staff?**
   A. Persons who are substance abusers
   B. Patients with complex wounds
   C. Patients who are infected
   D. Patients who do not adhere to care regimens

3. **Which of the following of Halldorsdottir's modes of being is seen as the highest level of caring?**
   A. Biocidic
   B. Biostatic
   C. Biogenic
   D. Bioactive

4. **Which of the following examples represents what patients mean by "caring for?" Select all that apply.**
   A. Feeling supported
   B. Having their wishes followed
   C. Feeling disregarded
   D. Feeling recognized

CHAPTER 2

Justifying Coercion in Patient Care

Beth Marie King, PhD,
APRN, PMHNP-BC

Objectives

1. Define the terminology associated with coercion.
2. Discuss the literature in relation to the use of coercion.
3. Identify the process/actions nurses utilize to justify the use of coercion.
4. Discuss three strategies nurses can employ to change use of coercion.

Critical Incident

As Mary arrived on the unit for the evening shift, she heard the hospital intercom announce a *Dr. Strong* for her unit, 6 South, the psychiatric unit. Mary hurried to the unit, in case more help was needed. John had been admitted earlier, was refusing to go into his room, and was being disruptive on the unit. He was being verbally abusive to both the staff and to other patients.

Mary's RN friend, Anne, was drawing up an IM injection to administer to John because he refused to take any oral medication. Mary knew Anne hated doing this, as this meant administering medication against the patient's will. But John was escalating, was beyond being talked down, and continued to refuse any medication. The call for *Dr. Strong* had brought security to the unit to offer assistance during medication administration. Ultimately John received his IM injection to help him de-escalate.

Four hours later, it was Mary's turn to offer John his oral medication. John's orders included an antipsychotic drug four times a day to help him with voices he heard in his head. Mary, accompanied by a psychiatric technician, approached John in his room, and informed him that it was time to take the medication prescribed by his doctor. John just looked at Mary and stated, "I don't want the medication." Mary informed him, "John, I don't want to call a *Dr. Strong,* but I will if I have to as I know you need this medication. This medication will help calm those voices in your head. I know you want to get better and taking this medication will help you do that." Mary continued to sit with John for about 15 minutes, but he still refused to take his medication. He was not verbally abusive or aggressive; he just did not want to take the medication.

Mary went back to the nursing office and asked the charge nurse what to do. Mary was informed to document refusal of medication and to document his behavior. Mary then asked the staff if anyone had developed a relationship with John during his short time on the unit. Frank, the psychiatric technician, indicated that he had "connected" with John. Mary asked him to talk with John about the need to take his medication. About 30 minutes later, Frank informed Mary that John had agreed to take his medication! When Mary asked him what he said, Frank indicated that he talked with him about what happened last time and that he knew he did not like being held down and given a shot, nor did the staff, but they just wanted to help him get better and get out of the hospital. Mary was relieved that John had finally agreed to take the medication orally and she did not have to call a *Dr. Strong*.

The use of coercion with medication administration occurs frequently in mental health settings. Patients often refuse medication for a variety of reasons, and it is the "relationship" between the nurse/staff and patient that can determine the outcome. But what other factors should be considered as we justify the use of coercion? What is best for the patient's well-being according to the staff, what is best for the unit's milieu, or what is best for the patient's well-being according to the patient and his or her right to determine what is best for them?

Background

An individual's decision regarding their own health care is considered a human right. The World Health Organization's (2013) *Mental Health Action Plan 2013–2020* recognizes the "need for services, policies, legislation, plans, strategies and programs to protect, promote and respect the rights of persons with mental disorders" (p. 7). Yet, Lavelle and Tusaie (2011) asserted that mental health is the only area of health care that "a person can make an adverse decision regarding their health and have that decision be challenged" (p. 274). A patient's decision to refuse medication or psychiatric treatment is often questioned and coercive techniques may be used, and if required, legally mandated.

The literature indicates that coercion is commonly used in health care settings, in particular psychiatric health care settings (Al-Maraira et al., 2019). However, there is not one common definition for coercion. Breggin defined coercion as "any action or threat of actions, which compels the patient to behave in a manner inconsistent with his own wishes" (as cited in Cutcliffe & Travale, 2013, p. 279); whereas Allison and Fleming (2019) defined coercion as "the action or practice of persuading someone to do something by using force or threats" (p. 2274). Most frequently, coercion is associated with the use of seclusion, restraints, and involuntary admission and treatment.

Coercion has been further delineated by Allison and Fleming (2019) as *hard coercion*, "legal measures, physical restraint, and enforced medication," *soft coercion*, "a perceived threat of punishment or force," or *subtle coercion*, "an interpersonal interaction wherein one person exerts his/her will on another and infers the potential to action a threat" (p. 2274).

Although coercion may be considered a common practice in psychiatric settings, the use of coercion can create ethical dissonance among health care professionals. The use of coercion violates the ethical principles of autonomy, respect, and a person's right to refuse treatment. The following codes, laws, and declarations articulate guiding principles for health care professionals caring for persons with mental health challenges and/or health issues: *Guide to the Code of Ethics for Nurses with Interpretive Statements: Development, Interpretation, and Application* (American Nurses Association, 2015); *Psychiatric-Mental Health Nursing: Scope & Standards of Practice* (American Nurses Association, American Psychiatric Nurses Association & International Society of Psychiatric Mental Health Nurses, 2014); *Patient Bill of Rights/The Patient Care Partnerships* (American Hospital Association, 1992, 2003); *Restatement of Bill of Rights for Mental Health Patients* (United States Code, 1991); *Convention on the Rights of Persons with Disabilities* (United Nations Human Rights, 2008); *Mental Health Action Plan 2013–2020* (World Health Organization, 2013); and *Mental Health Declaration of Human Rights* (Citizens Commission on Human Rights, 2019).

To justify the use of coercion, health care professionals must provide themselves with "sufficient lawful and ethical reasons for an act" (Vuckovich & Artinian, 2005, p. 371) and/or "the action to be taken must be considered beneficent and failing to act grossly maleficent" (Vukovich & Artinian, 2005, p. 373). The following review of the literature addresses research related to coercion from both the staff's and patient's perspectives, as well as the ethical issues that arise in relation to the use of coercion.

Literature

The literature discusses coercion in terms of the use of coercion, the health care staff's perspective of coercion, the patient's perspective of coercion, and the justification of coercion. However, underlying all discussions of coercion are the ethical principles related to coercion.

Coercion

The literature frequently associates the use of coercion with the use of seclusion and/or physical restraints (Al-Maraira et al., 2019; Ryan & Bowers, 2005). Ryan and Bowers (2005) attempted to categorize additional coercive measures utilized by psychiatric nurses in a psychiatric setting other than seclusion or restraints. Using the observational method, the researchers observed staff for six months on a psychiatric intensive care unit in an attempt to understand other coercive measures used by staff.

The findings indicated that serious conflict was addressed using time out, seclusion, and administration of prn medication (Ryan & Bowers, 2005). When nurses considered the patient was pushing boundaries or out of control, other coercive measures were used. For example, verbal warnings, guidance by contacting/touching the patient, negotiating with the patient, offering diversion, ignoring the patient, deceiving (making a promise but not following through) the patient, and overt denying the patient's requests were used. Body blocks, bear hugs, using imposing/confrontational behavior, and show of force were used as last-ditch efforts (Ryan & Bowers, 2005, p. 701). Although the effectiveness of the various coercive techniques was not studied, the authors clearly identified the various coercive techniques utilized by nurses in a psychiatric setting.

Defining coercion does not provide the full impact of the use of coercion on the client, the staff, or the ethical issues at stake with the use of coercion. The following discussion aids in further understanding the use of coercion from the staff's perspective.

Staff's Perspective: Use of Coercion

A grounded theory study was conducted by Lutzen in 1998, with 10 psychiatric nurses who were asked to "describe an incident in which a patient refused to comply with a nursing intervention, which they believed to be 'right,' and how they dealt with the patient's non-compliance" (p. 103). Examples of patient non-compliance included: wanting to leave the hospital; refusing to take medication, to wash, or to eat; voicing self-harm; and taking other patient belongings. The nurses described using acceptable ways to overcome the patient's non-compliance, which the researcher described as using subtle coercion. The researcher defined subtle coercion as a "dynamic activity, involving one person (or several) exerting his or her will upon another" (p. 103). Subtle coercive measures were termed by the nurses as: acting strategically, making trade-offs, using manipulation, and using persuasion. In conclusion, the researcher questioned the justification of coercion and emphasized the need for awareness of the patient's vulnerability and relational power.

Larsen and Terkelsen (2014) further examined the use of coercion in an inpatient locked psychiatric unit in Norway. They interviewed 22 staff—14 men and 8 women—consisting of nurses, psychiatrists, and social health workers. The staff had differing viewpoints as to the enforcement of house rules; some staff thought there should be more flexibility while others thought there should be discipline. In terms of the use of coercion, all the staff agreed that coercion was necessary, and utilized coercion when they feared violence, or for the benefit of the patient. Yet many of the staff shared the feeling expressed by one:

> Physical coercion, like forced medication, for instance, is absolutely the worst thing I do. Some patients believe I poison them. I feel like a perpetrator, it gives me a bad conscience. But I blame the system [p. 431].

Hutchinson et al. (2013) offered another view of coercive measures of nursing, more subtle measures which were used to marginalize, devalue, and label patients. The following statements by nurses exemplify the measures:

> he is just an attention seeker. If he was serious, he would not have pressed the [emergency] button [to call for help after attempting suicide] … he was attention seeking and we were not to give him attention … should not be on painkillers, he says that he is in pain to get drugs … he is a danger to others … [and is] so horrible even his mother doesn't love him … we'll do his observations every hour … just to annoy him [p. 477].

The researchers called for further investigation in the moral disengagement of nurses and resulting impact on patient care.

Most recently, Andersson et. al (2020) conducted a qualitative study in Sweden with 10 nurses working in psychiatric units. The study focused on the nurse's experience with informal coercion and associated ethical challenges. Results indicated that informal coercion is a process that includes the initiation of coercion, the coercive event, and the aftermath (p. 244), and factors that influence the event. The first domain identified—initiating informal coercion—described several motives for coercion: "for the good of the patient…, a way of adjusting to people's expectations…, to cope with the demands of everyday work, … a way to avoid formal coercion" (p. 747). The second domain—description of the coercive event—focused on how nurses exerted informal coercion. Descriptions included waiting for the patient to respond, persuading the patient, negotiating with the patient, and using professional power. The final domain—the aftermath—discussed how nurses rationalized their actions by scrutinizing their own actions and reflecting with peers and patients.

Yet what is the impact of exposure to patient aggression by the nursing staff? Jalil et al. (2017) conducted a cross-sectional, correlational, observational study to determine the impact of exposure to patient aggression and attitude toward use of coercive techniques. Several measurement tools were completed by 68 mental health nurses: Novaco Anger Scale, Positive and Negative Affect Schedule, Perception of Prevalence of Aggression Scale, and Attitude to Containment Measures. In addition, incident reports related to physical restraints and seclusion were reviewed for participant inclusion in restraint/seclusion incidents. The findings revealed that exposure to patient verbal abuse rather than physical aggression was positively associated with provoking anger of the nurse. In addition, the emotion of anger was associated with approval by the nurse for physical restraint use, but not seclusion, whereas guilt was negatively associated with seclusion.

Pawlowski (2018) questioned if the personality traits of the nurses and/or the organizational climate had any effect on the frequency of coercive techniques. He conducted a one-year observational study and analyzed all direct use of coercion by 83 members of the nursing staff in a 236-bed psychiatric unit. Members of the nursing staff completed the Gough's Adjective Check List (ACL), which consists of 300 adjectives correlating to 24 scales assessing the needs or wants, and attributes, potentials, and role characteristics (p. 288). In addition, participants completed the Kolb's Organizational Climate Questionnaire (KOCQ) which measures six areas (responsibility, requirements, rewards, organization, atmosphere, and leadership) using a 10-point scale. The findings indicated that *initiation of coercion* was significantly correlated with an individual with a low score on the Creative personality scale of Gough's ACL instrument and a low score on the KOCQ Leadership subscale. The Creative personality scale listed adjectives such as, "capable, skillful, humorous, individualistic, intelligent, having broad interests" (p. 290). The best predictor for the decision to *use coercion* was a low score on the KOCQ Requirements subscale. The best predictors for *participation in coercion* were high score on the KOCQ Leadership subscale and low score on the Requirements subscale. The Requirements subscale focused on the organization's skill development and encouragement to meet challenges. This study indicates that the organizational climate and personality traits of personnel can impact the use of coercive measures in a psychiatric unit.

Doeden et al's. (2020) recent systematic review of the literature found that psychiatric nurses' attitudes toward coercion have shifted over the last 20 years from a therapeutic focus to a safety focus. The review indicated that although nurses perceived coercive measures as "unwanted and harmful," they were "necessary to regain safety in the case of aggressive behavior" (p. 450). Yet, the literature review also indicated a need for "more gentle, humane" coercive measures to manage aggressive patient behavior (Doeden et al., 2020, p. 450).

Most recently, Laukkanen et al. (2019) conducted an integrative review of studies conducted from 2002 to 2017 to determine psychiatric nurses' attitudes toward containment (use of seclusion, restraints, and involuntary medication). Twenty-four studies from 13 countries were reviewed; no studies were from the United States. Twenty-three of the studies used quantitative measures; most frequently identified was the use of Survey of Nurses' Attitudes to Seclusion and Attitude to Containment Methods Questionnaire. Several studies indicated that nurses have an overall positive attitude toward containment, but nurses also expressed feelings of "frustration, helplessness, and regret" (p. 400). Unexpectedly, the review also indicated that alternative methods to containment were not frequently utilized.

Lastly, a study conducted by Motteli et al. (2020) examined the attitude of 110 staff members of a psychiatric hospital toward coercion using the Staff Attitude to Coercion Scale (SACS) and the Recovery Oriented Scale (RAQ-7). The findings indicated that 73.6 percent of the staff were critical of coercion, with 16.4 percent that identified coercion as offending, and 87.3 percent agreed with coercion as care and security. Yet, 5.5 percent of the staff had a positive attitude toward coercive measures. Furthermore, staff with optimistic recovery expectations for patients and who worked on open wards were more critical of coercive measures.

The literature offers varying viewpoints regarding nursing staff's use and attitudes toward coercive measures. But a nurse cannot understand the impact of the use of coercive measures without listening to the patient's view. The following discussion presents research related to the patient's perspective and the use of coercive measures by nursing staff.

Patients' Perspectives: Use of Coercion

A study by Larsen and Terkelsen (2014) examined the use of coercion in an inpatient locked psychiatric unit in Norway. Twenty-two staff and 12 patients were observed and interviewed regarding their perception of the use of coercion during their hospitalization. Staff's enforcement of corrections and house rules were noted in the field notes of the researchers, along with the patients' difficulty understanding the rules and feelings of inferiority and humiliation. One patient expressed, "It's of no use to protest, you just have to do what they say" (p. 430). In terms of the use of seclusion, a patient stated, "It was necessary, it was. But it wasn't good.... I understand why they have to remove everything in there" (p. 430). Another patient stated, "After a while it only makes you feel worse" (p. 430). Patients expressed the need to be treated as "ordinary people … as human beings" and "not as a diagnosis" (p. 343).

Staff presented conflicting viewpoints regarding coercion. One staff member thought, "It was necessary to correct more," yet another indicated, "We shouldn't humiliate people by correcting them all the time" (Larsen & Terkelsen, 2014, p. 430). This study reflected the value of understanding both the patients' and staff's views on coercion.

Newton-Howes and Mullen (2011) conducted a review of the literature of 27 articles and perceived coercion experience from the patients' perspective. The main theme identified in the qualitative articles was the feeling of being "dehumanized through a loss of normal human interaction and isolation" (p. 467). Newton-Howes and Mullen's results were confirmed by Tingleff et al. (2017). They analyzed 26 studies related to a patient's perception of coercion, before, during, and after coercion. Analysis revealed two themes related to *before coercion*: being subjected to a professional's control and protest behavior (p. 685). Before coercion was characterized by the patient's feelings of humiliation, powerlessness, anger, loss of power and control, and lack of communication with staff. *During coercion,* the main theme related to being subjected to professionals' control and impact of coercive measures (p. 690). Patients' perception of coercion was negative and represented strong feelings of humiliation, feeling abused, and traumatized.

Furthermore, patients indicated that communication with professionals was "insufficient, disrespectful, and degrading" (p. 691). *After coercion* themes consisted of interactions with professionals' communication, physical discomfort, and other consequences. Again, patients' feelings were anger, embarrassment, fear, powerlessness, pain, and feeling being punished, feeling vulnerable, feeling worthless, and feeling helpless. They also feared enclosed spaces, loss of trust, and being traumatized.

Recently, Allison and Fleming (2019) conducted a review of qualitative literature examining the patient's experience with subtle/soft coercion and impact on interactions with providers. Studies related to harder coercive techniques, such as physical restraints, were not included in the review. Thematic synthesis of findings from 11 articles was conducted by reviewing findings and expanding on original findings to devise new interpretations. Eleven articles were reviewed. Three analytical themes were identified: losing a sense of self, less than therapeutic relationship, and journey through treatment. *Losing a sense of self* was illuminated through discussion of several studies. A descriptor supporting the theme was presented in the Gault et al. (2013) study of medication adherence and provided an exemplar which clearly reflected the theme: "I used to be someone, went to college, had a job, now I'm just a patient" (p. 793). Another descriptor described by Allison and Fleming was from Duncan's (2013) qualitative study with 10 mental health users: "You're an underclass because you don't have the rights that anyone else in the society has. You know the right to refuse treatment for a start" (p. 68). The second theme, *less than therapeutic relationships,* had four sub-themes: brokerage of responsibility, lack of genuine choice, less than equal, and importance of feeling connected. Katsakou et al.'s (2011) study of 36 patients' perception of coercion during hospitalization offered a supporting descriptor of this theme: "There's a whole team there and they don't listen to you, they TELL you … it just made me feel like I wasn't human, and nobody actually took my point of view into consideration" (p. 279). The third theme, *journey through the system,* included two sub-themes: accepting illness-based explanations and playing the game. Duncan's (2013) study also provided a descriptor representing this theme: "You feel that, you know, the only way to get out is to cooperate, so in order to get out you cooperate with everything" (p. 77). Allison and Fleming's 2019 review provided more evidence of the need to listen to patients and to be cognizant of the use of softer and subtle coercion.

Jarrett et al.'s (2008) study aimed to offer a demographic overview of patients who were coerced and forcibly medicated by reviewing 14 published studies from seven countries, during 1980–2008. Results indicated that of the six studies that reported gender, two indicated that women experienced higher rates of coercion, and one study indicated that men had higher rates. No significant differences were noted in terms of diagnosis, but schizophrenia, bipolar disorder, or psychotic disorder were the most common diagnoses. Eight of the studies indicated a strong correlation between aggressive or threatening behavior and forced medication.

Jarrett et al. (2008) also reviewed the studies for patients' refusal to take medication. Reasons included: side effects, feeling better and not needing the medication, thinking the medication was poisonous, and fear of addiction. Patients' perspectives on being forced to take medication were also discussed in four studies and ranged from agreeing to the need for the forced medication, would be more likely to take medication in the future, to not agreeing that there was a need for the medication. Patients also expressed feelings of being frightened, angry, sad, panicked, helpless, embarrassed, and relieved. Interestingly, the patients' perspectives of coercion and the staff's perspectives are similar in some respects and dissimilar in others. This leads to the need for justifying the use of coercion.

Justifying Coercion

Justifying coercion first requires that nurses look at guiding ethical principles for the nursing profession and care of persons, as well as the nurse-patient relationship. Provision 1 of the *Guide to the Code of Ethics for Nurses* (American Nurses Association, 2015) states, "The nurse practices with compassion and respect for the inherent dignity, worth, and unique attributes of every person" (p. 1). Furthermore, the *Patient Bill of Rights/The Patient Care Partnerships* (American Hospital Association, 1992, 2003) states that the patient has the right to respectful care and right to refuse treatment. Both emphasize respect for the person cared for, which is further explained in Kant's writings, "A primary ethical principle; a moral attitude; a human value that addresses justice, honor and human dignity; an attitude necessary for justifiable ethical actions between people ... a core value of human rights" (Cutcliffe & Travale, 2013, p. 275).

The rationale for the use of coercion in psychiatric settings is frequently cited as what is "best for the patient ... best interest of others ... dangerous to themselves and others" (Wynn, 2006, p. 249). Yet, the use of coercion unmistakably violates a person's respect for autonomy and right for self-determination. The *Guide to the Code of Ethics for Nurses* defines respect for autonomy as "duty to respect the autonomous choices of others" (American Nurses Association, 2015, p. 16). The use of coercion denies this right.

Although there is a consensus by health care professionals as to the right and value of respect for all patients, in practice respect for autonomy, dignity, and compassion may not always be as evident. The following studies clarify the concept of justification of coercion and infringement on nurses' guiding principles.

A grounded theory study by Vuckovich and Artinian (2005) described the process nurses go through prior to the use of coercion. Seventeen nurses were interviewed and asked to discuss their experience of administration of medication to patients who were involuntarily admitted to a psychiatric unit. The findings revealed that to justify the administration of medication against the patient's desire, even when mandated by the courts or in an emergency situation, the nurses used a social process to come to the decision to use coercion.

The researchers identified three stages of the process: assessment of need, negotiation, and justifying and taking coercive action (Vuckovich & Artinian, 2005). When assessing need, the nurses recognized the importance of the patient's autonomy rights yet considered the "severity of the illness and the danger to the patient" (p. 374) and voiced "the problem is how you balance the patient's rights thing and how you balance someone's ability to make a decision for their own self" (p. 374). Moving to the next stage, negotiation indicated that the decision had been made to take coercive action, but also a desire for the "patient's understanding of himself or herself as having a mental illness that requires treatment" (p. 376). The final stage of justifying and taking coercive action involved documentation which supported the need or justification for coercive action and "mitigate[d] the coerciveness by caring interactions before, during, and after a coercive act" (p. 377). Underlying this process was the nurse's belief that the patient would improve with coercive action and eventual voluntary acceptance of medication.

Another study by Lind et al. (2004) examined the perspectives of 170 psychiatric nurses in Finland regarding the use of coercive measures and perceived ethical problems. Most of the nurses were female (63 percent) and 72 percent worked on an inpatient unit, with 94 percent having had less than five years of experience. The participants ($N = 126$) were asked to complete a questionnaire consisting of six questions using a five-point Likert scale response (*totally disagree* to *totally agree*). The questionnaire asked for nurses' opinion of a situation and if it was ethically problematic. Eighteen percent of the participants totally agreed/agreed that implementation of forced medication was ethically problematic, whereas 68 percent of the participants totally disagreed/disagreed that this was ethically problematic. The implementation of four-point restraints was considered ethically problematic by 16 percent of participants (totally agreed/agreed), and 66 percent totally disagreed/disagreed that this was ethically problematic. Implementation of patient seclusion was considered ethically problematic by 11 percent of the participants (totally agreed/agreed), and 72 percent of the participants totally disagreed/disagreed. Additionally, the nurses identified prohibiting or limiting patients from increasing their quality of life as ethically problematic.

These studies shed a unique light on the justification of coercion. While the literature indicates that nurses use a process to determine when to utilize and justify coercion, the ethical issues related to coercion are perceived differently.

Summary

The use of coercion in psychiatric settings has received attention over the years, ranging from descriptions of coercion, attitudes toward coercion, perceptions of coercion by patients and staff, to the justification of coercion. Many studies discuss the ethics of coercion, but there continue to be discrepancies in relation to acceptable use of coercion. Few studies offer strategies to change or impact the use of coercion. The following discussion offers several strategies to impact the use of coercion in psychiatric settings based on evidence in the literature.

Strategies to Effect Change

What can be done to change the use of coercion in psychiatric settings? The author recommends that all strategies be grounded in caring. Why caring? The caring nurse is one who focuses on the other and considers the welfare of the other which is a vital necessity to impact the use of coercion in psychiatric settings (Tuckett, 1999). The caring ingredients of trust, honesty, humility, hope, and courage (Mayeroff, 1971) and attributes of compassion, conscience, and competence (Roach, 2001) are illuminated in the evidence-based strategies below.

Communication

Tingleff et al.'s (2017) systematic review examined the patients' perception of situations before, during, and after a coercive experience. The findings indicated that patients called for more interactions with professionals during coercive experiences, a need to be present and treated with respect, and a need to hold a professional conversation after the coercive experience (p. 692). These findings indicate a call to change communication with patients and enhance caring within the nurse-patient relationship.

One of the first strategies to impact change should include establishing debriefings with patients after any coercive experience to discuss their perception of the experience as well as the staff's perception. Mayeroff's (1971) caring ingredients of courage, humility, and trust provide the groundwork for the debriefing strategy. He describes humility as "The man who cares is genuinely humble in being ready and willing to learn more about the other and himself" (pp. 29–30). Being open to debriefing strategies with patients leads to open and honest communication and enhances the development of trust and understanding in the nurse-patient relationship. Debriefing is currently standard procedure for staff and needs to be a standard procedure with patients. With increased understanding of behaviors and caring communication, reduction in coercive activities can be achieved.

Additional communication strategies include assessment and development of staff caring behaviors. Pawlowski's (2018) findings indicated that personality assessments and development may be a viable tool for staff recruitment/development and reduction of coercive techniques. Enhancement of staff's creativity personality trait and leadership skills through education and training may also lead to reduction in coercive activities.

Education and Training

Jalil et al.'s (2017) research demonstrated the need for additional education and training of staff in working with aggressive patients. Their findings indicated that staff's increased exposure to aggression by patients led to increased use of coercive measures by staff. In addition, Laukkanen et al. (2019) examined the attitudes of staff in relation to coercion and recognized the need for staff to change their views on coercive measures. Al-Maraira et al. (2019) also found that the use of coercive measures relates to lack of training about coercive measures, lack of knowledge of alternative approaches, and lack of knowledge about impact on patients. Based on these research findings, education and training are clearly needed, as well as development of staff's ability to increase their emotional regulation.

HeartMath® (Institute of HeartMath®, 2014) is an evidence-based technique that enhances emotional self-regulation, which is useful in stressful situations (Ratanasiripong et al., 2012; Thurber et al., 2010). Based on biofeedback technology and emotional shift in emotions, the HeartMath® technique teaches a person to control emotions and enhance coping skills in response to stressful situations. Learning stress reduction techniques assists nurses in controlling their emotions during stressful events, which could lead to reduction in coercive actions.

One training strategy described by Abma and Widdershoven (2006) is the CARE (Considerations, Actions, Reasons, Experiences) Model. The Care Model utilizes narratives related to coercion from both patients' and nurses' perspectives to facilitate dialogue. During discussion four questions are asked:

What are my core values and considerations and how do these relate to the situation presented? … How did I act in similar situations and what did I (not) like about my actions? … What kind of considerations do others use in similar situations, and what does our culture say about this situation? … What are the experiences of others when they find themselves in similar situations and what do I (not) like about their actions? [pp. 547–548]

Through discussions, participants enhanced understanding of the other's experience with coercive measures and developed understanding of their own practice values. This approach could easily be implemented in staff meetings and dialogues. By asking these questions, staff's own understanding of self can grow and lead to "trusting the other … trust my own capacity to care" (Mayeroff, 1971, p. 29).

Another teaching strategy is to engage in reflective activities with the staff, which is confirmed by Olofsson's (1998, 2005) studies. Olofsson et al. (1998) conducted a phenomenological hermeneutic study with 14 mental health nurses. Two themes emerged from the analysis: (1) no alternative to coercion and (2) need for reflection. The findings also revealed that the nurses wanted to be viewed as "doing good" by themselves and others.

Olofsson's (2005) study focused on the use of coercion with 21 psychiatric nurses who participated in reflection groups. The findings indicated that staff and supervisor support was important, especially the need for confirmation and endorsement that coercion was necessary and served patients' well-being. Nurses expressed the value of clinical supervision, having time for reflection, and being able to gain new perspectives. Although members of the reflection groups focused on the experience of using coercion, they identified a need to discuss other situations and the difficulty to find time for reflection. To successfully incorporate reflection strategies, both structured time and structured format would need to be in place. Johns (2001) offered a framework for reflection, which incorporates caring concepts. Through guided reflection, staff explore their own behaviors and meaning of coercive situations and come to develop effective practice techniques grounded in caring.

Patterson et al. (2014) recommended incorporation of mindfulness and reflection as another strategy to enhance staff's understanding of professional ethics. Mindfulness has been established as an evidence-based approach for self-care and self-growth. Through these strategies for the enhancement of one's conscience, a staff member commits to behaviors and actions that reflect love and caring (Roach, 2002). Nursing staff might benefit from incorporating mindfulness and reflection, as components of professional self-growth, to strengthen their ethical commitment to care for the patient's well-being.

Legal Regulations and Policy

The Department of Health and Human Services, Centers for Medicare & Medicaid Services (CMS), Federal Regulation, 42 CFR & 482.13, Condition of participation: Patient's rights, Standard: Restraint or seclusion (2012) states:

> All patients have the right to be free from physical or mental abuse, and corporal punishment. All patients have the right to be free from restraint or seclusion, of any form, imposed as a means of coercion, discipline, convenience, or retaliation by staff. Restraint or seclusion may only be imposed to ensure the immediate physical safety of the patient, a staff member, or others and must be discontinued at the earliest possible time.

A recent update to the regulation (84 FR 51817) addresses training of staff regarding restraints:

> Physician and other licensed practitioner training requirements must be specified in hospital policy. At a minimum, physicians and other licensed practitioners authorized to order

restraint or seclusion by hospital policy in accordance with State law must have a working knowledge of hospital policy regarding the use of restraint or seclusion [Federal Registrar, 2019, p. 5187].

This new regulation requires training to facilitate competence in the area of coercion, specifically seclusion and restraints. This training may address the threat to competence described by Roach (2002) as the "misconception and misuse of power" (p. 54). Misuse of power can lead to what Roach describes as "competence without compassion can be brutal and inhuman" (p. 54). Misuse of power and lack of compassion were evident in several studies which recounted the patient's fear of the staff and loss of personal dignity (Allison & Fleming, 2019). The Department of Health and Human Services, CMS regulations for mandated training related to seclusion and physical restraints offer the opportunity for training to focus on competence with compassion. Tuckett (1999) reminded us that "compassion requires a mutual flow of power" (p. 385) which could address the misuse of power in coercion.

Nurse practice acts offer another legal outlet for addressing the use of coercion. Collins and Mikos (2008) described five domains of the legal and professional regulation of nursing and offered a useful framework to evaluate conduct violations by nurses. The authors reviewed 500 cases of nurse practice violators represented by the authors. They identified six common categories of nurse practice violators: bad apples, impaired, incompetents, criminals, rule benders, and good nurses having a bad day. Violation of patient rights, such as using coercion, could be a violation of a nurse practice act.

Inherent in all nurse practice acts lies the caring attribute of conscience. Roach (2002) described conscience as the "voice where the claim of the one is asserted over the power and the persuasion of the many" (p. 58). In the review of the literature, a case study by Hutchinson, Jackson, Walter, and Cleary (2013) described nurse practice violators, yet what action has been taken to eliminate this type of coercive action in nursing? One strategy for change should be to review state-based nurse practice acts and to initiate adaptation including definitions of coercion, legal use of coercion, and consequences for aberrant use of coercion.

See Table 2 for practices to effect coercive interventions.

Table 2. Strategies to Effect Change on Coercion Supported by Evidence-Based Citations

Strategies to Effect Change	Evidence-Based Citations
Implement debriefing with patients and staff after coercive experience	Tingleff et al. (2017)
Implement personality assessment of staff with development of creativity and leadership skills	Pawlowski (2018)
Implement CARE Model for staff conferences and dialogues	Abma & Widdershoven (2006)
Implement guided reflective practice grounded in caring	Johns (2001)

Strategies to Effect Change	Evidence-Based Citations
Implement HeartMath®, mindfulness activities with staff	Ratanasiripong et al. (2012) Thurber et al. (2010)
Require DHS/CMS required training of staff—alternatives/coercive techniques grounded in competence and caring	Allison & Flemming (2019)
Review nurse practice acts	Collins & Mikos (2008)

The need to alter coercive experiences for patients and staff in psychiatric settings is evident. Strategies for development of communication grounded in caring, staff training and education, and policy change, all based on current research, can lead to a reduction in coercive experiences and enhance the well-being of both patients and staff.

Conclusion

Wolf (2012) described the justification of coercion as "nursing in the gray zone" (p. 17). Coercion can be ambiguous and is defined in a variety of ways. The more subtle, softer forms of coercion discussed in the exemplar often flourish in the gray zone of practice. The review of the literature depicts the lack of clear understanding of coercive activities practiced in psychiatric settings, as well as the lack of acknowledgment of the patient's voice when using coercive techniques. The ethical dissonance experienced by nurses when involved in coercive activities and subsequent justification of their actions also demonstrates the grayness of practice. Although there has been a regulatory call to address the coercive activities, such as seclusion and restraint, in a competent and compassionate manner, little has been addressed to change the subtle, softer techniques of coercion. The strategies for change offer approaches to address this issue and ultimately decrease the use of coercive measures. The grounding of all nursing practice in the caring ingredients of trust, honesty, humility, hope, and courage (Mayeroff, 1971) and attributes of compassion, conscience, and competence (Roach, 2001) will lead to compassionate care which respects human dignity and autonomy.

Discussion Questions

1. What are types of coercion as described in Allison and Fleming's (2019) article? Describe them.
2. What differentiates acceptable versus unacceptable use of coercion?
3. What behaviors do nurses show that suggest they are morally disengaged from patients with psychiatric disorders?
4. What are examples of "last-ditch efforts" that nurses and other providers use when caring for patients with psychiatric disorders?
5. How do nurses justify the use of coercion?

Author Selections

Berman. B., & Downer, J. (Executive Producers), & Fleder, G. (Director). (2001). *Don't say a word* [Film]. Regency Enterprises.

Bodie, C. (Executive Producer), & Mangold, J. (Director). (1999). *Girl interrupted* [Film]. Columbia Pictures.

Douglas, M., & Zaentz, S. (Producers), & Forman, M. (Director). (1975). *One flew over the cuckoo's nest* [Film]. Fantasy Films.

Lebel, J. (Producer), & Galvin, M. (Director). (2010). *Real danger: Restraints and our children* [Film]. Department of Mental Health, Boston, MA.

Reiner, R., & Scheinman, A. (Producers), & Reiner, R. (Director) (1990). *Misery* [Film]. Castle Rock Entertainment.

Ruefle, M. (2012). *On fear: Our positive capability* [Poem]. https://www.poetryfoundation.org/poetrymagazine/articles/69815/on-fear.

References

Abma, T.A., & Widdershoven, G.A.M. (2006). Moral deliberation in psychiatric nursing practice. *Nursing Ethics, 13*(5), 546–557. https://doi.org/10.1191/0969733006nej892oa.

Allison, R., & Flemming, K. (2019). Mental health patients' experiences of softer coercion and its effects on their interactions with practitioners: A qualitative evidence synthesis. *Journal of Advanced Nursing, 75*(11), 2274–2284. https://doi.10.1111/jan.14035.

Al-Maraira, O.A., Hayajneh, F.A., & Shehadeh, J.H. (2019). Psychiatric staff attitudes toward coercive measures: An experimental design. *Perspective in Psychiatric Care, 55,* 734–742. https://doi.10.1111/ppc.12422.

American Hospital Association (1992, 2003). *Patient Bill of Rights/The Patient Care Partnerships.* https://www.aha.org/other-resources/patient-care-partnership.

American Nurses Association, American Psychiatric Nurses Association, and International Society of Psychiatric Mental Health Nurses. (2014). *Psychiatric-mental health nursing: scope & standards of practice* (2nd ed.). https://www.apna.org/i4a/pages/index.cfm?pageid=5739.

American Nurses Association. (2015). *Guide to the Code of Ethics for nurses with interpretive statements: Development, interpretation, and application* (2nd ed.). https://www.nursingworld.org/practice-policy/nursing-excellence/ethics/code-of-ethics-for-nurses/.

Andersson, U., Fathollahi, J., & Gustin, L.W. (2020). Nurses' experience of informal coercion on adult psychiatric wards. *Nursing Ethics, 27*(3), 741–753. https://doi.org/10.1177/0969733019884604.

Citizens Commission on Human Rights. (2019). *Mental Health Declaration of Human Rights.* https://www.cchr.org/about-us/mental-health-declaration-of-human-rights.html.

Collins, S.E., & Mikos, C.A. (2008). Evolving taxonomy of nurse practice act violators. *Journal of Nursing Law, 12*(2), 85–91. https://doi.org/10.1891/1073-7472.12.2.85.

Cutcliffe, J.R., & Travale, R. (2013). Respect in mental health: Reconciling the rhetorical hyperbole with the practical reality. *Nursing Ethics, 20*(3), 273–284. https://doi.org/10.1177/0969733012462055.

Doedens, P., Vermeulen, J., Boyette, L.L., Latour, C., & de Haan, L. (2020). Influence of nursing staff attitudes and characteristics on the use of coercive measures in acute mental health services–a systematic review. *Journal of Psychiatric Mental Health Nursing, 27,* 446–449. https://doi.org/10.1111/jpm.12586.

Duncan, H. (2013). Experiences of coercion and treatment pressures amongst mental health service users. [Thesis, University of East London]. https://repository.uel.ac.uk/download/03b120b5ea06257e17f6d0ad9f28e8d10ae62b0cf36eb897bcb490451a5c3c47/3241252/2013_DClinPysch_Duncan.pdf.

Federal Register. (2019, September 30). Department of Health and Human Services, Centers for Medicare & Medicaid Services. *Section 482.13-Conditions of participation for patient rights, 84*(189), 51817. https://www.govinfo.gov/content/pkg/FR-2019-09-30/pdf/2019-20736.pdf.

Federal Regulations. (2012). Title 42. Chapter IV, Subchapter G Part 428 Section 428.13 https://www.law.cornell.edu/cfr/text/42/482.13.

Gault, I., Gallagher, A., & Chambers, M. (2013). Perspectives on medicine adherence in service users and carers with experience of legally sanctioned detention and medication: A qualitative study. *Patient Preference and Adherence, 7,* 787–799. https://doi.10.2147/PPA.S44894.

Hutchinson, M., Jackson, D., Walter, G., & Cleary, M. (2013). Coercion and the corruption of care in mental health nursing: Lessons from a case study. *Issues in Mental Health Nursing, 34*(6), 476–480.

Institute of HeartMath®. (2014). *The resilience advantage: Skills for personal and professional effectiveness.* http://www.trio-consulting.com/wp-content/uploads/2014/07/The-Resilience-Advantage-consolidated-flyer1.pdf.

Jalil, R., Huber, J.W., Sixsmith, J., & Dickens, G.L. (2017). Mental health nurses' emotions, exposure to patient aggression, attitudes to and use of coercive measures: Cross sectional questionnaire survey. *International Journal of Nursing Studies, 75,* 130–138. https://doi.org/10.1016/j.ijnurstu.2017.07.018.

Jarrett, M., Bowers, L., & Simpson, A. (2008). Coerced medication in psychiatric inpatient care: Literature review. *Journal of Advanced Nursing, 64*(6), 538–548. https://doi.org/10.1111/j.1365-2648.2008.04832.x.

Johns, C. (2001). Reflective practice: Revealing the [he]art of caring. *International Journal of Nursing Practice, 7*, 237–245. https://doi.10.1046/j.1440-172x.2001.00283.x.

Katsakou, C., Marougka, S., Garabette, J., Rost, F., Yeeles, K., & Priebe, S. (2011). Why do some voluntary patients feel coerced into hospitalization? A mixed methods study. *Psychiatry Research, 187*, 275–282. https://doi.10.1016/j.psychres.2011.01.001.

Larsen, I.B., & Terkelsen, T.B. (2014). Coercion in a locked psychiatric ward: Perspectives of patient and staff. *Nursing Ethics, 21*(4), 426–436. https://doi.org/10.1177/0969733013503601.

Laukkanen, E., Vehvilainen-Julkunen, K., Louheranta, O., & Kuosmanen, L. (2019). Psychiatric nursing staffs' attitudes towards the use of containment methods in psychiatric inpatient care: An integrative review. *International Journal of Mental Health Nursing, 28*, 390–406. https://doi.10.1111/inm.12574.

Lavelle, S., & Tusaie, K.R. (2011). Reflecting on forced medication. *Issues in Mental Health Nursing, 32*(5), 274–278. https://doi.org/10.3109/01612840.2011.552749.

Lind, M., Kaltiala-Heino, R., Suominen, T., Leino-Kilpi, H., & Valimaki, M. (2004). Nurses' ethical perceptions about coercion. *Journal of Psychiatric and Mental Health Nursing, 11*, 379–385. https://doi.10.1111/j.1365-2850.2004.00715.x.

Lutzen, K. (1998). Subtle coercion in psychiatric practice. *Journal of Psychiatric and Mental Health Nursing, 5*, 101–107. https://doi.10.1046/j.1365-2850.1998.00104.x.

Mayeroff, M. (1971). *On caring*. Harper Perennial.

Motteli, S., Hotzy, F., Lamster, F., Horisberger, R., Theodoridou, A., Vetter, S., Seifritz, E., & Jager, M. (2020). Optimistic recovery expectations are associated with critical attitudes toward coercion among mental health professionals. *International Journal of Mental Health, 49*(2), 157–169. https://doi.org/10.10 80/00207411.2019.1699338.

Newton-Howes, G., & Mullen, R. (2011). Coercion in psychiatric care: Review of correlates and themes. *Psychiatric Services, 62*(5), 465–470. https://doi.10.1176/ps.62.5.pss6205_0465.

Olofsson, B. (2005). Opening up: Psychiatric nurses' experience of participating in reflecting groups focusing on coercion. *Journal of Psychiatric and Mental Health Nursing, 12*, 259–267. https://doi.10.1111/j.1365-2850.2005.00827.x.

Olofsson, B., Gilje, F., Jacobsson, L., & Norberg, N. (1998). Nurses' narratives about using coercion in psychiatric care. *Journal of Advanced Nursing, 28*(1), 45–53. https://doi.org/10.1046/j.1365-2648.1998.00687.x.

Patterson, B., Bennet, L., & Bradley, P. (2014). Positive and proactive care: Could new guidance lead to more problems. *British Journal of Nursing, 23*(17), 939–941. https://doi.org/10.12968/bjon.2014.23.17.939.

Pawlowski, T. (2018). Personality traits of nurses and organizational climate in relation to the use of coercion in psychiatric wards. *Perspectives in Psychiatric Care, 54*, 287–292. https://doi.10.1111/ppc.12236.

Ratanasiripong, P., Ratanasiripong, N., & Kathalae, D. (2012). Biofeedback intervention for stress and anxiety among nursing students: A randomized controlled study. *International Scholarly Research Network, 2012*, 1–5. https://doi.10.5402/2012/827972.

Roach, M.S. (2002). *Caring, the human mode of being: A blueprint for the health professions*. (2nd ed.). CHA Press.

Ryan, C.J., & Bowers, L. (2005). Coercive manoeuvres in a psychiatric intensive care unit. *Journal of Psychiatric and Mental Health Nursing, 12*, 695–702. https://doi.10.1111/j.1365-2850.2005.00899.x.

Thurber, M.R., Bodenhamer-Davis, E., Johnson, M., Chesky, K., & Chandler, C. (2010). Effects of heart rate variability coherence biofeedback training and emotional management techniques to decrease music performance anxiety. *Biofeedback, 38*(1), 28–39.

Tingleff, E.B., Bradley, S.K., Gildberg, F.A., Munksgaard, G., & Hounsgaard, L. (2017). "Treat me with respect." A systematic review and thematic analysis of psychiatric patients' reported perceptions of the situations associated with the process of coercion. *Journal of Psychiatric Mental Health Nursing, 24*, 681–698. https://doi.10.1111/jpm.12410.

Tuckett, A. (1999). Nursing practice: Compassionate deception and the good Samaritan. *Nursing Ethics, 6*(5), 383–389. https://doi.org/10.1177/096973309900600504.

United Nations Human Rights. (2008). *Convention on the Rights of Persons with Disabilities*. https://www.ohchr.org/Documents/Publications/AdvocacyTool_en.pdf.

United States Code. (1991). *Restatement of Bill of Rights for Mental Health Patients*. (U.S. Code, Title 42, Section 10841). https://www.law.cornell.edu/uscode/text/42/10841.

Vuckovich, P.K., & Artinian, B.M. (2005). Justifying coercion. *Nursing Ethics, 12*(4), 370–38. https://doi.10.1191/0969733005ne802oa.

Wolf, Z.R. (2012). Nursing practice breakdowns: Good and bad nursing. *MEDSURG, 21*(1), 16–36. http://web.a.ebscohost.com.dbproxy.lasalle.edu/ehost/detail/detail?vid=1&sid=c29b43f1-3cb1-4d69-96dc-5d9b17669289%40sdc-v-sessmgr01&bdata=JnNpdGU9ZWhvc3QtbGl2ZSZzY29wZT1zaXRl#AN=7183 9591&db=asn.

World Health Organization. (2013). *Mental health action plan 2013-2020*. https://www.who.int/publications /i/item/9789241506021.

Wynn, R. (2006). Coercion in psychiatric care: Clinical, legal, and ethical controversies. *International Journal of Psychiatry in Clinical Practice, 10*, 247–251. https://doi.10.1080/13651500600650026.

Multiple-Choice Questions

1. What is the common element of coercion in health care as noted in various definitions of the construct?
    A. Persuasion
    B. Threat
    C. Exertion of will
    D. Disrespect

2. Last-ditch efforts, as described by Ryan and Bowers (2005), involve which of the following actions?
    A. Body blocks
    B. Seclusion
    C. Touch
    D. Warnings

3. A patient's behavior is escalating. The nurse recognizes the patient's need for medication and attempts to persuade the patient to take the medication. Which of the following types of coercion does the nurse use?
    A. Physical
    B. Hard
    C. Subtle
    D. Soft

4. Which of the following strategies used by nurses and other health care providers in psychiatric settings, following management of patient escalation and coercion actions, promotes trust and understanding between staff and patients?
    A. Debriefing
    B. Being creative
    C. Training
    D. Being mindful

CHAPTER 3

Lying to Patients
for Therapeutic Ends

Maureen Donohue-Smith, PhD, PMHNP

Objectives

1. Compare three functions of lies in health care settings.
2. Describe the role of deception in the effectiveness of placebos.
3. Identify at least two reasons for lying about medical mistakes.
4. List three reasons for the use of the "compassionate lie" in dementia care.

Critical Incidents

Dementia

A 70-year-old patient with dementia had difficulty urinating due to bladder cancer. His family requested that he not be reminded repeatedly of his cancer diagnosis, since this caused an increase in anxiety and agitation every time he had to go to the bathroom. In this case, being reminded of the truth led to the patient's re-experiencing being given a cancer diagnosis many times a day (Butkus, 2014). Staff and family agreed that the medical care team would tell the patient his difficulty urinating was secondary to other problems until he was discharged.

Psychosis

Psychosis also impairs patients' ability to accurately perceive and process reality. *Out of the Shadow* (Smiley, 2007) is a documentary film chronicling the life of Millie, the filmmaker's mother, and Millie's lifelong struggle with schizophrenia. One scene describes a disagreement between the filmmaker and her sister regarding the mother's refusal to take psychiatric medication. Susan, the filmmaker, learns that, without medication, her mother's exacerbation of symptoms (acute paranoia, aggressiveness, and inability to care for herself) requires psychiatric hospitalization that Millie refuses. Susan learns that her sister, Tina, has convinced Millie to sign a form, that Millie believes is a discharge form, but is a consent to treatment, including psychiatric medication. The following dialogue clearly articulates both sides of the ethical dilemma the sisters face, one that is common in families with a mentally ill member.

SUSAN: I can't imagine lying like that, though, Tina. It's so deeply deceitful. I just—I am not capable of lying that badly to her. I mean, she signed a paper that was completely false to her. I mean, you had her sign something that she thought was her ticket to freedom.

TINA: Well, it is her ticket to freedom. She doesn't realize that in order to have the life she wants, she has to be medicated to get her brain straight…. I figure lying to her is a sweet thing to do, other than letting her go homeless and die a horrid death like that. I'd rather her die in a situation where at least she has a roof over her head, she has people around her who love her, even though she doesn't figure it out. Do you understand where I'm coming from? So, if I have to lie, I'm going to f**king lie.

SUSAN: Deceiving her to sign that piece of paper, a ticket to freedom, because it's going to continue the cycle, of the medication, the housing, the end of medication, the losing the housing and it's going to go on and on and on. I guess that's the point I'm trying to make.

TINA: That's true. But that's where my conscience would bother me.

SUSAN: Each of us has to do what we can live with in our own conscience, right? You know, we do what we feel is best. I know you're doing what you feel is best; I know I'm doing what I feel is best.

There is no reference in the film to the provider who would have had to review the informed consent with Millie and to witness the signature. That Millie was hospitalized and medicated suggests the provider accepted her signature as valid. The viewer must decide for themselves whether the cost of violating the ethical principle of veracity should be superseded by the potential benefits of achieving remission of psychotic symptoms and return to community living.

Placebo

A nurse caring for individuals with AIDS in sub–Saharan Africa lacks access to effective medications to treat HIV, since there is neither adequate funding nor means to obtain them. The nurse instead gives her patients iron pills, which she assures them will help them to *feel better.*

In this case report, Ambrose (2006) observed that the nurse believed her patients did experience some relief due to the expectation of the patient for improvement as a result of taking a pill. The nurse believed that, in the absence of retroviral treatment, the benefit provided to the patients through the use of a placebo takes precedence over concerns about deception.

Lying About Medical Errors

I am affected not because you have deceived me,
but because I can no longer believe in you.
—Friedrich Nietzsche

The nurse was asked to administer several medications to a 49-year-old woman who had just arrived in the emergency department suffering an acute allergic reaction to a bee sting. The physician ordered two medications to be administered via IV, along with a subcutaneous injection of epinephrine. The nurse, who was caring for several critically ill patients at the same time, mistakenly injected the epinephrine into the IV instead of administering the dose subcutaneously. The patient experienced increased, bounding pulse, numbness in her fingers, and intense anxiety. The nurse, recognizing her error, attempted to calm the patient by telling her these symptoms commonly occur in allergic reactions and that she would recover quickly. The patient gradually experienced a return to normal heart rate without experiencing any adverse events. The nurse breathed a sigh of relief and never informed the doctor, patient, or family of the error.

Background

Nursing has been ranked as the most trusted profession for over 17 years. Nurses are the team members who work most closely and continuously with patients and their families, and nurses are team members from whom patients and family frequently seek information. Nurse-client interactions grounded in truth and openness are basic elements of the nurse-patient relationship and essential to establishing trust. In addition to the ethical principle of veracity (honesty), beneficence (the responsibility to promote good), nonmaleficence (the responsibility to avoid doing harm), and respect for autonomy (patient self-directed care) are also ethical principles that guide nursing practice (Alfano, 2015). Although nurses are expected to adhere to each of these principles, clinical realities create competing and often conflicting demands that may require honoring the commitment to certain principles ahead of others.

According to Cantone et al. (2019), nurses are the professionals who most often must deal with these ethical decisions. Nurses are confronted daily with situations where they must decide what information to provide, when to provide it, and to whom. In making these determinations, nurses may find themselves caught on the horns of an ethical dilemma. What if telling patients the truth not only fails to promote good, but results in harm? Although nurses' primary responsibility is to patients, there are situations where competing interests also require consideration of the family's wishes and involvement of other members of the health care team. What decision-making guidelines can nurses use to determine the most ethical, yet effective, nursing intervention? Are there cases where avoidance of harm or promotion of good may take higher priority than veracity?

One challenge to truth-telling is the nature of truth itself. Truth has been the Holy Grail of philosophers, poets, and ethicists across time, and success in establishing objective, incontrovertible truths has been elusive. Determining what is "true" may present providers with clinical conundrums. Consider the nurse who engages in a sensitive conversation about end-of-life issues with a hospice patient who has been coping with being told his or her life expectancy is less than six months. With supportive treatment, the patient recovers and is being discharged because they are no longer considered appropriate for hospice services. Does this mean the patient was lied to about their prognosis?

The nurse's ability to provide completely accurate or *truthful* information to their patients is constrained by their own individual level of knowledge and expertise, the extent of current knowledge in the field, and their ability to interpret and communicate medical information unambiguously. According to a Medicare report (Medicare Payment Advisory Committee, 2019, p. 330), 16.9 percent of hospice patients recover sufficiently to be discharged from hospice services. When talking about potential outcomes with patients, statistical probability, as well as the degree of variability in the symptoms and outcomes of their condition, further complicate the making of accurate predictions for a particular condition or patient. Fallowfield et al. (2002), in a discussion on predicting survival in palliative care settings, pointed out that what the provider knows (foresees) may be different from what they communicate to the patient (foretells). This may lead to intentionally or unintentionally misleading the patient about their prognosis.

Even when nurses provide clear, fact-based information to patients, there is no assurance that patients understand the full implications of what is being communicated. To hear a nurse accurately, the patient must have sufficient background knowledge to interpret the information. The patient may be processing this information under conditions of anxiety that may further impair comprehension and prevent information processing. That is, characteristics of the sender, the receiver, the message, and the context in which the information is delivered, all affect the likelihood that what the nurse said is what the patient heard. Where does the truth reside? In the content of the message? In the words chosen by the sender? In the perception of the receiver?

The term *brutal honesty* describes communication in which the truth itself is hurtful. Without considering the potential impact on the patient, transmission of unpleasant truths or poorly timed revelations can irreparably damage personal and professional relationships, as well as the patient's emotional well-being. Levine et al. (2020) noted that the degree of potential harm caused by unpleasant news is often overestimated, as the messenger frequently focuses more on the short-term outcome without considering the context or potential long-term benefits. If information is delivered prematurely, without the professional and emotional support the patient may need to cope, patients may respond to the "bad news" by avoiding their health care provider, withdrawing from treatment, or even becoming suicidal (Agronin, 2010). In this litigious age, providers may feel they are limiting their legal liability by giving patients more information, but this is often more than the patient could be expected to understand and interpret. An excess of potentially confusing and superfluous information is provided to address liability risks of the provider, with little consideration of the patient (Agronin, 2010). Nurses need the knowledge and skills to provide information in an understandable form, in a sensitive manner, and in a setting where the patient has time to reflect, clarify, and explore their options.

If defining *truth* is challenging, determining what constitutes a *lie* can present its own complexities. A deliberate misstatement of fact is perhaps the clearest example of a lie. However, in clinical practice, the lie takes several forms and is perpetrated from various motives. A lie may be one of omission (e.g., intentionally failing to inform a patient about potential negative side effects of an antipsychotic medication) or commission (e.g., telling the patient that they will not experience pain following a major surgical procedure). A lie may be told to ease a patient's anxiety, to please the family, to make the nurse's job easier, or to otherwise serve the interests of the provider or health care system, sometimes taking priority over the interests of the patient.

Gray areas in defining truth-telling certainly exist. For example, at what point do delays in communicating information become lies of omission? Consider the patient admitted to the emergency department in critical condition following a car accident in which two family members were killed. The patient, suffering from severe injuries, repeatedly asks the nurse about what happened to the others in the car. The health care team, believing the shock of learning of these deaths will interfere with effective treatment of the patient, withholds the information while the patient undergoes emergency treatment. Have the staff lied to the patient by not responding immediately to the patient's questions? If this is considered a lie, was the staff right to do so?

Therapeutic, compassionate, or respectful lying is defined as "deliberately deceiving patients for reasons considered to be in their best interest" (Sperber, 2015, p. 43). That is, the nurse intentionally chooses to misstate facts when the nurse believes that disclosing information will be harmful, based on assessment of the patient's emotional state, physical condition, or cognitive competence. Given the ethical obligation to be honest with patients (veracity), some have said that the term *therapeutic lying* is an oxymoron. However, if *therapeutic* means to heal or produce a positive outcome, a strategic lie may accomplish the goal. The question is whether the use of a lie is ever an ethical option to bring about a positive, therapeutic outcome.

Data that describe intentionally misinforming a patient about their condition or treatments are limited. With the advent of electronic health care records, patients have ready access to medical information through their provider's internet portals, so overt lying to patients about their conditions or test results may now be less common. Among some cultural groups, such as Korean, Chinese, and Mexican Americans, and among the elderly, patients themselves or their families may request that the patient not be given too many details or any "bad news" (Fallowfield, 2002; Tuckett, 2012), either to protect the patient or because there are cultural conventions regarding who is responsible for informing them. In this case, the request comes from the patient or family.

Literature

Three forms of lying or misrepresentation are more commonly encountered in nursing practice and will be discussed here. The first example of a "compassionate lie" is in cases where individuals suffer from cognitive impairment, particularly dementia. The example of lying for therapeutic ends in psychiatric care is included above for illustrative purposes. However, the individual with schizophrenia is expected to recover the ability to comprehend, while individuals who suffer from dementia typically do not. Therefore, the argument for the use of the therapeutic lie in psychiatric care has less support. Placebos represent another form of deception to achieve a therapeutic outcome, with the third example being the lie of self-interest, the deliberate failure to disclose medical errors.

Deception in Dementia Care: The "Compassionate Lie"

A truth that's told with bad intent
Beats all the lies you can invent.
—William Blake, "Auguries of Innocence"

Opinions vary regarding the use of the therapeutic lie in working with individuals with dementia. Dementia, or major cognitive disorder, is a "broad term used to describe progressive deterioration of cognitive functioning and global impairment" (Varcarolis, 2018, p. 435). A cardinal symptom of dementia is memory impairment, particularly in moderate-advanced stages. Patients are often unable to remember significant events from their past or to recall information provided to them in the present. Terms such as compassionate lying, benevolent deception, white lies, and fiblets are used to describe those lies told to minimize or avoid anxiety and distress.

Cantone et al. (2019) stated that a lie becomes nontherapeutic when it serves the interests of the nurse rather than the patient. Nurses who misinform patients in order to exert control over the patient, or for the convenience of the nurse, would be violating the ethical principle of veracity. Making decisions for patients without their input is infantilizing and paternalistic when the patient is sufficiently able to understand and process the information provided. Some also argue that causing increased distress or anxiety by repeatedly reminding patients of painful realities they have forgotten, and will be forgotten again in five minutes, violates the principle of nonmaleficence.

Knowledge is power and, without knowledge, the patient cannot fully understand the implications of their health care choices or participate actively in treatment planning. Carter (2016) cautioned against the use of deceit as a method to control or exercise power in the clinical setting. Nurses empower patients and respect their autonomy by providing the needed information, and any additional explanations, to allow the patient to make informed choices. To be able to exercise autonomy, however, patients must "have the capacity for setting personal goals, the ability to establish moral principles and values, and to act on them" (Butkus, 2014, p. 1390).

An overvaluation of autonomy when the patient's ability to understand is compromised fails to meet the needs of the patient "where they are" and does not represent need-based care. Limitations on patient autonomy are common. For patients in advanced disease states, nurses often impose restrictions that are generally accepted as being in the patient's best interest. In fact, the nurse would be found negligent if restrictions that assure patient safety were not enforced. For example, patients with dementia in long-term care residences are commonly restricted to the facility, and they may not be permitted to go for walks, indoors or outdoors, unaccompanied. Patients may be asked to surrender their driver's license. They may even be unable to choose when they wake up, when they eat, what they eat, or with whom. The nurse may be obligated to suspend the principle of autonomy under certain conditions, such as acute psychosis, advanced dementia, or delirium in the interest of patient safety.

Cantone et al. (2019) administered a questionnaire to 106 nurses from 12 geriatric facilities in Italy, finding that only a small minority believed it was never acceptable to lie to a patient (12.3 percent) and only 10.4 percent had never done so. Nurses may have the most contact with the patient, but they may not be the primary decision maker about disclosing diagnoses or test results. Since nurses may be expected to refer certain questions to the physician, nurses are more likely to engage in deception through lies of omission, half-truths, evasion of questions, and the use of euphemism (Tuckett, 2004). Interestingly, patients in hospice were seen as less anxious and depressed than those in hospitals or long-term care facilities, where communication regarding their illness was more open and direct than in hospitals or long-term care facilities (Tuckett, 2004).

Cantone et al. (2019) summarized the arguments for and against therapeutic lying by nurses providing dementia care. Advantages may include more effective pain management, a more positive outlook, more active engagement in treatment, less distress, and fewer incidents of physical acting out or aggression. On the other hand, lying may be unethical if used to control the patient or to ease management of routines of daily care. Lying also limits the patient's autonomy by limiting information needed for decision making. If detected, even the lie told with good intentions may damage the nurse-patient relationship in the present and deter the patient from developing positive relationships with health care providers in the future. According to Benn (2001), trust in the provider is more likely to suffer if the lie is an overt or direct lie, rather than other types of deception.

Discussions of the ethics regarding the use of therapeutic lying are predicated on the assumption that the patient is competent. Butkus (2014) proposed that, in cases of dementia, it is the disease itself that has deprived the individual of autonomy. Caiazza and James (2015) endorsed the adoption of the concept of a dementia-oriented reality that would provide an organizing framework for ethical decision making. This approach suggests that the nurse should respond to the patient with compassion and respect for the patient's perceptions and personal reality, a response that may include elements of deception. If therapeutic lying is the treatment of choice, then practice guidelines should be established to provide both a specific guide to create a shared understanding of the issues related to ethical decision making and a formally endorsed algorithm that could be followed and agreed to by all those involved in the patient's treatment. Two proposed sets of guidelines that attempt to maintain a patient-centered, ethical decision-making process which preserves individual dignity while taking into account the patient's current level of functioning are described below.

Sokol (2007) offers a flowchart based on six deceptively simple questions to determine whether a given act of deception, therapeutic lying, would meet the moral and ethical standards of care.

The six questions to be addressed are:

1. Is the act deceptive?
2. What justifications exist for engaging in deception?
3. Is the deception likely to succeed in light of the patient's mental state, and is it possible for us to meet our objective without the deception?
4. Do the justifications for deception outweigh the objections that can be raised?
5. Can we defend this decision to a professional board or court of law?
6. Would the patient consent to the lie in advance? (Adapted from Sokol, 2007)

The flowchart includes both specific examples of acceptable evidence to support deception, as well as a set of similar examples of common objections to lying to be considered. Reasons to consider deception include preventing physical or psychological harm; maintaining hope; ameliorating stress or anxiety; respecting the patient's wishes not to be informed; and supporting autonomy in the long term. Objections to deception include possible loss of trust, violation of professional ethics, and increased distress if truth is uncovered. Personal bias may affect the provider's ability to accurately weigh potential advantages and disadvantages of lying. Once the provider engages in deception, they may have to repeat, or even elaborate on, their original disinformation narrative in their ongoing interactions with the client and family. Sokol's (2007) model suggests an additional caveat—that deception might be a slippery slope in that, once engaged in, lying may become a more easily selected option.

Another set of ethical guidelines proposed by James et al. (2006) overlaps with and extends Sokol's framework. In a survey of the incidence of lying among staff in dementia settings, the authors found that only 1.8 percent of ($N = 112$) respondents said they were unaware of any lying to patients, either by coworkers or themselves. In this sample, 93.3 percent supported the statement that lying might be helpful to reduce negative emotional reactions and to increase adherence to medications and routines. On the other hand, 88.5 percent were aware that lying could also present problems, such as creating confusion when all staff did not provide the same information, mistrust between patients and staff, and friction between staff and family members. To assure ethical and consistent application of decision rules for determining when/whether to engage in therapeutic lying, the authors developed the following recommendations for use by the health care team in providing care for individuals suffering from dementia:

1. Lies should only be told if they are in the best interests of the resident (to ease distress).

2. Specific areas, such as covert medication and aggressive behavior, require individualized policies that are documented in the care plan.

3. A clear definition of what constitutes a lie should be agreed upon in each setting.

4. Mental capacity assessments should be performed on each resident/patient prior to use of therapeutic lies.

5. Communication with family should be required and family consent gained if a lie is to be told to the patient.

6. Once a lie has been agreed on, it must be used consistently across people and settings.

7. Lies told should be documented to ensure they are told in residents'/patients' best interests.

8. An individualized approach should be adopted toward each case, that is, the relative costs and benefits established relating to the lie.

9. Staff should feel supported by management and the resident's/patient's family. They should not feel at risk of being accused of misconduct by telling lies if they have been agreed using these guidelines.

10. Circumstances in which lies should not be told need to be outlined and documented.

11. The act of telling lies should not lead to staff disrespecting the patient. The lies should be seen as a strategy to enhance the resident's/patient's well-being, rather than an infringement of their basic rights.

12. Staff should receive training and supervision on the potential problems of lying and taught alternative strategies to use when lies are not appropriate [James et al., 2006, p. 800].

Research supports the conclusion that although nurses value truth-telling and recognize its importance in establishing strong patient relationships, reports from the field indicate that deception is common in the care of patients experiencing dementia.

Placebos: Deception as Treatment

The use of charms to treat the soul as well as the body can be documented as far back as the time of Socrates and Plato (Papakostas & Daras, 2001). In the Middle Ages, placebo singers were engaged to provide solace and comfort at funerals, but the term began to take on negative connotations (Rawlins, 2018). In Chaucer's *The Merchant's Tale*, Placebo is a poor advisor to his friend, the consummate yes man, full of false flattery. Placebo became a pejorative used to describe sycophants and people pleasers (Rawlins, 2018). While some view placebos in contemporary medical practice as quackery, other researchers endorse the placebo effect as a multi-dimensional phenomenon which draws not only upon physiology, but upon culture, social norms, and psychological characteristics to improve health (Greener, 2018).

According to the American Medical Association (AMA), a placebo is "a substance provided to a patient that the physician believes has no specific pharmacological effect upon the condition being treated" (AMA, 2020, para. 1). Alfano (2015) summarizes Grumbaum's description of the placebo effect as "any effect on the target disorder caused by factors of treatment that are not identified by the dominant theory as efficacious" (p. 4). Some researchers differentiate between the *pure* placebo, which is a pharmacologically inactive substance, and the *impure* placebo, a substance that is physiologically active (e.g., vitamins), but is not known to have any impact on the target illness (Jutte, 2013).

Three major mechanisms of action have been advanced to account for the efficacy of treatment with placebo (Alfano, 2015). The most popular explanation is that the patient's expectation of an outcome, whether of a positive (placebo) or negative (nocebo) outcome, produces the anticipated response, a type of self-fulfilling prophecy. Patients who believed their intravenous infusion contained pain medication reported lower pain levels and requested less pain medication (Alfano, 2015). Of course, the state of anticipation itself creates neurophysiological changes in the brain, and an increase in the release of dopamine has been found in studies of patients with Parkinson's disease who were administered a placebo (de la Fuente-Fernandez, 2001). Studies have found activation of the nucleus accumbens and the ventral striatum, key components of the reward pathway, that supports the involvement of neurotransmission in reactions to placebo (Czerniak, 2016).

Another potential explanation for the effect of placebos is classical conditioning. That is, once someone has experienced an effect of taking a pill, they are more likely to respond in the same way when they are given a similar pill (Alfano, 2015). If people experience pain relief following an injection, they may be more likely to experience reduced pain when given an injection of a placebo. In Italy, women tended to respond better to blue pills (sedatives), the color associated with Mary, the Blessed Mother; Italian male subjects responded better to red pills, the color associated with the national soccer team.

A third hypothesis proposes the development of an attention-somatic feedback loop. When the placebo is administered, the individual focuses on the target area, with an expectation of change. As the person's attention centers on that area, any changes in feeling are interpreted as a positive response. The experience of relief is fed back to centers of the brain which decrease tension, thus reducing physiological tension and anxiety and confirming the medication is working. Benedetti et al. (2018) reported that the neurochemical response to placebos has, in some cases, been found to be similar to the same neural pathway activated by active substances. Benedetti et al. (2018) noted that there may not be a single mechanism for explaining placebo effectiveness. For example, the giving of a placebo involved both symbolic behavior (giving a pill) and brain activation, a result of the expectations of the result of taking the pill.

The current debate over the ethical uses of placebos continues a discussion started over 200 years ago (Blease et al., 2016). The use of placebos as controls is common in randomized clinical trials; however, placebo effects have sometimes been comparable to the results of the active intervention. In reviews of randomized control trials, Greener (2018) and Blease (2015) both described positive responses to placebo for conditions including epilepsy, neuropathic pain, dental pain, fibromyalgia, migraine, pancreatic pain, Crohn's disease, and asthma. In a report of Cochrane Library's review of 158 clinical trials, no response was found for depression, obesity, smoking, or hypertension (Greener, 2018) nor for allergies (Leibowitz, 2019). To better understand the placebo response, Enck and Klosterhalfen (2018) called for refinement of research protocols that involve placebos. Since those in the treatment group may also experience a certain degree of placebo response in addition to effect of active treatment, research must include designs that minimize the level of placebo response in the treatment group.

In contrast, patients may experience an increase in pain or distress after receiving the nonspecific substance or *nocebo*. Greener (2018) cited an example of a Maori woman who ate fruit that was taken from a taboo area. When she learned of the fruit's source, the woman firmly believed the cursed fruit would kill her, and she died by the following day. Patients reading the long list of side effects included with medications may anticipate unpleasant or dangerous side effects that are, in fact, quite rare. The provider must decide how much, or how detailed, the information provided to a specific patient will be, balancing the right of patients to truly informed consent against needless distress over rare, but significant, negative sequelae of treatment. Blease (2015) noted that blind randomized control trials of antidepressant medication are often confounded by the presence of side effects of the active medication which suggests which medication that subject is taking. On the other hand, there are cases where the expectation of side effects results in the subject experiencing the side effects for no physiologically based reason.

Although including the nurse-patient relationship in a discussion may overly broaden the concept of placebo, it is important to note that the quality of provider-patient interactions can also influence placebo effectiveness (Papakostas & Daras, 2001). The nature of the content and the manner it is presented both affect treatment efficacy. Czerniak et al. (2016), in a randomized control study, found that patients experienced greater relief from a placebo topical cream when treated by physicians who were more personally interactive, who moved about the room, who made frequent eye contact, and who employed more physical touch. Thus, a complex interaction among physiological and psychological factors influences treatment response—whether to a pill, to a somatic intervention, or to characteristics of the provider.

Current advances in neuroscience, such as the fMRI, positive emission tomography and SPECT analysis, have created new avenues for research into the neurological processes which mediate the response to placebos (Frisaldi et al., 2018). Work continues to create ways of identifying those individuals who are more likely to be placebo responders, which may lead to more standardized protocols for using placebos in clinical practice. Individuals who are genetically homozygous for COMT Val158 met polymorphism, which is involved in dopamine metabolism, were more likely to be positive responders to placebo in a study of IBS (Frisaldi et al., 2018). Studies continue to use advanced neuroimaging and assessment tools to explore whether patients' expectations of symptom relief, like Dumbo's belief in the power of his feather, reduce pain or discomfort.

In addressing the ethics of patient deception, the AMA (2008) supported *authorized ignorance* and asserted that placebos can be effective, even when the patient is aware of what they are receiving. According to AMA guidelines, the provider should obtain agreement for the use of placebo, but they are not obligated to reveal its specific composition or when it is being used during treatment (Blease et al., 2016). Thus, patients know they will be given a placebo; however, they anticipate it will lead to improvement. This is further supported by Ambrose (2007) who confirmed that the creation of optimism for efficacy can be accomplished without lying, noting that classical conditioning produces conditioned responses, even when the individual participates knowingly in the conditioning. In making the request of the patient for permission to use a placebo, Blease et al. (2016) suggested that when informing patients and there is no known specific mechanism of action, research suggests that the substance has affected brain functioning in ways that have been found to produce relief of symptoms. In this approach, the patient determines whether they choose to participate. In the psychotherapy of depression, Blease (2010) described findings that individuals suffering depression have a more realistic appraisal of reality and that therapy relies to a significant extent on the development of a different cognitive frame which allows for a more optimistic view of the future.

In addition to authorized ignorance, in which the patient agrees to administration of a placebo, the provider may also consider *authorized concealment*. In this case, the patient agrees to have certain information withheld. Alfano (2015) advised against "making autonomy a sacred value" (p. 3), with careful consideration of potential benefits to the patient. Blease et al. (2016) found that most patients (85 percent) supported the use of open label placebos and a small majority (53.9 percent) indicated that deception would be damaging to the patient-provider relationship. From the provider's perspective, 55 percent of providers in internal medicine or rheumatology used placebos, while in the United Kingdom lifetime prevalence for placebo use was 97 percent.

In evaluating the effectiveness of placebos, several alternative explanations must be considered. Are effects due to statistical functions, like regression to the mean? Are patients simply following the typical course of recovery? Are there other variables, such as provider concern and attention that produce positive response?

Strong arguments are made both for and against the use of placebos. Patients may benefit by avoiding adverse events, drug dependence and decreased cost. Although some authors suggested that the value of patient autonomy may be overridden by the need to promote good and avoid harm (Alfano, 2015), others argued strenuously that such practice is unethical (Golomb, 2009). New avenues of research are being pursued that may provide new paradigms for understanding the mechanisms of placebos and stronger evidence for incorporating them into evidence-based practices. Nurse practitioner prescribers, especially those who take a holistic approach to meeting the needs of their patients, can follow the current research on complementary and alternative therapies to expand their range of therapeutic options (Mendes, 2019).

Lying About Medical Errors: Self-Serving Deception

When truth is replaced by silence, the silence is a lie.
—Yevgeny Yevtushenko

Medical errors are the third leading cause of death in the United States (Makary & Daniel, 2016), with 1.5 million patients experiencing 400,000 adverse events each year (Rogers et al., 2017). The consequences of making a medical error can be severe. In addition to termination of current employment, nurses who make serious medical errors suffer significant emotional distress and may choose to leave nursing entirely.

In extreme cases, nurses' subsequent guilt and depression can lead to a lifetime of self-recrimination or even suicide (Aleccia, 2011). How, or whether, nurses choose to disclose the error, presents another challenge to the ethical principle of veracity. Medical errors are those actions that involve failure to meet standards of best practice, either by commission (e.g., administering the wrong dose of medication) or omission (e.g., failing to give medication as ordered or patient neglect). When a particular action or lack of action is defined as a medical error, this presumes a violation of the standard of care and potential harm to the client resulting from an intentional breach of this standard. Grossman et al. (2020) pointed out the subjective nature of error and the inherent risks that are unavoidable in the practice of medicine.

Errors may occur as the result of the nurse's lack of knowledge, lack of skill in carrying out a procedure, poor clinical judgment, or non-adherence to evidence-based protocols (Hannawa, 2009). According to nurses (Hammoudi et al., 2017), the most common causes for medication errors were: (1) confusing labeling on medication packages, (2) poor legibility and clarity of physician orders, (3) incorrect dosages sent by the pharmacy, and (4) errors in transcribing of orders. Poor nurse-patient ratios and caring for clinically complex patients may also increase the likelihood of error.

As in earlier examples, several principles compete in shaping the nurse's decision to tell a patient an error has been made: (1) the degree to which disclosure results in improvement to the patient's circumstances (beneficence) or an avoidance of harm (maleficence) versus (2) an overriding commitment to veracity, that to tell the truth is always *the right thing to do*. If the error did not cause physical harm to the patient, the nurse may choose not to disclose, believing that such disclosure would destroy the patient's trust in the nurse, increase the patient's anxiety, and perhaps result in the patient's refusal to continue in treatment. On the other hand, the nurse may believe that the patient's right to know supersedes potential risks, regardless of the impact on the patient. It is difficult to disentangle the degree to which concerns about personal repercussions may affect the interpretation of whether disclosure is in the patient's best interest.

It is not surprising that errors in medical settings often go unreported. Hannawa (2009) found that among physicians, the pattern of disclosure is curvilinear; that is, doctors are more likely to tell patients about the most trivial and the most serious errors, with considerable variation in the decision to reveal those mistakes that resulted in moderate risk. Nurses report a failure to report medication errors out of fear of disciplinary action by the hospital, fear of being sued by the patient or family, concern over the negative response by physician, patients, or families, and the long-term impact on their career (Hammoudi, 2017). The disagreement of what constitutes an error also contributed to non-reporting in this study as well.

Arguments have been made on both sides, that is, both for disclosing errors and for withholding such incidents from the patient, with both benefits and limitations to disclosure for both patient and nurse. Disclosure benefits patients by providing them with important information should they experience any negative effects. Knowing the potential risks resulting from the error may increase patients' willingness to monitor their symptoms more carefully. Symptoms resulting from the error can then be attributed to the correct source and treated appropriately. The patients themselves may be relieved to know the true origins of their new symptoms, rather than fearing they have worsened or developed a new condition. Patients may be compensated for any marginal increase in cost of treatment accruing from treatment of error-related conditions. Disclosure may result in an increase in trust in nurses and an increased engagement in participating in their own treatment (Hannawa, 1997). For the nurse, benefits of disclosing include a sense of relief, since the stress of a cover-up, especially if it is ultimately uncovered, may result in even greater distress and legal liability.

Effective verbal and nonverbal communication in the disclosure of errors were both associated with less distancing from the provider by client and family, as well as a decreased likelihood of pursuing litigation (Hannawa, 2009; Hannawa & Frankel, 2018). Disclosure may create an opportunity to be forgiven by the patient and to increase trust in the nurse by the patient, by coworkers and by administration. Long-term advantages of sharing the circumstances contributing to the error may promote system changes or create educational opportunities for other nurses so they may reduce the likelihood of similar errors in the future.

On the other hand, disclosure carries with it the potential for harm, both to patient and nurse. Obvious adverse consequences of error for the patient include any increase in pain and suffering, lost time from work or permanent disability, or the added cost in both time and money needed for continuing treatment. In addition, the patient may no longer see medical treatment as safe and reliable, thereby failing to seek needed care in the future. Mansouri et al. (2019) found that fear of reprisal, lack of clarity surrounding reporting procedures and inadequate feedback, or punitive climate were associated with nonreporting of errors.

The nurse also faces negative consequences from disclosing practice errors. The nurse may have been confronted with anger and humiliation, both when disclosing to the patient and to coworkers and supervisors. The patient may sue the nurse, or a history of malpractice may be reported to the state board of nursing and affect the nurse's license. With the rise in social media, a patient may provide a negative review on provider-rating websites, expanding the scope of the potential audience and intensifying the humiliation.

Several authors emphasized the responsibility of health care educators and supervisors to teach students and staff appropriate ways of dealing with practice errors. It is not a question whether a nurse will commit an error, but when. Both nursing faculty and nurse administrators can transform commission of an error into a critical learning experience for students and staff. The development of a disclosure protocol, embedded in a framework that recognizes error as inevitable, provides both the tools and motivation for students and staff to present this unpleasant news to their patients (Hannawa, 2009; Noland, 2012).

Noland (2015) noted that nursing students are rarely taught systematically about what to report, how to report, or to whom to report, whether this is an error they themselves make or an error they have seen made by a coworker. Providing students and practitioners with training in the most helpful, least harmful ways to tell patients about a practice error increases the likelihood of the patient being treated appropriately, that trust in the provider is affirmed, that the professional integrity of the individual committing the error is maintained, and the safety and the legal responsibilities of the institution are respected.

Creating effective responses to medical error necessitates changes to institutional climate and its attitude toward medical error, as well as promotion of transparent and respectful communication by nurses when errors occur. Institutional adoption of the

Just Culture model for managing practice errors establishes a systematic, non-punitive approach which shifts the emphasis from *blame and shame* to professional accountability and competence (Rogers et al, 2017). By categorizing caregiving actions resulting in clinical mistakes into "human error, at-risk behavior, and reckless behavior" (Rogers et al., 2017, p. 309), supervisory responses to errors can be tailored to the specific situation. This framework recognizes that errors are inevitable and have varying causes and provides suggestions for performance monitoring that supports staff accountability and, in doing so, creates an organization that grows and changes in response to its needs.

Communicating about a medical error is a delicate and difficult conversation for any health care provider. The Massachusetts Alliance for Communication and Resolution following Medical Injury (n.d.a.) created a four-step response to medical errors which encourages "competent disclosure" and minimizes the negative impact on patient and provider alike of extended litigation. MACRMI's website describes the CARe Model, which has been adopted by several institutions. This model offers the following recommendations:

- proactively identify adverse events
- distinguish between injuries caused by medical negligence and those arising from complications of disease or intrinsically high-risk medical care
- offer patients full-disclosure and honest explanations
- offer an apology with rapid and fair compensation when standards of care were not met [MACRMI, n.d.b].

At the level of the organization, having a specific institutionalized response, one which would ideally be embedded in an overarching atmosphere of professional respect and understanding, would provide a structure that may overcome some of the barriers to disclosure described above.

Competent disclosure to the patient should include being clear that an error occurred and providing specific information about the error. Patients want (and need) to know the nature of the error, why it occurred, its implications for their present physical condition, and any future concerns that may result. Especially significant is the explicit apology for the event, accompanied by what will be done to assure that it does not happen again in the future (Hannawa, 2009). Providing this information in a sensitive, empathic manner in terms the patient can understand is essential. This difficult conversation should also be held at a time and place that allows the patient to express their anger, fear or disappointment. The nurse should also be prepared to manage these difficult emotions that the patient may express and to answer any questions the patient may have (Wu, 1997).

Disclosure is not considered competent when characterized by defensiveness, denial that an error occurred, or denial that the action was an error. Minimizing the importance of the error, blaming external circumstances, the patient's condition or the patient themselves are also nontherapeutic responses.

Reliance on a protocol does not eliminate the challenges to decision making about disclosing errors to patients in all circumstances. The nurse may still have to determine when to disclose, based on the patient's psychological and physical condition, and how disclosure might affect the treatment and recovery process. In complex cases, referral to the ethics committee of the hospital may be the appropriate action.

Conclusion

The wise thing is for us diligently to train ourselves to lie thoughtfully, judiciously; to lie with a good object, and not an evil one; to lie for others' advantage, and not our own; to lie healingly, charitably, humanely, not cruelly, hurtfully, maliciously; to lie gracefully and graciously, not awkwardly and clumsily; to lie firmly, frankly, squarely, with head erect, not haltingly, tortuously, with pusillanimous mien, as being ashamed of our high calling.
—Mark Twain, "On the Decay of the Art of Lying"

Although studies of nurses' attitudes toward deception do not support directly lying to patients, the literature suggests that patient deception, particularly in several specific areas, is common. Culley et al. (2016) found that, although psychiatrists did believe that lying to patients could have therapeutic advantages, they also did not believe lying was ethical. Nurses in long-term care facilities reported that they valued the principle of autonomy; however, in practice, staff frequently engaged in deception both to minimize patient distress and to encourage compliance with routines. While some authors support full directness with individuals experiencing dementia, others prioritize principles of beneficence and maleficence in cases where the provided information is likely to fade quickly from memory. To reconcile these views, one might think of the cognitive impairment associated with dementia as a form of disability. From this perspective, by avoiding distressing reminders that are quickly forgotten, the nurse is interacting within the patient's dementia-oriented reality and meeting the patient *where they are.*

The literature also describes the controversy surrounding the use of placebos. Again, ethical dilemmas are posed by the potential for enhancing response to treatment at the cost of patient deception. The significance of patients' expectations in predicting response to placebos has implications for the way in which nurses provide medication teaching. The nurse's biases, as well as the content of the information provided, may facilitate or inhibit the patient's response. In this case, the effect of treatment relies on deception; however, there are interesting options, such as *authorized ignorance*, that informs the patient without losing the potential placebo effect. Placebos may benefit the patient who is then able to forego expensive medications and reduce the possibility of any untoward side effects. It is interesting to note that, when patients believe they are taking an active medication, some of the side effects anticipated in the treatment group are also experienced by those in the placebo group.

When medical errors are made, nurses must decide about how, or whether, to tell the patient. Arguments for disclosure include adherence to the principle of veracity, affirming the patient's trust in being properly informed, minimizing the patient's emotional distress, and avoiding potential withdrawal from treatment due to a loss of confidence. Withholding information about a medical error may avoid unnecessarily upsetting the patient, especially when the error does not have significant consequences. The nurse may also fail to report the error to protect their professional reputation, out of fear of lawsuits, or concern about termination of employment.

Strategies

The following table includes evidence-based strategies to inform nurses about the complexities associated with lying for therapeutic ends.

Table 3. Strategies to Address Complexities Associated with Lying for Therapeutic Ends

Strategies to Effect Change	Evidence-Based Citations
Incorporate education about ethics into the nursing curriculum	Langone (2007) Noland & Carmack (2015) Noland & Carmack (2014)
Provide guidelines for having difficult conversations with patients in the nursing curriculum and reinforce through supervision in the workplace	Agronin (2010) Papakostas & Daras (2001) Tuckett (2012)
Develop and document a consistent, interdisciplinary approach to communication with patients experiencing cognitive impairment, such as dementia and psychosis	Butkus (2014) Caizza & James (2015) Cantone (2019)
Employ established guidelines for the use of deception in the clinical setting	AMA (2008) Butkus (2014) James et al. (2006) Sokol (2007)
Identify alternatives to deception where possible, such as obtaining authorized ignorance	AMA (2008) Blease et al. (2016) Gold & Lichtenberg (2015)
Teach nursing students how to competently disclose medical errors, including strategies for reporting	McKenzie et al. (2020) Noland (2012) Noland (2015)
Adoption of the Just Culture model as a proactive and nonpunitive approach to medical errors	Dimond (2018) Rogers (2017) Trossman (2019)

Conclusion

In general, nurses' support for honesty and directness in communicating with patients is highly valued. However, the complexities of clinical practice create ethical dilemmas that are not easily addressed, with issues that are situation specific. Development of protocols and guidelines for handling both institutional and individual responses to medical errors have been developed. Providing education to both nursing students as part of the undergraduate curriculum and to working nurses through in-service sessions and continuing education are encouraged.

Discussion Questions

1. Describe what is meant by an ethical dilemma. What are the competing ethical principles that the nurse caring for the patient with dementia must confront?

2. What is the rationale for telling the patient a compassionate lie? Under what conditions might lying to a patient be therapeutic? What are the arguments against the compassionate lie?

3. Describe a situation in which you or a colleague lied to a patient. What

were the reasons for the lie? Did the lie accomplish the desired outcome? Was there another way the situation could have been dealt with to achieve the outcome?

4. Should nurses always inform the patient when a medical error has occurred? Can withholding information about a medical error ever be in the patient's best interest? What are the potential benefits and liabilities for the nurse who conceals information about a medical error?

5. Have you ever seen examples in your practice of the placebo effect? In what ways can nurses enhance the placebo effect of evidence-based nursing interventions?

AUTHOR SELECTIONS

Ariely, D. (Producer), & Melamede, Y. (Director). (2015). *(Dis) Honesty: The truth about lies* [Film], Netflix.

Braschi G., & Ferri, E. (Producers), & Benigni, R. (Director). (1997). *Life is beautiful* [Film]. Miramax.

Ekman, P. (2009). *Telling lies.* W.W. Norton & Company.

Glass, I. (Host). (2016, April 22). What you don't know [Audio podcast episode]. In This American Life. https://www.thisamericanlife.org/585/in-defense-of-ignorance.

Melia, D., Saraf, P., Turtletaub, M., Miano, A., Weitz, C.,...Gou, A. (Producers), & Wang, L. (Director). *The farewell* [Film]. Ray Productions, Big Beach, Depth of Field, Kindred Spirit.

Smith, D.D. (2007). *Why we lie.* St. Martin's Griffin.

REFERENCES

Agronin, M. (2010). How we age: A doctor's journey into the heart of growing old. *Publishers Weekly, 257*(48), 42.

Aleccia, J. (2011, June 27). *Nurse's suicide highlights twin tragedies of medical errors.* Healthcare on NBC-NEWS. https://nbcnews.com/id/43529641/ns/health-health_care/t/nurses-suicide-highlights-twin-tragedies-medical-errors/#.Xhoa8FNKiRs.

Alfano, M. (2015). Placebo effects and informed consent. *American Journal of Bioethics, 15*(10), 3–12. https://doi.org/10.1080/15265161.2015.1074302.

Ambrose, E.G. (2007). Placebos: The nurse and the iron pills. *Journal of Medical Ethics, 33*(6), 325–328. https://dbproxy.lasalle.edu:6149/10.1136/jme.2006.016915.

American Medical Association. (2020). *Code of Medical Ethics Opinion 2.1.4: Use of placebos in clinical practice.* https://www.ama-assn.org/delivering-care/ethics/use-placebo-clinical-practice.

Benedetti, F., Piedimonte, A., & Frisaldi, E. (2018). How do placebos work? *European Journal of Psychotraumatology, 9,* Article 1533370. https://doi.org/10.1080/20008198.2018.1533370.

Benn, P. (2001). Medicine, lies and deceptions. *Journal of Medical Ethics, 27*(2), 130. https://dbproxy.lasalle.edu:6149/10.1136/jme.27.2.130.

Blake, W. (2017, December 22). *The Pickering manuscript/Auguries of innocence.* https://en.wikisource.org/wiki/The_Pickering_Manuscript/Auguries_of_Innocence.

Blease, C. (2010). Deception as treatment: The case of depression. *Journal of Medical Ethics, 37*(1), 13–16. https://dbproxy.lasalle.edu:6149/10.1136/jme.2010.039313.

Blease, C. (2015). Authorized concealment and authorized deception: Well-intended secrets are likely to induce nocebo effects. *American Journal of Bioethics, 15*(10), 23–25. https://dbproxy.lasalle.edu:6149/10.1080/15265161.2015.1074310.

Blease, C., Colloca, L., & Kaptchuk, T.J. (2016). Are open-label placebos ethical? Informed consent and ethical equivocations. *Bioethics, 30*(6), 407–414. https://dbproxy.lasalle.edu:6149/10.1111/bioe.12245.

Butkus, M.A. (2014). Compassionate deception: Lying to patients with dementia. *Philosophical Practice: Journal of the American Philosophical Practitioners Association (American Philosophical Practitioners Association), 9*(2), 1388–1396. http://dbproxy.lasalle.edu:2057/login.aspx?direct=true&db=asn&AN=97373078&site=ehost-live&scope=site.

Cantone, D., Attena, F., Cerrone, S., Fabozzi, A., Rossiello, R., Spagnoli, L., & Pelullo, C.P. (2019). Lying to patients with dementia: Attitudes versus behaviours in nurses. *Nursing Ethics, 26*(4), 984–992. https://dbproxy.lasalle.edu:6149/10.1177/0969733017739782.

Carter, M. (2016). Deceit and dishonesty as practice: The comfort of lying. *Nursing Philosophy, 17*(3), 202–210. https://dbproxy.lasalle.edu:6149/10.1111/nup.12129.

Culley, H., Barber, R., Hope, A., & James, I. (2013). Therapeutic lying in dementia care. *Nursing Standard, 28*(1), 35–39. https://dbproxy.lasalle.edu:6149/10.7748/ns2013.09.28.1.35.e7749.

Czerniak, E., Biegon, A., Ziv, A., Karnieli-Miller, O., Weiser, M., Alon, U., & Citron, A. (2016). Manipulating the placebo response in experimental pain by altering doctor's performance style. *Frontiers in Psychology, 7*(874). Article 874. https://doi.org/10.3389/fpsyg.2016.00874.

De la Fuente-Fernández, R., Ruth, T.J., Sossi, V., Schulzer, M., Calne, D.B., Stoessl, A.J. (2001). Expectation and dopamine release: Mechanism of the placebo effect in Parkinson's disease. *Science, 293*(5532), 1164–1166.

Dimond, V. (2018, July 22). The terror of medical errors. *Healthcare Purchasing News.* https://jackson-medical.com/the-terror-of-medical-errors-healthcare-purchasing-news-august-2018-issue/.

Enck, P., & Klosterhalfen, S. (2013). The placebo response in clinical trials–The current state of play. *Complementary Therapies in Medicine, 21*, 98–101.

Fallowfield, L., Jenkins, V., & Beveridge, H. (2002). Truth may hurt but deceit hurts more: Communication in palliative care. *Palliative Medicine, 16*(4), 297–303. https://dbproxy.lasalle.edu:6149/10.1191/0269216302pm575oa.

Farag, A., Lose, D., & Gedney-Lose. (2019). Nurses' safety motivation: Examining predictors of nurses' willingness to report medication errors. *Western Journal of Nursing Research, 41*(7), 954–972.

Frelick, M. (2019, January). Physicians, nurses, draw different lines for when lying is OK. *Medscape.* https://www.medscape.com/viewarticle/908418_print.

Frisaldi, E., Shaiban, A., & Benedetti, F. (2018). Placebo responders and nonresponders: What's new. *Pain Management, 8*(6), 405–408.

Gold, A., & Lichtenberg, P. (2015). Clinical placebo can be defined positively: Implications for informed consent. *American Journal of Bioethics, 15*(10), 25–27. https://dbproxy.lasalle.edu:6149/10.1080/15265161.2015.1074305.

Golomb, B. (2009). Doctoring the evidence: The case against lying to patients about placebos. *American Journal of Bioethics, 9*(12), 34–36. https://dbproxy.lasalle.edu:6149/10.1080/15265160903244242.

Greener, M. (2018). Taboos, worms and prophecies: Insights into the placebo enigma. *Progress in Neurology & Psychiatry, 22*(2), 30–32. https://dbproxy.lasalle.edu:6149/10.1002/pnp.503.

Grossman, S.A., Gurley, K.L., & Wolfe, R.E. (2020). The ethics of error in medicine. *Rambam Maimonides Medical Journal, 11*(4), e0033. https://doi-org.dbproxy.lasalle.edu/10.5041/RMMJ.10406.

Hammoudi, B.M., Ismaile, S., & Abu Yahya, O. (2018). Factors associated with medication administration errors and why nurses fail to report them. *Scandinavian Journal of Caring Sciences, 32*(3), 1038–1046. doi: 10.1111/scs.12546.

Hannawa, A. (2009). Negotiating medical virtues: Toward the development of a physician mistake disclosure model. *Health Communication, 24*(5), 391–399. https://dbproxy.lasalle.edu:6149/10.1080/10410230903023279.

Hannawa, A.F., & Frankel, M. (2018). "It Matters What I Think, Not What You Say": Scientific evidence for a Medical Error Disclosure Competence (MEDC) Model. *Journal of Patient Safety.* Advance online publication. doi: 10.1097/PTS. 0000000000000524.

James, I.A., Wood-Mitchell, A.J., Waterworth, A.M., Mackenzie, L.E., & Cunningham, J. (2006). Lying to people with dementia: Developing ethical guidelines for care settings. *International Journal of Geriatric Psychiatry, 21*, 800–801.

Kerfoot, K. (2006). The art of truth telling: Handling failure with disclosure and apology. *Nursing Economics, 24*(4), 216–217.

Langone, M. (2007). Promoting integrity among nursing students. *Journal of Nursing Education, 46*(1), 45–47.

Leibowitz, K.A., Hardebeck, E.J., Goyer, J.P., & Crum, A.J. (2019). The role of patient beliefs in open-label placebo effects. *Health Psychology, 38*(7), 613–622. https://dx.doi.org/10.1037/hea0000751.

Levine, E., Roberts, A., & Cohen, T. (2020). Difficult conversations: Navigating the tension between honesty and benevolence. *Current Opinion in Psychology, 31*, 38–43.

Makary, M.A., & Daniel, M. (2016). Medical error–the third leading cause of death in the US. *BMJ (Clinical Research Ed.), 353*, i2139.

Mansouri, S.F., Mohammadi, T.K., Adib, M., Lili, E.K., & Soodmand, M. (2019). Barriers to nurses reporting errors and adverse events. *British Journal of Nursing, 28*(11), 690–695. https://dbproxy.lasalle.edu:6149/10.12968/bjon.2019.28.11.690.

Massachusetts Alliance for Communication and Resolution Following Medical Injury. (n.d.). *About CARe.* https://www.macrmi.info/about-macrmi/about-dao/.

Massachusetts Alliance for Communication and Resolution Following Medical Injury. (n.d.) *About MACRMI.* https://www.macrmi.info/about-macrmi/.

McKenzie, K., Taylor, S., Murray, G., & James, I. (2020). The use of therapeutic untruths by learning disability nursing students. *Nursing Ethics, 27*(8), 1607–1617. doi: 10.1177/0969733020928130.

Medicare Payment Advisory Commission. (2019). Ch. 12: Hospice Services. *Report to the Congress: Medicare and the health care delivery system.* MedPAC. http://www.medpac.gov/docs/default-source/reports/mar19_medpac_ch12_sec.pdf.

Mendes, A. (2019). The power of placebo. *British Journal of Community Nursing, 24*(4), 196–97. doi: 10.12968/bjcn.2019.24.4.196.

Nietzsche, F. (1907). *Beyond good and evil.* (H. Zimmem, Trans.). Macmillan. (Original work published in 1886).

Noland, C.M. (2012). Baccalaureate nursing students' accounts of medical mistakes occurring in the clinical setting: Implications for curricula. *Journal of Nursing Education, 53*(3), Suppl. S34-S37. https://doi.org/10.3928/01484834-20140211-04.

Noland, C.M., & Carmack, H.J. (2015). "You never forget your first mistake": Nursing socialization, memorable messages, and communication about medical errors. *Health Communication, 30*(12), 1234–1244. https://dbproxy.lasalle.edu:6149/10.1080/10410236.2014.930397.

Papakostas, Y.G., & Daras, M.D. (2001). Placebo effects and the response to the healing situation: The evolution of a concept. *Epilepsia, 42*(12), 1614–1625.

Rawlins, R. (2015). On the ethical use of placebos. *Focus on Alternative and Complementary Therapies, 20*(2), 97–101.

Rogers, E., Griffin, E., Carnie, W., Melucci, J., & Weber, R.J. (2017). A Just Culture approach to managing medication errors. *Hospital Pharmacy, 52*(4), 308–315. https://dbproxy.lasalle.edu:6149/10.1310/hpx5204-308.

Sokol, D. (2007). Can deceiving patients be morally acceptable? *BMJ, 334*(7601), 984–986. doi: 10.1136/bmj.39184.419826.80.

Sperber, M. (2015). Therapeutic lying: A contradiction in terms. *Psychiatric Times, 32*(4), 43–47.

Trossman, S. (2019). Preventing harm: Reporting, recognition, and just culture can make a difference. *American Nurse Today, 14*(2), 30–32.

Tuckett, A.G. (2004). Truth-telling in clinical practice and the arguments for and against: A review of the literature. *Nursing Ethics, 11*(5), 500–513.

Tuckett, A.G. (2012). The experience of lying in dementia care: A qualitative study. *Nursing Ethics,19*(1), 17–20.

Twain, M. (1880). *On the decay of the art of lying* [Essay]. Historical and Antiquarian Club of Hartford Connecticut. Odins Library Classics.

Wu, A., Cavanaugh, T., McPhee, S., Lo, B., & Micco, G. (1997). To tell the truth: Ethical and practice issues in disclosing medical mistakes to patients. *Journal of General Internal Medicine, 12*, 770–775.

Yevtushenko, Y. (n.d.). *Quote*. Goodreads. https://www.goodreads.com/quotes/101004-when-truth-is-replaced-by-silence-the-silence-is-a-lie.

MULTIPLE-CHOICE QUESTIONS

1. Which of the following indicators point to deciding that therapeutic lying violates moral and ethical standards of care?
   A. The patient consents to the lie in advance
   B. The lie is upheld in a court of law
   C. The lie meets the needs of the nurse, not the patient
   D. Objections to the lie can be made based on mental state of the patient

2. Which of the following has been proposed as an acceptable reason for lying to patients?
   A. Misstatement of facts is necessary for the nurse to carry out care efficiently
   B. Positive effects of drugs outweigh harmful effects
   C. Nursing staff think the lie protects the patient
   D. The aggressive behavior of the person with dementia decreases

3. Which of the following medications is an example of an impure placebo?
   A. Sugar-filled capsule
   B. Vitamin capsule
   C. Lactose-filled capsule
   D. Cornstarch-filled capsule

4. Which of the following findings of James et al.'s (2006) survey research was a conclusion?
   A. Most staff caring for persons with dementia lie
   B. Lying does not improve residents' emotional reactions
   C. Lying does not present any problems whatsoever
   D. Staff agree on the same information presented as lies

CHAPTER 4

Blurred Lines

Professional Boundary Violations

Doris C. Vallone, PhD, RN, PMHCNS-BC,
and Zane Robinson Wolf, PhD, RN,
CNE, FCPP, ANEF, FAAN

Objectives

1. Distinguish boundary crossing from boundary violation.
2. Identify risk factors for boundary violations.
3. Provide examples of boundary violations.
4. Discuss strategies for preventing boundary violations.

Critical Incident

Marisa was 19 years old when admitted to a private psychiatric clinic following a suicide attempt by overdose that occurred following the death of her mother. She was working as a cashier at a local drug store and was living with her mother prior to her mother's death. She was not partnered and had no children. Marisa was diagnosed as depressed with borderline personality features, prescribed antidepressant medication, and treated with both group and individual therapy. She responded well to the milieu and readily attached to staff and unit peers. She was very bright, took a leadership role among her peers and sometimes questioned the rules, pitting staff against each other. She was attractive and likeable and made no secret about which staff were her favorites.

Ms. Curry was a part-time nurse working the evening shift. She was 45 years old with two preteen daughters. She also had an older daughter who lived with her ex-husband. Ms. Curry took an interest in Marisa and spent much time with her on the days she was working. She sometimes came to work early to meet with Marisa during a free hour. Marisa said that Ms. Curry was the only nurse who understood her, and she demonstrated insight and control around Ms. Curry. In response, Ms. Curry allowed her extra privileges and advocated with other staff for level increases. Marisa stabilized, was no longer suicidal, and was discharged after 20 days' hospitalization. Her follow-up plan consisted of outpatient therapy, a grief support group, and medication management.

Ms. Curry resigned about six months later. Shortly thereafter, a staff member encountered Marisa and Ms. Curry at a supermarket and learned that Marisa was employed by Ms. Curry, babysitting her children and doing household chores. It appeared that Marisa was living with Ms. Curry. When asked, Ms. Curry told the staff member to mind her own business.

In this critical incident, Ms. Curry may have missed her older daughter, which might pre-dispose her to take an interest in Marisa. Because of her vulnerability, Marisa might have welcomed the extra attention. Ms. Curry embarked on a slippery slope when she spent extra time with her, giving her extra privileges and acting more as a friend. The progression to hiring Marisa and keeping it a secret put her at professional risk. Marisa was at personal risk as she was being exploited.

Background

This case illustrates the progression toward a serious professional boundary violation. It shows that a shift occurred in the nurse-patient relationship, from the nurse's professional responsibility to serving a personal need. Furthermore, the distinction between social and therapeutic relationships is a core concept of professionalism and is emphasized in nursing fundamentals classes (Potter et al., 2017) prior to students meeting their first patients. This distinction focuses the center of nursing practice. Regardless of setting, the nurse-patient relationship and professional boundaries are core to developing and sustaining therapeutic interventions (Slobogian et al., 2017). The nurse-patient relationship is maintained to benefit the patient, not the nurse. This chapter is framed by psychiatric nursing practice and broad principles of professional nursing practice. Nonetheless, boundary violations confront nurses in many settings, such as long-term care (Thys et al., 2018), as they care for patients.

Professional behavior is included in the nursing standards of practice (American Psychiatric Nurses Association, 2014) and American Nurses Association's (ANA's) Code of Ethics (2019). When nurses do not act in the patients' or residents' best interest and gain personally at a patient's expense, professional boundary violations occur (Hudspeth, 2006). Furthermore, the National Council of State Boards of Nursing (NCSBN) defined boundary violations as "the phenomena that occur when there is confusion of the professional's needs with the client's needs" (NCSBN, 1996, p. 11). The NCSBN champions education regarding boundaries and offers a wide variety of multimedia resources.

Guthiel and Gabbard (1993) first used the phrase boundary crossing in describing the sometimes-blurred edge between professional behavior and behavior approaching a boundary violation. Boundary crossings were further defined in the literature as "brief excursions over the line with a return to the established limits of the professional relationship" (Sheets, 2001, p. 37).

In *A Nurse's Guide to Professional Boundaries* (2018), there are three useful definitions:

- Professional boundaries are the spaces between the nurse's power and the patient's vulnerability.
- Boundary crossings are brief excursions across professional lines of behavior that may be inadvertent, thoughtless, or even purposeful, while attempting to meet a special therapeutic need of the patient.

• Boundary violations can result when there is confusion between the needs of the nurse and those of the patient [p. 4].

The document also offered a conceptual continuum of professional behavior that defines under-involvement, therapeutic relationship, and over-involvement (p. 5).

The inherent risks involved in nurses' close proximities to patients have prompted professionals to offer explicit guidance to nurses regarding professional boundaries. The Code of Ethics of the American Nurses Association (2019) defined boundaries in provision 2.4 and acknowledged the risk of boundary violations. Explicitly stated are prohibitions of gift acceptance, dating, and sexual relationships.

The NCSBN (2018a) suggested a continuum for evaluating professional behavior in which there are zones for a therapeutic relationship, including a horizontal zone of helpfulness in the center, adjacent to the extremes of under-involvement (left) to over-involvement (right). The boundary of the therapeutic zone is not a clear edge, but often a fluid line depending on context. The range of behaviors within the zone of therapeutic relationship differs, depending on the context of care and role. Brief boundary crossings may be intentional and acceptable when they occur in service to clients (College & Association of Registered Nurses of Alberta, 2020).

Nurses are held in esteem by the public and are considered the most trusted profession (Forbes, 2019). They are among a handful of professionals who are licensed to touch patients to provide care and to support the most intimate of bodily functions. They are privy to intimate details of a patient's life and are often the first to learn about trauma and pain. Investment in the patient's well-being and caring are critical to the therapeutic role. The strength of the nurse-patient dyad has been found to improve patient satisfaction (Tejero, 2011).

Professional Intimacy, Nurses' Bodywork, and Boundaries

Nursing work involves direct contact with the bodies of patients and with bodily products (Wolf, 2009). Because of this proximity, nurses are often considered unclean and their work profane by association. However, nursing's bodywork is defined as the "work that nurses do in managing their own bodies in carrying out their work as professionals" (Shakespeare, 2003, p. 47). Bodywork suggests that "nurses use themselves—body, mind, and spirit—to improve patients' welfare along with scientific (objective) and personally developed (subjective) clinical knowledge" (Wolf, 2009, p. 178). The embodied nature of nursing work involves the nurse and the patient in relationship. Nurse-patient relationships and the knowledge, skills, and values of nurses are mediated by their bodies and patients' responses. They perform a wide-ranging assembly of bodywork in cooperation with nurses and other professional colleagues (Shakespeare, 2003).

Nurses use their bodies to connect with and care for patients. Patient care is bidirectional (Sumner, 2006), in that nurses respond to patients in the moment during care episodes and patients respond to them in turn. The practice of nursing is defined by the expertise developed by this experience over a nursing career and "the somological character of nursing ... remains its greatest asset and liability" (Sandelowski, 2002, p. 61). Although nurses' work is emotionally demanding (Liaschenko, 2002; Stayt, 2009) and gendered and risky (Holder & Schenthal, 2007), it necessitates physical labor. Nurses witness suffering and alleviate it. Physical, psychological, social, and spiritual suffering are inherent in nursing work (Leary, 2006).

Nurses occupy a unique societal role. Bodywork distinguishes nursing practice, and the way nurses respond to it may well give nursing its charism (Hughes, 1971). Perhaps this is because patients and families appreciate that nurses not only work in emotionally stressful environments (Stayt, 2009), but also recognize its coexistence via nurses' contact with intimate parts of patients' bodies. When patients and their families witness the comfort realized by the bodywork nurses perform, they value it. Nursing bodywork is "profoundly important to patients" (Wright, 2008, p. 26).

The physical dimensions of nursing work involve touching body parts that are private for patients and residents of health care settings and homes. The professional intimacy accomplished by nurses, in the context of patients' lived illness experiences, provides atypical access that family members often do not have. Bodily care is assumed by nurses based on patients' clinical situations and is relinquished as they return to autonomous function and privacy in providing self-care. Bodywork affords nurses a unique place in the hierarchy of health care professionals (Savage, 1995; 1997), because of their shared common space with patients. Nurses' bodies and use of their bodies, for example, their posture, encourages relational closeness with patients just as they are physically close.

Bodywork also brings forth sexuality concerns (Twigg, 2000). Consequently, nurses' work has been linked to speculation about their immorality. Nurses learn to manage this misconception despite patients who might assume them to be morally loose. In contrast, patients and families may react to nurse gender due to religious or other rules (Zang et al., 2008). Some cultural prohibitions restrict contact between opposite sexes.

Considering the complex issues of gender, culture, sexuality, bodywork, and other factors, nurses establish professional intimacy to increase patient comfort (Huebner, 2007). They develop such skill over time and attribute this kind of work to helping patients heal, keeping patients' wishes in mind. In protecting patients' during intimate care, they strive to promote the privacy and dignity of patients and family members.

Professional intimacy is more than a theoretical exercise for nurses (Dowling, 2006) as experienced during bodywork. It is negotiated with patients and family members and functions in complex health care organizations and other settings as nurses manage intimate care daily. They carefully disclose personal information to patients and family members, balancing personal and professional distance (Dowling, 2006). Intimacy is also an attribute of connectedness in patient-provider relationships (Phillips-Salimi et al., 2011). Intimate nurse-patient relationships are established and maintained and transitory. Bodywork, proximity to patients, and intimate nursing care provide numerous situations that challenge professional boundary maintenance. The complexity of the therapeutic work that nurses perform requires them never to enact boundary violations that are personal, self-disclosing, and physical and oppose the creation of professional, therapeutic relationships (Fischer, 2020).

Boundary Violations and Boundary Crossings

Holder and Schenthal (2007) defined a *slippery slope* toward boundary violation as that which has as precedent *boundary drift*, which is the presence of thoughts or fantasies that occur prior to actions. The boundary drift progresses toward a boundary crossing, then to transgression, and finally to a boundary violation. This progression model accounts for individual nurse and patient factors. The authors suggested that a catalytic event, for example, divorce, can increase the nurse's violation potential that can result in the nurse crossing the line to transgression. The model further posits two critical factors: nurse violation potential and patient vulnerability. The presence of these factors can result in boundary violations if not mediated by professional accountability and resistance factors.

Manfrin-Ledet et al. (2015) described the following seven common themes associated with boundary violations, and point to how nurses could go outside therapeutic relationships:

- dual relations/role reversal
- gifts and money
- excessive self-disclosure
- secretive behavior
- excessive attention/over-involvement
- sexual behavior
- social media [Manfrin-Ledet et al., 2015].

They differentiated boundary violations from boundary crossings. A boundary crossing takes place when nurses deviate from an established boundary for a perceived therapeutic purpose. The authors also shared that one or more boundary crossing may precede a boundary violation. They pointed out that home settings are opportunities for increased boundary blurring and emphasized that nurses' responsibility is the maintenance of professional boundaries. Like Manfrin-Ledet et al. (2015), Guthiel and Gabbard (1993) considered the dimensions or themes of role, time, place and space, money and gifts, and services to represent boundary violations. To this they added clothing, language, and physical contact.

Boundary crossings can be considered innocent. Purchasing toiletries for a patient and accepting a gift are examples (Hudspeth, 2006). Patient exploitation is missing. In contrast, boundary violations exploit patients. Behavioral cues suggesting the potential for boundary violations proposed by Hudspeth include:

- excessive self-disclosure by the nurse, talking about personal or intimate issues including their feeling or sexual attraction
- secretive behavior between the patient and the nurse
- feeling that only the nurse can fully understand the patient's complex needs
- excessive patient attention whereby the nurse is overly attached to the patient, trades assignments to provide care, comes in to visit on off time and spends greater than normal amounts of time with the patient
- selective communication whereby the nurse fails to fully relate all necessary information to others, thereby retaining some control over the care
- flirting with the patient
- overly protective behavior whereby the nurse assumes the attitude of you and me against the world
- failure to protect the patient by not recognizing a boundary issue, not seeking peer or supervisor consultation, and not transferring care to others [p. 376].

Literature

Literature on boundary violations consists of examples of theoretical literature on professional boundary situations and research, such as self-report surveys, examination of disciplinary decisions related to boundary violations, and characteristics of violators.

Schafer (1997) explored the challenges of boundary violations for correctional nurses. Because of the unique environment, challenges to maintaining the therapeutic relationship were at risk because of prisoner isolation from family and friends, history of poor interpersonal relationships, and gratitude toward nurses. Nurses may assume responsibility for prisoner behavior, feel battered, and not resolve problems. They may tolerate sexual comments and feel an obligation to tolerate unacceptable behavior. Tolerance of abusive behavior does not allow nurses to accept responsibility for the behavior. Consequently, nurses need to develop self-awareness and maintain the professional boundaries of the correctional nurse. Noting the impact of feelings and behavior on therapeutic relationships is key to understanding the countertransference of prisoners and to preventing boundary violations by nurses. Schafer attributed female socialization, application of caring concepts that may blur boundaries, hierarchical and paternalistic health care organizations, and the medical model to influence nurses' behavior. Schafer (1997) also noted that nurses' objectivity, acceptance of offensive behavior, and nonjudgmental approaches to caring for patients further contributed to the challenges of correctional nursing practice and may mirror the societal context of professional nursing. Nurse managers and staff nurses need to increase awareness of boundary issues. Schafer recommended accomplishing understanding of reactions to clinical situations and therapeutic relationships through peer review and support groups.

Campbell et al. (2005) surveyed 2,009 nurses in Alberta, Canada, who were actively working in the mental health field; 923 responded (476 RNs, 44 RPNs, 6 no role identified). The survey's 37 items queried their knowledge, attitudes, and behaviors regarding the common themes of role, intimacy, and sexual conduct. Most subjects responded that sexual contact and dating were inappropriate, both in treatment and following discharge. No respondents admitted to having sex with active patients, and six nurses reported having relationships with patients following discharge. The authors acknowledged the limitations of a convenience sample and an instrument lacking reliability and validity. They also suggested that a socially desirable response set may have been a factor influencing responses. Routine, professional boundary training and education about effects of sexual relationships with patients were advocated.

The frequency of boundary violations of nurses was examined by Jones et al. (2008); they compared complaints against nurses on boundary violations. Violations of nurses with basic associate degree preparation were compared to those with baccalaureate degrees. They analyzed the Ohio Board of Nursing's disciplinary reports from 1999 to 2006 for those charges related to boundary violations. Jones et al. found 27 cases meeting the criteria and used licensure data to determine whether nurses' basic preparation was ADN or BSN. The ADN group had a statistically higher frequency of boundary violations than the BSN-educated group. The researchers did not report if the nurses had education beyond their basic program. They concluded that more content was presented in BSN curricula relating to legal and ethical issues.

The National Practitioner Data Bank (NPDB) was analyzed by AbuDagga and associates (2019) for sexual misconduct identified in both board violations and malpractice insurance payments. They reviewed the data from 2004 to 2016 and found 882 sexual misconduct discipline reports. Males comprised the majority with 63.2 percent, while 30.1 percent were female, and 6.8 percent reporting no gender. They additionally reported 47 sexual misconduct malpractice payment reports for 33 nurses. AbuDagga et al. noted that there were 16 malpractice cases in which there was no corresponding disciplinary action by boards of nursing. Sexual misconduct consisted of only .06 percent of all reports. They cautioned that the incidence might be higher because it is not known how many violations go unreported.

The factor of gender was the focus of a study by Chiarella and Adrian (2014). They examined 175 disciplinary decisions registered in New South Wales, Australia, from 1999 to 2006 and found 29 cases that related to boundary violations. Violations ranged from gift giving, compliments, and inappropriate self-disclosure to out-of-hospital meetings and sexual contact. All cases involved registered nurses and the majority (65.5 percent) were male. The researchers acknowledged that nursing work involves intimacy, and that the bodywork and gender association pose challenges for male nurses. The issue of gender stood out and stereotyping might have played a role, because only 9 percent of nurses in Australia are male. The researchers suggested that female patients might be anxious about men who are nurses. They proposed that patients may see male nurses' behavior as predatory, when compared to that of female nurses. Female nurses engaged in many of the same behaviors that were in the complaints against males. Disciplinary cases showed that female nurses' involvement with patients mostly showed passionate and risky sexual relationships. The researchers invited a larger discourse on the nature of nursing work, especially bodywork, and the effect of gender on boundaries.

A literature review by Manfrin-Ledet et al. (2015) reviewed a qualitative study on boundary violations that occurred between faculty and students. Major themes paralleled those violations encountered in patient care and included personal disclosure, time factors, and touch. They found touch was a common dilemma and considered taboo by their sample. Some faculty had a policy of never touching a student; others found it sometimes appropriate in the clinical setting.

Classification and Examples of Boundary Violations

Role Blurring

A fundamental question to ask is *whose needs are being met*? Role reversal occurs when the nurse is gaining personal satisfaction from being in the relationship with the patient, such as discussing personal problems and asking for advice. With excessive self-disclosure, the relationship becomes more like friendship and the nurse begins to seek the company of a patient. The progression to violation occurs when the boundaries of time and place are expanded. Examples are giving out a cell phone number, friending on social media, and meeting outside the clinic setting or in the community after discharge. There is no agreement as to when social contact can occur after discharge. Proper use of social media can be guided by nursing literature and professional nursing organizations. Advice is provided, for example, do not friend patients or former patients or post sexually explicit material (Catlin, 2013).

Gifts and Money

Patients often want to give gifts to their providers. Offering a small gift can be therapeutic for a patient, but nurses should proceed with caution in accepting these gifts. For example, patients on mental health units will often give their staff member an item they made in a crafts class. Accepting gifts can lead to the appearance of preferential treatment. There is a general agreement (CARNA, 2011; NCSBN, 2018) that money should not change hands. Conversely, giving gifts to patients can result in misunderstanding about the nature of the relationship (Guthiel & Gabbard, 1993).

SEXUAL BEHAVIOR

It is inevitable that nurses and patients will be attracted to each other. The intensity of interactions can create a strong bond and can result in a drive to satisfy an unmet need. Sexual behavior often follows a predictable course that begins with a series of increasing boundary crossings, role reversals, and secrets. Casual language, increased use of touch, and seductive clothing on either part can indicate assent to sexual involvement (Gutheil & Gabbard, 1993). These signals can be exchanged within the bounds of the treatment episode with a plan to engage in a relationship following discharge.

SOCIAL MEDIA

Social media provides opportunities for sharing, professional networking, and dissemination of information. Inevitably, patients can invite nurses to friend them on various platforms. Additionally, the openness of such platforms can result in unintended self-disclosure.

Privacy of both patients and nurses was emphasized by Slobogian et al. (2017). Although unintended exposure of patient information is most often cited, photographs and details of nurses' private life can be open to public examination. This can tarnish a nurse's professional image and cause additional scrutiny of family and friends. The authors also reported survey results indicating that nurses did not employ adequate security settings and were unaware if their employers had such a policy. Nurses also lacked understanding of the legal and ethical implications of their social media behavior, including potential disciplinary action.

NCSBN (2011) surveyed 46 state boards in 2010 and received responses from 33 who indicated that they received complaints of violations of privacy on social media. Of the 33, the majority took disciplinary actions ranging from letters of concern to license suspension.

Protecting Boundaries

ORGANIZATIONAL AND REGULATORY SAFEGUARDS

Boundary safeguards from broad to narrow include legal statutes, licensure regulations, professional organization standards, agency policies, peer evaluation and education in the academic setting and the health care agency. Because boundary violations are very serious, they could result in loss of professional licensure. Such disciplinary action signifies that a nurse violated a boundary with a vulnerable patient and departed from accepted standards (Virine & Lawyers, 2014).

Most nurse practice acts have references to boundary violations and sexual misconduct; however, Holder and Schenthal (2007) noted a disparity in reporting trends as well as lack of clarity regarding the nature of sexual misconduct, with some including sexual harassment and use of foul language in the reports. Although whistleblower laws exist, nurses are reluctant to report colleagues who are seen or who disclose inappropriate behavior (Peternelj-Taylor, 2003). Whistleblowers may be viewed as troublemakers and traitors or guardians of professional standards. However, nurses abide by the ethical principle of nonmaleficence which creates a dilemma when observing a patient exploited by a colleague. There is not always a clear reporting path.

Sheets (2001) suggested that hiring procedures be thorough enough to capture reports of infractions from boards in different states and public and private agencies. She recommended a structure with more than one reporting channel for complaints to be instituted, including a vehicle for anonymous reporting. After complaints are received, the staff member is suspended pending investigation and a confidential inquiry is conducted. Once the investigation is completed, appropriate action is taken and, if warranted, the behavior is reported to the appropriate regulatory agency. The trust and safety in the reporting system are key to promoting a culture of accountability.

EDUCATION

As stated in their study, Jones et al. (2008) suggested that boundary management education was lacking, and students may not understand the difference between boundary crossing and boundary violation. Holder and Schenthal (2007) recommended that undergraduates be educated regarding the concepts of power differentials and the slippery slope toward boundary violations. The College & Association of Registered Nurses of Alberta published a guideline (2020) that expanded the content promoted by the NCSBN and includes teaching anecdotes and discussion scenarios that can be used in the classroom.

New employee orientation is an opportunity to connect agency and regulatory guidelines with professional boundary concepts. NCSBN (2019) offered an online video that explains the continuum of professional behavior and the distinctions between boundary crossings and boundary violations. Vignettes depict the continuum of the therapeutic relationship and the progression from boundary crossing to boundary violations. Examples of boundary violations are found in Table 4.

Table 4. Examples of Boundary Violations

Boundary Violation	Example
Dual relationships	The nurse and patient discuss their experiences with various dating sites.
Gifts and money	The patient offers the nurse a discount on a new car at a dealership he owns and the nurse accepts.
Excessive self-disclosure	The nurse shares an experience of child sexual abuse by a priest.
Secretive behavior	The nurse promises to keep a secret and the patient shares that he has been saving pills to overdose.
Excessive attention	The nurse switches assignments to be with a particular patient. The nurse stays an hour past quitting time.
Sexual behavior	The patient invites the nurse to engage in intimate contact and they agree to get together following discharge.
Special privileges	The nurse allows a patient to vape in his room.
Social media	The nurse invites the patient to friend her on Facebook.

In addition to in-service education, organizations must provide a culture where professional ethics are valued and there is accountability at every level. A safe reporting mechanism needs to be in place so that colleagues can confidently report incidents without fear of reprisals. Supervisors need to be aware of resources to support staff who experience challenges. Employee assistance programs can provide confidential counseling.

The unique approach proposed by Holder and Schenthal (2007) acknowledged boundary violation as an occupational risk. They noted that boundary violations can be considered inherent in nursing practice due to therapeutic contexts including the perceived powerful nurse and vulnerable patient. Holder and Schenthal (2007) produced a list of key terms and definitions.

They recommended using their Boundary Formula to assist staff to assess their violation potential by examining the interaction between personal factors and external elements that may predispose them to over-involvement and recognize their own warning signs. The slippery slope formula included the constructs of violation potential, risk factors, vulnerabilities, accountability, resistance, and catalyst. Educators might also use the formula to describe nurses' and nursing students' relative violation potential.

Strategies

A summary of strategies to promote change is listed in Table 5.

Table 5. Strategies for Change: Boundary Violations

Strategies to Effect Change	Evidence-Based Citations
Pre-licensure education Modules on professional boundaries early in curriculum	Manfrin-Ledet et al. (2015) Jones et al. (2008)
Hiring procedures that include verification of licenses from all states Comprehensive reference checks	Sheets (2001)
Guidance and clear policies on the use of social media	Tarimen (2010)
Zero tolerance policy on sexual misconduct	NCSBN (2009)
Use Boundary Formula teaching tool to self-assess violation potential	Holder & Schenthal (2007)
Mandatory review of NCSBN professional boundary guidelines	NCSBN (2018)
Establish whistleblower protections for reporting boundary violations	Peternelj-Taylor (2003)

The examples of boundary violations and the strategies to effect change and eliminate them could assist nurses challenged by a boundary drift after self-reflection. The strategies above provide evidence-based citations on strategies to support actions that support the continuance of professional boundaries.

Conclusion

Boundary violations can result in significant distress for patients who place trust in nurses who care for them when they are most vulnerable. Exploitation of that vulnerability can be a traumatic experience that lasts well beyond the treatment episode. Nurses' role, as direct care providers who operate in personal, intimate space, positions them for boundary crossings and boundary violations.

Education about therapeutic relationships, boundary crossing, and boundary violations must occur at all career levels. Regulations that exist currently are clear and must be enforced to protect the public. Organizations need to promote a culture of ethical responsibility, disseminate expectations, and provide a vehicle for reporting violations.

Discussion Questions

1. What are the differences among boundary drift, boundary crossing, and boundary violation?
2. What factors increase a nurse's violation potential?
3. What are some strategies to increase reports of serious boundary violations?
4. What are some warning signs of a boundary violation?
5. How might nurse managers foster communication among nursing staff on boundary violations?

Author Selection

National Council of State Boards of Nursing. (2019). *Boundary Violations: Professional Boundaries in Nursing* [Video]. https://www.ncsbn.org/professional-boundaries.htm.

References

AbuDagga, A., Wolfe, S., Carome, M., & Oshel, R.E. (2019). Crossing the line: Sexual misconduct by nurses reported to the National Practitioner Data Bank. *Public Health Nursing, 36*, 109–117.

American Nurses Association. (2019). *Guide to the Code of Ethics for Nurses.* https://www.nursingworld.org/practice-policy/nursing-excellence/ethics/code-of-ethics-for-nurses/.

American Psychiatric Nurses Association (2014). *Psychiatric mental health nursing: Scope and standards of practice.* https://www.apna.org/i4a/pages/index.cfm?pageid=5739.

Campbell, R.J., Yonge, O., & Austin, W. (2005). Intimacy boundaries between mental health nurses and psychiatric patients. *Journal of Psychosocial Nursing, 43*(5), 32–39.

Catlin, A. (2013). Considering boundaries in nursing: What the staff nurse needs to know. *Advances in Neonatal Care, 13*(5), 331–334. doi:10.1097/ANC.0b013e3182a3fe16.

Chiarella, M.A., & Adrian, A. (2014). Boundary violations, gender and the nature of nursing work. *Nursing Ethics, 21*, 267–277.

College & Association of Registered Nurses of Alberta. (2020). *Professional boundaries: Guidelines for the nurse-client relationship.* https://nurses.ab.ca/docs/default-source/document-library/guidelines/rn_professional-boundaries.pdf?sfvrsn=cc43bb24_24.

Dowling, M. (2006). The sociology of intimacy in the nurse-patient relationship. *Nursing Standard, 20*, 48–54.

Erickson, A., & Davies, B. (2017). Maintaining integrity: How nurses navigate boundaries in pediatric palliative care. *Journal of Pediatric Nursing, 35*, 42–49.

Fisher, M.J. (2020). Navigating professional boundaries: The use of the therapeutic self in rehabilitation nursing. *Journal of the Australasian Rehabilitation Nurses' Association, 23*(1), 2–3. https://doi.org/10.33235/jarna.23.1.2-3.

Guthiel, T.G., & Gabbard, G.O. (1993). The concept of boundaries in clinical practice: Theoretical and risk-management dimensions. *American Journal of Psychiatry, 150*, 188–196.

Holder, K.V., & Schenthal, S.J. (2007). Watch your step: Nursing professional boundaries. *Nursing Management, 38*(2), 24–29.

Hudspeth, R. (2006). Professional boundary crossings and boundary violations and their implications. *Nursing Administration Quarterly, 30*(4), 375–376.

Huebner, L.C. (2007). *Professional intimacy: An ethnography of care in hospital nursing* [Dissertation, University of Pittsburgh].

Hughes, E.C. (1971). *The sociological eye: Selected papers*. Aldine.

Jones, J.S., Fitzpatrick, J.J., & Drake, V.K. (2008). Frequency of postlicensure registered nurse boundary violations with patients in the state of Ohio: A comparison based on type of prelicensure registered nurse education. *Archives of Psychiatric Nursing, 22*(6), 356–363.

Leary, A. (2006, December 11). Nursing a secret. *The Guardian.* http://www.theguardian.com/society/2006/dec/11/publicsectorcareers.health.

Liaschenko, J. (2002). Thoughts on nursing work. *JONA, 32,* 69–70.

Manfrin-Ledet, L., Porche, D.J., & Eymard, A.S. (2015). Professional boundary violations: A literature review. *Home Healthcare Now, 33*(6), 326–332.

National Council of State Boards of Nursing. (1996). Raising awareness of professional boundaries and sexual misconduct: Nursing faculty are encouraged to take a proactive role. *Issues, 17*(2), 11–13.

National Council of State Boards of Nursing. (2009). *Practical Guidelines for Boards of Nursing on Sexual Misconduct Cases.* https://www.ncsbn.org/Sexual_Misconduct_Book_web.pdf.

National Council of State Boards of Nursing. (2011, August). *White paper: A nurse's guide to the use of social media.* https://www.ncsbn.org/Social_Media.pdf.

National Council of State Boards of Nursing. (2018). *A nurse's guide to professional boundaries.* https://www.ncsbn.org/ProfessionalBoundaries_Complete.pdf.

National Council of State Boards of Nursing. (2018). *A nurse's guide to the use of social media* [Brochure]. https://www.ncsbn.org/3739.htm.

National Council of State Boards of Nursing. (2019). *Boundary violations: Professional boundaries in nursing* [Video]. https://www.ncsbn.org/professional-boundaries.htm.

Patternelj-Taylor, C. (2002). Professional boundaries: A matter of therapeutic integrity. *Journal of Psychosocial Nursing and Mental Health Services, 40*(4), 22–29.

Patternelj-Taylor, C. (2003). Whistleblowing and boundary violations: Exposing a colleague in the forensic milieu. *Nursing Ethics, 10*(5), 526–537.

Phillips-Salimi, C.R., Haase, J.F., & Kooken, W.C. (2011). Connectedness in the context of patient-provider relationships: A concept analysis. *Journal of Advanced Nursing, 68*(1), 230–245.

Potter, P.A., Perry, A.G., Hall, A., & Stockert, P.A. (2017). *Fundamentals of nursing* (9th ed.). Mosby Elsevier.

Sandelowski, M. (2002). Visible humans, vanishing bodies, and virtual nursing: Complications of life, presence, place, and identity. *Advances in Nursing Science, 24*(3), 58–70.

Savage, J. (1995). *Nursing intimacy: An ethnographic approach to nurse-patient interaction.* Scutari Press.

Savage, J. (1997). Gestures of resistance: The nurse's body in contested space. Nursing Inquiry, 4, 237–245. https://doi.org/10.1111/j.1440-1800. 1997.tb00109.x.

Schafer, P. (1997). When a client develops an attraction: Successful resolution versus boundary violation. *Journal of Psychiatric and Mental Health Nursing, 4,* 203–211.

Shakespeare, P. (2003). Nurses' bodywork: Is there a body of work. *Nursing Inquiry, 10,* 47–56.

Sheets, V.R. (2001). Professional boundaries: Staying in the lines. *Dimensions of Critical Care Nursing 20*(5), 36–40.

Slobogian, V., Giles, J., & Rent, T. (2017). Social media: #Boundaries: When patients become friends. *Canadian Oncology Nursing Journal, 27*(4), 394–400.

Stayt, L.C. (2009). Death, empathy and self-preservation: The emotional labour of caring for families of the critically ill in adult intensive care. *Journal of Clinical Nursing, 18,* 1267–1275.

Sumner, J. (2006). Concept analysis: The moral construct of caring in nursing as communicative action. *International Journal for Human Caring, 19*(1), 8–16.

Tariman, J.D. (2010). Where to draw the line: Professional boundaries in social networking. *ONS Connect, 25*(2), 10–13.

Thys, K., Mahieu, L., Cavolo, A., Hensen, C., Dierckx de Casterlé, B., & Gastmans, C. (2018). Nurses' experience and reactions towards intimacy and sexuality expressions by nursing home residents: A qualitative study. *Journal of Clinical Nursing, 28,* 836–849. https://doi.org/10.1111; jocn.14680.

Twigg, J. (2000). Carework as a form of bodywork. *Ageing and Society, 20,* 389–411.

Valente, S. (2017). Managing professional and nurse-patient relationship boundaries in mental health. *Journal of Psychosocial Nursing, 55*(1), 45–51.

Virine, J., & Lawyers, H.P. (2014). Boundary violations: Sexual relationships with patients. *TQN, 33*(1), 26–27.

Wolf, Z.R. (2009). Knowing patients' bodies: Nurses' bodywork. In R.C. Locsin, & M.J. Purnell, *A contemporary nursing process: The (un)bearable weight of knowing in nursing* (pp. 177–203). Springer Publishing.

Wright, S. (2008). Be proud to wash. *Nursing Standard, 22*(17), 26–27.

Zang, Y-L., Chung, L.Y.F., & Wong, T.K.S. (2008). A review of the psychosocial issues for nurses in male genitalia-related care. *Journal of Clinical Nursing, 17,* 983–998. https://doi.org/10.1111/j.1365-2702.2007. 02067.x.

Multiple-Choice Questions

1. Which of the following descriptions represents a boundary crossing for a nurse?
   A. Accepting a gift
   B. Pointing out risky health behaviors
   C. Teaching preventive health strategies
   D. Investing in therapeutic interventions

2. Which of the following aspects of nursing practice consistently challenges nurses to adhere to professional boundaries?
   A. Nurse autonomy
   B. Intimate care
   C. Situational context
   D. Caring behaviors

3. Which of the following opportunities provides a context for institutions to present the continuum of the therapeutic relationship with staff?
   A. During employee orientation programs
   B. On receipt of boundary violation complaints
   C. Seeing news accounts of professional infractions
   D. Throughout institutional investigations

4. Which of the following strategies might staff nurses and nurse managers engage in to recognize and manage boundary problems consistent with everyday nursing practice?
   A. Yearly experiential learning forums
   B. Monthly vignette postings of violations
   C. Quarterly self-awareness discussion groups
   D. Yearly whistleblowing campaigns

CHAPTER 5

"Difficult" Patients

Deborah Byrne, PhD, RN, CNE

Objectives

1. Examine the vulnerable situations of patients labeled difficult.
2. Describe challenges for nurses when interacting with patients judged as difficult.
3. Explore the ethical and legal principles violated by negative interactions with patients labeled difficult.
4. Analyze nursing interventions to improve the nurse-patient relationship.

Critical Incident

A home care nurse was assigned to care for a client well known to the agency. This situation was the client's fifth time using the home health agency's services over two years. The client was a 78-year-old female with a stage 4 pressure injury, type 2 diabetes, heart failure, and impaired mobility. The client required wound care three days a week and education on diabetes and heart failure. She also received physical therapy and assistance from a medical social worker.

The client lived in a poorly maintained home that was cluttered and often infested with mice. The social worker had been investigating resources for the client to help with cleaning and to obtain an exterminator. The client was disheveled and often belligerent with nurses. During the nurse's last visit, the client attempted to remove a clean dressing and yelled at the nurse. She had not complied with the treatment plan and often refused to allow the nurse to perform wound care, leading to further skin breakdown.

The home care nurse attempted to get the case reassigned, to no avail. The nurse arrived at the home and knocked lightly on the door one time. Because of the nurse's knowledge of the client's behavior and condition of the home, the nurse documented that the client was not at home at the assigned visit time. The nurse did not attempt to call the client, the emergency contact, nor did she call her office.

The client's daughter found the client unconscious in her home that evening. The client was transported to an emergency room with a diagnosis of a cerebral infarction. The emergency room physician could not aggressively treat the cerebral infarction due to an unknown onset of symptoms. This resulted in the client having right-sided weakness and visual and speech problems. As a result of the client's co-morbidities, the prognosis was poor. It was not known when the cerebral infarction occurred, but had the nurse seen the client that day, the nurse's assessment could have prevented the client's acute situation and early treatment might have affected positive outcomes. The nurse avoided the client that day by stating the client was not at home, after a feeble attempt to have the client answer the door.

This critical incident illustrates numerous problems when the nurse-patient relationship fails. The nurse missed opportunities to care for the client. Labeling the client as difficult contributed to the missed opportunities to provide nursing care that could have been called patient centric. The nurse should have called the client via phone, knocked harder, called the client's emergency contact, and alerted the home care agency's office. Home care nurses frequently call police for a home check. The nurse did not contact the police. Any one or more of these actions could have resulted in a better outcome for the client.

Home care nurses work alone most often. Like nurses in other settings, they encounter clients they and their colleagues characterize as difficult. Behaviors clients display that are associated with the difficult patient label can include hostility, refusal to comply with a plan of care, or allowing their hygiene to deteriorate. To avoid these clients is not an option because of the consequences for patients' health and well-being.

Nurses can confront tendencies to avoid clients and reconsider each situation from the perspectives of clients. It is essential to accept that avoidance might have serious outcomes for clients and to assess clients to evaluate their health problems (Michaelsen, 2020). Also, the challenge for nurses may lie in problems in the nurse-patient relationship (Michaelsen, 2020). Complicating the relationship are differences in the cultural norms and values of clients and nurses and nurses' work situations.

Nurses could use self-reflection techniques (Olson et al., 2016) on why they feel patients are difficult, perhaps considering differences in the cultures of both. Through self-reflection, nurses might increase understanding of their thoughts, feelings, and behaviors and expand their awareness of underlying patient issues. For example, if a client is non-compliant with medication adherence, nurses need to question if it is because they cannot afford the medication.

The labels non-compliant and non-adherent may also impede nurses from thinking critically about nursing situations in which they are embedded. The nurse acting in the critical incident violated the ethical principle of beneficence by not increasing her attempts to check on the well-being and health status of her client. Such violation of duty might result in complaints of neglect or negligence by home care agency administrators or relatives to state boards of nursing.

Background

Avoiding difficult patients or communicating poorly with them can lead to civil torts against nurses. Avoidance of difficult clients or patients is not a cause of negligence, but a breach of duty for nurses (18 Del. C. 6801[7]). Nurses are expected to typically perform nursing services according to a standard of skill and care in the field of nursing and to do this diligently. The Pennsylvania Nursing Law, Section 2, defines the practice of professional nursing:

Section 2. Definitions. When used in this act, the following words and phrases shall have the following meanings unless the context provides otherwise: (1) The "Practice of Professional

Nursing" means diagnosing and treating human responses to actual or potential health problems through such services as case finding, health teaching, health counseling, and provision of care supportive to or restorative of life and well-being, and executing medical regimens as prescribed by a licensed physician or dentist. The foregoing shall not be deemed to include acts of medical diagnosis or prescription of medical therapeutic or corrective measures, except as performed by a certified registered nurse practitioner acting in accordance with rules and regulations promulgated by the Board [Professional Nursing Law, The Act of May 22, 1951, P.L. 317, No. 69 Cl. 63].

In the Pennsylvania Code, standards of nursing conduct are also listed. One standard is that a registered nurse may not "knowingly abandon a patient in need of nursing care. Abandonment is defined as the intentional deserting of a patient for whom the nurse is responsible" (§ 21.18 Standards of Nursing Conduct [2] [7] [b]). The critical incident in the home care setting highlights the risk of harm for patients when nurses label them difficult and avoid them. In addition to legal problems, patient suffering is a serious concern to nurses whose practice is framed by caring behaviors and legal and ethical obligations.

Rather than focusing on fear of litigation, it is important that nurses carry out the altruistic values of nursing practice. These values stand for nurses' obligation to not harm patients (nonmaleficence) and a desire to help (beneficence) them (Sitzman & Watson, 2014). The shift in the nurse-patient relationship toward caring in nursing by practicing lovingkindness with self and others fosters compassion, gentleness, and mercy. Nurses need to commit to ongoing development of lovingkindness through "attitude, intentions, and a stance" (Sitzman & Watson, p. 43–44):

> The temperament of the nurse, the temperament of the patient, and other situation-specific factors will influence what the outward expression of caring lovingkindness will be, while the inner resolve of the nurse to care and to love remains constant [p. 44].

The dignity and individuality of patients are respected in caring encounters. Their autonomy and self-determination to make decisions about their lives and health care are valued. Noncaring behaviors, such as distancing, withdrawal, or punitive behaviors, are a persistent nursing concern (Maupin, 1995) and counter to nursing values.

In challenging situations, for example, when patients suffer from fecal incontinence, a difficult patient label can be assigned. Incontinence is difficult to manage, and basic nursing care is required. Although nurses need to be professional, non-judgmental, and caring, incontinent patients' situations may lead nurses to detach themselves from patients in attempts to manage their disgust and revulsion (Butcher, 2020). Patients might be shamed and suffer emotionally and psychologically in these situations, because control of bowels connects to a sense of competence developed as a child. Nurses caring for patients that are often incontinent might physically distance themselves, wear protective equipment, and blame patients for deliberately being incontinent because they need attention from staff (Butcher, 2020). They might chastise patients. In contrast, the importance of maintaining therapeutic relationships with patients experiencing fecal incontinence or in other difficult patient care situations can be recognized through the self-reflective practices of nurses. Becoming self-aware of their own coping strategies and attitudes can assist them to better meet the needs of patients. Whether or not nurses' personal and professional values correspond or conflict needs to be examined and addressed during patient care.

Courvoisier et al. (2014) developed the Care-Related Regret Coping Scale for Health-Care Professionals (RCS-HCP). The researchers acknowledged clinicians' common experience of regret about clinical practice activities. Although coping style varied among providers, such as problem- or emotion-focused coping, the researchers pointed out that no single approach might fit in all situations. Of concern were negative outcomes associated with self-blame behaviors and depression among providers. The researchers developed a scale for measuring habitual coping style addressing care-related regret. They established initial and subsequent reliability and validity characteristics and separated nurse ($N = 240$) from physician ($N = 220$) scores. Items were reduced to 13, and the three types of strategies consisted of problem-focused strategies, trying to find solutions, and talking to colleagues. Problem- and emotion-focused coping strategies were positively correlated with increased quality of life, decreased sleep problems, and decreased depression in health care providers. An instrument, such as the RCS-HCP, that measures the overall regret experience can be used to assist nurses and other providers to self-assess their coping strategies, including those experienced in difficult patient situations. They could seek support from professionals skilled in counseling health care professionals and share concerns with managers and administrators.

A therapeutic nurse-patient relationship is critical to achieve quality patient care. However, several factors can threaten and disrupt this relationship. The phrases "difficult patient" or "bad patient" can have different meanings, such as difficult to treat and difficult based on behavior and interactions (Koekkoek et al., 2011). However, the meaning of the difficult patient label is complex and situated in the perspectives of health care providers, patients, family members, health care administrators and institutions, and society. The judgments and perceptions of nurses and other authority figures who provide health care services impose the notion of difficulty onto patients, further complicating clinicians' concerns about diagnostic categories and other clinical findings. Additionally, patients and providers of care are separated by the social distance (Creary & Eisen, 2013) and the power differentials of caregiver and care receiver.

The power differential between nursing staff and patients suggests that staff are seen as having greater power than patients (Kangasniemi, 2010). To facilitate the nurse-patient relationship and address the power in it, nurses need to recognize that this type of power is temporary. Although temporary power is evident in the relationship, the imbalance of power does not mean inequality. Nurses need to share sufficient information with patients to empower them because insufficient information disempowers. As nurses make decisions and choices for patients unable to do so at the time, paternalism is evident. As nurses show that they respect patients' will or values and respect their autonomy, beneficence is seen, patients' behavior might change, and difficult patient situations resolve (Kangasniemi, 2010).

Perhaps by enacting caring behaviors, nurses and other health care providers might change the imbalance between them through improved interactions (Duffy, 2013). Such behaviors, demonstrated verbally and nonverbally through words, timing, facial expressions, touch, eye contact, and active listening, and by clarifying information and other indicators of caring, can equalize the authority gradient. Patients might then feel cared for and change their behaviors, thus eliminating the difficult patient label. Nurses might also find themselves more centered on carrying out professional values (Duffy, 2013).

For some time, nurses have been frustrated by patients they judge as difficult;

nurses decide that some patients' care requires more time than their conditions warrant. They perceive patients' behavior as demanding, manipulative, complaining, and uncooperative, particularly when attempting to carry out interventions intended to help them (Ujhely, 1967). Additionally, terminally or chronically ill patients and those needing complex physical care and skilled pain management challenge nursing competencies during care encounters.

Difficult patients' litany of characteristics includes abusive, violent, demanding, aggressive, recalcitrant, lying, angry, frightened, confused, seductive, moody, bullying, irrational, sexually provocative, or easily agitated. They challenge nursing staff by spitting, refusing hygienic care, reporting confusing symptoms, refusing to follow plans of care, disrupting professionals' routines, being overweight, addicted, and hostile, and being difficult to treat or diagnose (Michaelsen, 2011; Wolf & Robinson-Smith, 2007). Designations or characteristic types also differ by types of health care providers caring for patients during challenging clinical encounters (Marcum, 2015).

Like Ujhely's (1967) classic work, Stockwell (1972), a nurse researcher, published a brochure over 45 years ago titled *The Unpopular Patient*. Stockwell divided the factors that influenced nurses' view of patients into four areas, including personality, communication, attitudes, and factors related to nursing. In Stockwell's view, personality pertains to a patient being happy or uncooperative. A patient who is happy and compliant is perceived as a good patient. Communication is centered on whether the patient is grateful or unappreciative. Attitude refers to whether the patient is open to accepting treatment; factors relating to nursing include whether patients are interesting to the nurse. Any negative component in these areas can lead to the nurse ignoring patients or disconnecting from them. These problematic issues affect not only patients but can add to the emotional labor of nurses. They suppress their feelings to help patients feel cared for (Michaelsen, 2011, citing Smith). Consider the expectation when at work nurses "have to always be positive with their patients" (Kasdovasili & Theofilou, 2016, p. 539), despite the adversities of patient care. Although positivism is important, it is also important to consider effective strategies that promote skilled communication and to examine creative, evidence-based alternatives.

Building nurse-patient relationships has been connected to strategies that focus on increasing patient participation, essential to promote patient-centered care. To explore how actions and behaviors foster patient participation in clinical environments, researchers (Tobiano et al., 2016) conducted an observational study in an Australian public hospital. Part of a larger ethnography, the researchers observed 28 dyadic interactions between nurses and diverse adult patients during morning and afternoon shifts throughout the week. Field notes, audiotaped researcher observations, and audiotaped researcher reflections comprised data organized in a categorization matrix. The unit of analysis was the encounter, with nurse and patient together. Patients' knowledge was respected during dialogues; patient preferences were considered, and approval of nurse-performed activities was sought by nurses. Nurses shared knowledge of symptoms, issues, and procedures. Vital signs that were outside of normal were reported. Directions about how patients were able to move and carry out activities of daily living were elicited from patients. Nurses explained procedures while performing them. In turn, patients shared information about symptoms and showed understanding of their situations. Few instances were described in which patients carried out self-care activities.

In contrast, nurses controlled their work when facing pressures by being task-oriented, by administering physical care, and by limiting communication (Tobiano et al., 2016). Nurses' time constraints, task completion, and set routines restricted patients' ability to choose some care activities. Maintaining control over the environment was more frequent for nurses than encouraging patients to participate in planning care and self-care. The researchers suggested developing strategies to optimize nurse-patient interactions and communication to achieve patient-centered nursing care.

When nurses recognize that the therapeutic characteristic of the nurse-patient relationship begins to deteriorate and positive outcomes and patient safety are threatened, the delivery of quality care is compromised. Nurses are professionally responsible for identifying problems in the relationship, investigating implicit or explicit causes, and determining how to maintain or reestablish caring relationships. It may be difficult for them to practice lovingkindness in the intimate, personal space of an especially problematic interaction (Watson, 2010); nonetheless, this may be what is required so that encounters do not escalate and result in patient harm.

When the relationship between patients and nurses becomes difficult, nurses can practice enhanced communication by directly inviting patients to an open interaction place, created by both parties (Boykin et al., 2014). The nurse then makes clear why he or she was there to care for the patient and creates openness so that what matters most in the moment is discussed. In the caring space created between patient and nurse, the patient's voice may be better heard.

A number of nursing theoretical and conceptual frameworks place the nurse-patient relationship at the center of health care services. As applied to clinical settings, they have the power to transform institutions and interpersonal interactions. For example, the Relationship-Based Care Model (Koloroutis, 2004), implemented in numerous nursing service departments, identifies three crucial relationships: "care provider's relationship with patients and families, care provider's relationship with self, and care provider's relationship with colleagues" (p. 4). Everyday experiences with vulnerable patients in health care environments are emphasized. As such a model permeates an organization, nursing staff and other providers have opportunities to step back, reflect, strategize, and implement change in the moments when direct care is provided to patients.

In the critical incident described in this chapter, the home care nurse perceived the patient as difficult, which led her to avoid the client, resulting in harm. Had the nurse investigated the reason for the client's belligerence and failure to follow the plan of care, a different outcome may have resulted. The next section of this chapter discusses difficult patients, effects of being labeled difficult, nurses' responses to difficult patients, ethical and legal implications, and interventions to improve the nurse-patient relationship. As the chapter progresses, case examples are interspersed, so solutions to the difficult patient stories inform nursing interventions and alternate strategies.

Literature

Different databases were searched to locate studies on nurse's interactions or lack of interactions with difficult patients. The search discovered a plethora of research on defining the difficult patient, causes for the difficult patient, and interventions to improve the interactions between the nurse and difficult patient.

"Difficult" Patients

Nurses are charged with providing quality patient care. A threatened nurse-patient relationship can impede this care and affect negative health outcomes for patients. Many terms describe patients whom nurses are more likely to avoid than others, such as difficult patients, offensive patients, unpopular patients, and so on. What determines the makeup of difficult patients is often debated with no consistent definition or cause. The judgment of difficult is subjective, based on nurses' personal experiences and background. Often patients are termed difficult if they are not complying with the plan of care or if they ask too many questions (Michaelsen, 2012). They may also be labeled as difficult if they threaten nurses' competence and control. Michaelsen conducted a qualitative study exploring the relationships between nurses and patients they perceived to be difficult. Nurses and patients in a nursing home unit in Denmark were interviewed. Three different strategies were identified including persuasion, avoidance, and compromise.

Persuasion refers to the nurse attempting to encourage the patient to be compliant, and this can occur on a scale from giving advice to threatening the patient (Michaelsen, 2012). Nurses in the study described the strategy of persuasion to elicit compliance from patients but included the threat of keeping patients in the hospital if they did not listen to advice or instructions (Michaelsen, 2012). Nurses have many demands and time constraints in giving care to patients. Although persuasion can be a benign strategy, to have patients comply with a nursing intervention, it can easily lead patients to feeling threatened.

Avoidance refers to emotional distance and is considered a survival mechanism nurses employed when they felt they could no longer care for patients (Michaelsen, 2012). This avoidance could either be appearing cold toward patients or asking another nurse to take over care. Nurses can safely and professionally hand off care of patients, but emotionally distancing themselves or avoiding patients may lead to patient harm. Compromise meant that nurses relinquished the idea of compliance, but they were not at the point of avoidance. Depending on the interactions, relationships could improve or lead to avoidance. Michaelsen (2012) concluded that avoidance did not have to be a terminal stage, but rather could be improved with effective communication. It is important for nurses to self-reflect on erosion of nurse-patient relationships and attempt to make improvements or report the potential problem to a supervisor for guidance. Nurse managers need the tools to help navigate problematic nurse-patient relationships.

The home health setting is vastly different from the acute care setting. Normally nurses work independently in patients' homes without the immediate benefit of coworkers. It is in this intimate setting where nurses have a broader view of patients' complete environment. Falkenstrom (2017) conducted a qualitative study exploring nurse-patient relationships in the home care setting. Two of the themes that emerged from the analysis relating to the encounters between home health nurses, patients, and their caregivers include objective language and navigating the unknown. Objective language referred to nurses' desire to use objective language to describe patient encounters. Nurses did not use the word "difficult" when describing a patient, but rather labeled an action or occurrence as difficult. They considered the word difficult as subjective. It is well documented that objective language is preferable in documentation of care. Its intention is to give all the members of the health care team an accurate account of the progress of patients. Nurses preferred the word "challenging" when describing problem patient behaviors and environments. Navigating the unknown was interpreted to mean that home health nurses may not know what they may encounter in the home. One of the most challenging factors in home care is the unknown. Although phone calls establish communication prior to a first visit, there remains an element of the unknown. A home environment that is cluttered, unclean, or vermin-infested could prompt nurses to want to leave quickly or avoid a patient.

In one study, difficult patients were perceived as being able but unwilling to change; staff's pessimism of the patients' ability to change was acknowledged (Koekkoek et al., 2011). This study also found that patients who required frequent monitoring or high levels of care were judged difficult. Further, the stigmatization associated with mental illness and addiction could lead nurses to have implicit bias toward patients with psychiatric diagnoses.

The phrase "difficult patient" is seen frequently in the literature related to psychiatric nursing where labeling can often occur. Mental health services are complex, and compliance with treatment plans is often challenging. Patients with a mental health diagnosis can often be labeled difficult and seen as aggressive, disruptive, and prone to self-harm (Breeze & Repper, 1998).

Often complex or hard-to-treat psychiatric conditions lead to long hospitalizations or frequent outpatient treatment in comparison to acute medical conditions. Some psychiatric conditions stem from a lifetime of neglect, abuse, or lack of love (Manos & Braun, 2006). Nurses may feel the stress of caring for complex patients with psychiatric conditions. Previous nursing experience caring for them may contribute to strain in nurse-patient relationships.

Nurses are challenged to reflect on patients' behavior and assess it for indicators of depression. For example, a clustered and unclean home environment can be a red flag for clinical depression. Nurses need to evaluate if patients had a previous psychiatric consult and if other nurses performed a standardized depression screening. They might consider if their feelings, whether explicit or implicit toward clients, may have led them to overlook assessment and neglect discussing alternate planning options with patients. It is imperative that nurses' use standardized tools to assess clients despite personal bias.

To measure depression in adult patients that demonstrate depressive symptoms, nurses can administer the Center for Epidemiologic Studies Depression Scale (CES-D) (U.S. Department of Health and Human Services, National Institute of Mental Health, n.d.). The instrument has 10- and 20-item versions, is free, and has been frequently administered to diverse groups; it continues to be tested for validity (Carleton et al., 2013). It compares with the well-established Beck Depression Inventories.

In contrast, nurses are charged with the task of assessing their own stereotypes and biases when caring for patients (Campinha-Bacote, 2007). The persistence of stereotypes and biases can lead to charges of negligence. The failure to perform self-reflection can reduce the quality of care nurses give patients. Recognition of stereotypes and biases is essential for giving quality care. Because implicit biases can affect the way nurses communicate with patients and provide other nursing care services, nurses need to assess their biases. An important step for nurses is to complete a self-assessment of stereotypes and biases. After identifying issues, nurses can put those feelings aside to care for patients.

Cultural competence, appreciation of cultural differences, not being judgmental by understanding that being different is not bad and being open to cultural encounters help to address implicit biases (Greenwald et al., 1998). Implicit biases could affect the treatment of patients ultimately judged as difficult.

The unconscious attitudes and associations of nurses toward patients of various racial and ethnic groups can be measured by tests such as the Implicit Association Test (Project Implicit, 2011). Also, providers might benefit by self-assessing implicit bias on the different tests available within the Harvard University instrument. Additionally, cultural competence has been a major agenda in the education of many health care providers. Sessions are provided in health care organizations to continue the focus on employee development.

Non-Compliance and "Difficult" Patients

Non-compliance is a common descriptor for patients termed difficult. Patients described as non-compliant with established nursing and medical interventions are often called difficult. Thus, they receive two labels. Most of the nursing literature focuses on improving communication and increasing patient education to increase compliance with the health care plan. However, a study by Russell et al. (2003) suggested that nurses should assess patients' social environments and adapt interventions to their actual needs. For instance, it is not realistic to recommend a daily increase in fresh vegetables, if the patient has limited financial resources, or to suggest they walk daily in their neighborhoods, if they fear for their safety. This alternative approach, in conjunction with traditional methods to increase compliance, might yield more positive results.

When recognizing that clients seem to be always upset or non-compliant, nurses can stop to reflect and then investigate the causes of these issues. Nurses then act to resolve such problems and reassess behaviors on an ongoing basis. An example is patients with co-morbid conditions. Nurses that label clients as belligerent could have missed assessing that they were in pain. A client's non-compliance could indicate that a responsible caregiver needs to listen to clients' concerns. However, some nurses may have been available to clients or clients did not share their perspectives with the caregivers.

The literature suggests that non-compliance with the health care plan is a reason for labeling a client as difficult. In the critical incident at the beginning of this chapter, the nurse saw non-compliance as a reason for labeling the client as difficult. This led to the nurse avoiding the client and subsequent injury. Had the nurse assessed possible clinical problems when determining the reason for the non-compliance? It is imperative that nurses look beyond difficult patients' actions and personality to strategize so that improved compliance is achieved.

Factors that contribute to the label of difficult patient include personality, physical and mental illnesses, socioeconomic status, and attitudes. It is critical that nurses reflect on factors underlying difficult behavior and get to the root of patients' problems.

Nurses' Responses to "Difficult" Patients

Nurses spend a considerable amount of time, energy, and resources when caring for difficult patients (Bos et al., 2011). However, difficult nurse-patient relationships often cause nurses to feel emotionally and morally distressed. They can feel pessimistic, emotionally distant, and stressed and may experience burnout (Bos et al., 2011; Breeze & Repper, 1998; Manos & Braun, 2006).

Nurses are educated and trained to be caring, compassionate, confident, and professional. Nonetheless, they may not consider the power gradient patients and family members perceive nurses to represent. Being a competent authority can benefit the nurse-patient relationship and not be interpreted as power over patients and relatives. For example, nurses' sharing of knowledge and expertise can persuade patients to comply with a treatment plan. On the other hand, if nurses' authoritative personality combines with no patient involvement, patients may perceive nursing care negatively.

To shape this perception, nurses can accept that patients appreciate feeling part of care planning, interventions, and decisions made for them (Manos & Braun, 2006). Nurses recognize that they must prepare to deal with difficult patients and use opportunities to improve patient outcomes rather than avoiding the nursing challenge.

When patients' perceptions about nursing care differ from nurses', other complications follow. For example, in a study by Khalil (2009), nurses reported that even when they judged their care as good, difficult patients reported them to supervisors. The study's findings revealed that nurses avoided or delayed care for patients known as difficult. However, other respondents refuted that claim by stating short staffing as the reason for only giving some patients essential care.

Many factors contribute to nurses' work stress: short staffing, lack of support, conflict with physicians and other nurses, working conditions, and the constant changes with technology. The challenges of caring for difficult patients can substantially increase their stress. It is critical that nurses use coping mechanisms to prevent burnout and avoidance of difficult patients. Coping mechanisms include stress management practices, mindful meditation, exercise, reflection, and relaxation response training. Alerting and seeking support from administrators about very challenging situations might result in de-escalating situations. Many hospital facilities offer resources to staff nurses, and the use of these services should be encouraged.

Nurses might reflect on their own responses to patients labeled difficult. They can question if they avoided caring for patients due to that label. Other options are available to eliminate staying away from these clients. For example, did nurses in that home care agency receive training in how to deal with difficult patients; did clinical case managers recognize that nurses failed to visit certain patients and intervene? It is important for nurses to practice self-care and self-reflection to avoid giving substandard patient care or miss giving care altogether.

Ethical and Legal Concerns

The American Nurses Association (ANA, 2015) Scope of Practice includes the standards of professional nursing practice that state the duties that all registered nurses are expected to perform competently. Standard 11 pertains to communication and charges nurses to assess their own communication skills as well as continuous improvement of communication between nurses and patients (ANA, 2015). Nurses that avoid difficult patients violate this standard. Nurses need to evaluate their communication competencies regarding stereotypes, judgments, and tone of delivery to deliver competent care.

ANA's Code of Ethics (2015) is another authoritative guide for nurses developing and maintaining ethical behavior. Provision 1 charges nurses to practice with compassion and respect for every patient. Labeling patients as difficult can inhibit nurses from acting with compassion and respect toward those patients.

Nurses that avoid or fail to deliver care to patients labeled difficult are in jeopardy of violating the ethical principle of beneficence. Nurses potentially harm patients by avoiding them. The literature supports the belief that patients labeled difficult often receive substandard care or care is missed, so that the ethical principle of justice is not upheld.

Nurses are obligated to respect patients' autonomy. A client who refuses to take a medication or allow an intervention, and is then labeled difficult, has the right to refuse. This right needs to be honored (Juliana et al., 1997; Wolf et al., 1997). Moreover, nurses' responsibility includes ensuring that clients are educated about pertinent information on their health status and consequences for not following treatment plans. However, refusal of care and lack of adherence can lead to compromised nurse-patient relationships.

In the critical incident at the beginning of this chapter, the nurse's previous communication experiences with the client contributed to avoidance. The nurse did not take additional steps to check that the client was home nor contact other responsible parties. Also, describing a patient using words such as belligerent is judgmental. This behavior conflicts with the Standards of Professional Practice (ANA, 2015), ANA Code of Ethics (2015), and ethical principles of beneficence, nonmaleficence, justice, and autonomy.

It is evident in the previous case scenario that the nurse violated or potentially violated ethical values. The nurse's failure to reach the patient was inconsistent with beneficence (doing good). The patient needed care that day; it was not provided due to the nurse's inaction. The nurse did not treat the patient equally as compared to other patients, based on past, frustrating interactions with her (violation of justice).

Nurses are challenged to look at the difficult patient situation in another way. At times there are difficult nurses and other problematic health care providers. Conway (2000) presented types of difficult patients by organizing them under the major category of difficult to nurse. Perhaps by changing perspectives and then creating alternative strategies, nurses can remove difficult patient labels. See Table 6 for patients seen as difficult to nurse.

Table 6. Patients Considered Difficult by Nurses*

Difficult to Nurse	Examples
Difficult by diagnosis	Stroke Alcoholic Back pain Munchausen's syndrome
Antisocial behavior	Abusive alcoholic Glue sniffer Child abuser
Breaks social conventions	Nasty Abusive Rude Bad mannered

Difficult to Nurse	Examples
Threats to professional autonomy	Litigators Involving staff in litigation Record keepers Complainers Second opinion request
Manipulator	Sets staff against each other Provokes others
Patient in charge	Expects to be boss "To the manor born" Treated like royalty Overlooks others Selfish
"I want to be first"	Perceived as trivial request Bellringer Demanding
Breaks the unwritten rules	Non-conforming Defeatist Does not attempt to improve Non-compliant Sexual overtones
"Knows the score"	Acts like one of the staff Regular attender
Aggression	Screaming Shouting Violent

*This table was adapted from the "Categorizing the 'Difficult' Patient" table in the paper, "Characteristics or Traits of Patients Which May Result in Their Being Considered as 'Difficult' by Nurses," delivered at the Qualitative Evidence–based Practice Conference, Coventry University, May 15–17, 2000, and posted to the Education-Line database May 11, 2000. Dr. Conway died in 2012 from cancer and was employed at University College Dublin (http://www.ucd.ie/news/2012/10OCT12/061012-padraic-conway.html).

Interventions to Improve Nurse-Patient Relationship

It is essential that nurses avoid assumptions, meet patients' expressed needs, and prioritize interventions. If nurses provide opportunities for communication, listen to patients' needs, and invite them to participate in care planning, a possible difficult encounter may be prevented. Effective communication techniques enhance nurse-patient relationships. The following patient situation challenged a nurse to examine feelings about caring for a prisoner, taken from an anecdote by a student:

> Prior to admission, a nurse reflected on her feelings about caring for a prisoner. The nurse resolved to care just as she would care for any patient. She acted according to the ethical value of justice and paid attention to treating the patient respectfully and being attentive during the nurse-patient interaction. Her attitude may have helped the patient to feel comfortable and communicate with the nurse, resulting in better patient outcomes.

After self-assessment and reflection, nurses could establish open communication and work on being nonjudgmental about patients that challenge them.

Therapeutic communication techniques are designed to invite responses from patients that encourage expressions of feelings and ideas and signal acceptance and respect. Fundamentals of nursing textbooks consistently describe therapeutic communication strategies: active listening, using silence, and sharing empathy, hope, and feelings (Potter & Perry, 2017). By reviewing these often-used techniques, nurses may be able to center again on communication basics and intentionally use them when caring for challenging patients.

Perhaps one of the most effective approaches to eliminating the difficult patient label and situation is to encourage patients to ask questions (Judson et al., 2013). Although fear of consuming health care providers' time and fear of being labeled difficult might prevent patients from asking questions, this approach might help them ask their questions and share in decision making with health care providers. In addition to promoting patient safety, it could improve nurse-patient communication and empower patients.

Difficult patients and nurses caring for them may be anxious, and thus might benefit from relaxation response techniques (Calisi, 2017). Nurses can teach patients relaxation techniques that could help to manage their unique situations. When interacting with patients who are screaming or visibly upset, nurses need to listen and show concern and empathy; however, they must set limits on unacceptable behavior when safety is threatened.

Crary (2016) emphasized the complexity of current nursing practice in hospitals, noting short lengths of stay, increased patient workloads, and increased technologies. The author asserted that hospital settings have barriers that inhibit relatedness, and advocated education and self-awareness. Crary (2016) reiterated the impact of the nurse-patient relationship on patient outcomes.

Crary (2016) compared relatedness during nurse-patient interactions to a many-faceted gemstone. Relatedness was defined as "people's inherent need to feel connected and connected to and accepted by others, to care for and be cared for by others, and to have a sense of belongingness both with other individuals and with one's community" (Crary, 2016, p. 349 citing Black & Deci). Crary's gemstone image placed relatedness in a center facet, with autonomy, empathy, presence, competence, acceptance, active listening, and genuineness surrounding it. Genuineness demonstrated by clinicians shows feelings and attitudes through verbal and nonverbal messages. Acceptance establishes a climate within which patients grow; nurses are caring and have unconditional regard for patients. Nurses are willing for patients to demonstrate their immediate feelings. As far as empathy, nurses are active listeners and sense feelings and personal meanings of patients' experience. They acknowledge patients and show understanding. Presence shows nurses' availability to patients by being there and sharing the experiences together, nurses and patients.

Crary (2016) connected relatedness to Self-Determination Theory (SDT), describing its person-centeredness and focus on motivation and the benefits of mutual respect. The SDT concepts of autonomy and competence were added to the gem's facets. Crary's model of relatedness can be applied to nurse-patient relationships. The gem figure could be posted in patient units as a reminder to nurses of core caring behaviors.

De-escalation techniques are used to prevent violent behaviors in patients becoming increasingly upset. The Joint Commission (TJC, 2018) developed a set of guidelines on de-escalation techniques. One expected outcome of effective de-escalation techniques is improved nurse-patient connections. The Crisis Prevention Institute (2020) developed 10 de-escalation tips to use in any health care setting and reflects the literature. Techniques include: 1. Be empathetic and non-judgmental; 2. Respect personal space; 3. Use non-threatening non-verbals; 4. Avoid overreacting; 5. Focus on feelings; 6. Ignore challenging questions; 7. Set limits; 8. Choose wisely what you insist upon; 9. Allow silence for reflection; 10. Allow time for decisions (para. 2).

When nurses fail to show empathy regarding patients' physical conditions or home environments and make judgments based on feelings, patients' negative behavior may escalate and endanger themselves and caregivers. When patients show belligerence or anger, nurses can initiate an exploration of their feelings and concerns or provide sufficient time to make decisions on their care. Any of the above de-escalation techniques could lead to a better patient outcome.

Threatened nurse-patient relationships can leave nurses feeling insecure about their professional ability. Breuner and Moreno (2010) discussed strategies for minimizing threats to nurses' feelings of self-efficacy. Shielding, keeping one's cool, taking a timeout, and seeking peer support were strategies suggested to care for difficult patients. Shielding was a form of emotionally distancing from patients involved with problematic relationships; shielding is often ineffective and leads to further breakdown in relationships. This study found that keeping cool was effective. Rather than avoiding patients or appearing angry, keeping a calm exterior allowed patients to see nurses in control of their emotions. Taking a timeout referred to taking time to cool off and physically disconnecting from patients. Timeouts allowed nurses to collect their thoughts and to revise action plans. It is important for nurses to take time to reflect and to report off to another nurse. Seeking peer support was deemed very positive for nurses in the study. Peer support helped relieve feelings of anger, guilt, and self-blame (Breuner & Moreno, 2010). Nurses understood that these situations can happen to any nurse.

In addition to nursing staff, difficult patients have challenged other members of the health care team, such as physicians and nurse practitioners. For example, the term heartsink (difficult patient) appeared in British literature over 20 years ago (Edgoose et al., 2015). Adding to the various patient characteristics leading in the label, poor functional status, unmet expectations, and high utilization of health care service were listed (Edgoose et al., 2015). In one study, issues around physician-patient relationships were reported and a structured intervention, consistent with a patient-centered care model, was implemented. A randomized, prospective controlled trial included reflection on clinicians' own biases and agendas. Prior to entering examination rooms for clinic visits, clinicians huddled and identified difficult patients, paused and breathed (BREATHE), carried out the visit, and then left the room (OUT). Satisfaction with difficult patient encounters improved in the experimental group following patient encounters. The BREATHE OUT protocol adds to options for experienced and inexperienced clinicians on the front lines to practice when caring for difficult patients (Edgoose et al., 2015).

Strategies

Strategies to mitigate difficult patient situations were identified in literature cited. However, more complex, interprofessional bundles of interventions are needed. See Table 7.

Table 7. Strategies to Effect Change
for Patients Labeled Difficult

Strategies to Effect Change	Evidence-Based Citations
In interprofessional sessions, practice reflective skills using simulated cases to understand unique health care professions' roles and cultural competence.	Olson et al. (2016)
Practice assessment of the potential for violence using a checklist and demonstrate de-escalation techniques to care for patients termed difficult.	Joint Commission (2018)
Practice basic nursing therapeutic communication techniques identified in fundamentals of nursing texts.	Potter et al. (2017)
Self-administer the Implicit Association Test choosing specific cultures represented in patient populations served.	Project Implicit (2011)
Reemphasize listening skills and the multifaceted nature of nurse-patient interactions.	Crary (2016)
Break the silence by encouraging patients to ask questions.	Judson et al. (2013)

Conclusion

Dealing with difficult patients has been a topic of discussion in nursing for decades. Many variables lead nurses to label patients as difficult, including behaviors, attitudes, non-compliance, psychiatric and addiction illnesses, and refusal of treatment. They can lead to deterioration of the nurse-patient relationship and result in patient harm. Several strategies are available for nurses to use that might improve the relationship with patients labeled difficult. Examples include de-escalation techniques, active listening, encouraging questions, and inviting patients to plan their care. Nurses are obligated to improve their competencies when communicating with patients and performing nursing interventions. Nursing and interprofessional interventions need to be created, tested, and compared across patient groups.

Discussion Questions

1. What are factors that lead nurses to label a patient difficult? Describe them.

2. What types of legal and ethical issues may arise out of interactions with a difficult patient?

3. What are 10 nursing actions or interventions nurses can use to modify approaches to caring for difficult patients?

4. How does labeling a patient as difficult affect the patient? How does it affect the nurse?

5. Outline interventions for the nurse to implement to improve the nurse-patient relationship with a challenging patient.

AUTHOR SELECTIONS

Falkenstrom, M.K. (2017). A qualitative study of difficult nurse-patient encounters in home health care. *Advances in Nursing Science, 40*(2), 168–183. doi: 10.1097/ANS.0000000000000156.

Manos, P.J., & Braun, J. (2006). *Care of the difficult patient: A nurse's guide.* Routledge.

References

American Nurses Association. (2015). Code of ethics for nurses with interpretive statements. https://www.nursingworld.org/practice-policy/nursing-excellence/ethics/code-of-ethics-for-nurses/.

American Nurses Association. (2015). Nursing: Scope and standards of practice (3rd ed.). https://www.nursingworld.org/practice-policy/scope-of-practice/.

Bos, M., Kool-Goudzwaard, N., Gamel, C.J., Koekkoek B., & Van Meijel, B. (2012). The treatment of 'difficult' patients in a secure unit of a specialized psychiatric hospital: The patient's perspective. Journal of Psychiatric and Mental Health Nursing, 19(6), 528–535. doi: 10.1111/j.1365–2850.2011.01827.x.

Boykin, A., Schoenhofer, S., & Valentine, K. (2014). Transforming leadership structures and process. In Health care system transformation for nursing and health care leaders: Implementing a culture of caring (pp. 147–174). Springer Publishing.

Breeze, J.A., & Repper, J. (1998). Struggling for control: The care experiences of 'difficult' patients in mental health services. Journal of Advanced Nursing, 28(6), 1301–1311. doi: 10.1046/j.1365–2648.1998.00842.x.

Breuner, C.C., & Moreno, M.A. (2011). Approaches to the difficult patient/parent encounter. Pediatrics, 127(1), 163–169. doi: 10.1542/peds.2010–0072.

Butcher, L. (2020). Psychological issues surrounding faecal incontinence: Experiences of patients and nurses. British Journal of Community Nursing, 25(1), 34–38. doi: 10.12968/bjcn.2020.25.1.34.

Calisi, C.C. (2017). The effects of the relaxation response on nurses' level of anxiety, depression, well-being, work-related stress and confidence to teach patients. Journal of Holistic Nursing, 35(4), 318–327. doi: 10.1177/0898010117719207.

Campbell, C., Scott, K., Skovdal, M., Madanhire, C., Nyamukapa, C., & Gregson, S. (2015). A good patient? How notions of 'a good patient' affect patient-nurse relationships and ART adherence in Zimbabwe. BMC Infectious Diseases, 15(1), 404. doi: 10.1186/s12879–015–1139-x.

Campinha-Bacote, J. (2007). The process of cultural competence in the delivery of healthcare services: The journey continues (5th ed.). Transcultural C.A.R.E.

Carleton, R.N., Thibodeau, M.A., Teale, M.J., Welch, P.G., Abrams, M.P., Robinson, T., & Asmundson, G.J. (2013). The center for epidemiologic studies depression scale: a review with a theoretical and empirical examination of item content and factor structure. PLOS ONE, 8(3), e58067. doi: 10.1371/journal.pone.0058067.

Conway, P. (2000). Characteristics or traits of patients which may result in their being considered as 'difficult' by nurses. Paper presented at Qualitative Evidence-based Practice Conference, Coventry University, England: United Kingdom. http://www.leeds.ac.uk/educol/documents/00001415.htm.

Courvoisier, D.S., Cullati, S., Ouchi, R., Schmidt, R.E., Haller, G., Chopard, P., Agoritsas, T., & Perneger, T.V. (2014). Validation of a 15-item Care-related Regret Coping Scale for Health-care Professionals (RCS-HCP). Journal of Occupational Health, 56, 430–443.

Crary, P. (2016). Relatedness matters. Holistic Nursing Practice, 30(6), 345–349. doi:10.1097/HNP.0000000000000177.

Creary, M., & Eisen, A. (2013). Acknowledging levels of racism in the definition of "difficult." American Journal of Bioethics, 13(4), 16–18.

Crisis Prevention Institute. (2020). CPI's top 10 de-escalation tips. https://www.crisisprevention.com/Blog/October-2017/CPI-s-Top-10-De-Escalation-Tips-Revisited.

Duffy, J.R. (2013). Quality caring in nursing and health systems (2nd ed.). Springer Publishing.

Edgoose, J.Y., Regner, C.J., & Zakletskaia, L.I. (2015). BREATHE OUT: A randomized controlled trial of a structured intervention to improve clinician satisfaction with "difficult" visits. Journal of the American Board of Family Medicine, 28, 13–20. doi: 10.3122/jabfm.2015.01.130323.

Falkenstrom, M.K. (2017). A qualitative study of difficult nurse-patient encounters in home health care. Advances in Nursing Science, 40(2), 168–183. doi: 10.1097/ANS.0000000000000156.

Grant, A.M., Franklin, J., & Langford, P. (2002). The Self-reflection and Insight Scale: A new measure of private self-consciousness. Social Behavior and Personality, 30(8), 821–836.

Greenwald, A.G., McGhee, D.E., & Schwartz, J.L. (1998). Measuring individual differences in implicit cognition: The Implicit Association Test. Journal of Personality and Social Psychology, 74(6), 1464–1480.

Joint Commission. (2018). Physical and verbal violence against health care workers. Sentinel Event Alert, 59. https://www.jointcommission.org/assets/1/18/SEA_59_Workplace_violence_4_13_18_FINAL.pdf.

Judson, T.J., Detsky, A.S., & Press, M.J. (2013). Encouraging patients to ask questions: How to overcome "white-coat silence." JAMA, 309(22), 2325–2326.

Juliana, C.A., Orehowsky, S., Smith-Regojo, P.S., Sikora, S.M., Smith, P.A., Stein, D.K., Wolf, Z.R. (1997). Interventions used by staff nurses to manage "difficult" patients. Holistic Nursing Practice, 11(4), 1–26. https://doi.org/10.1097/00004650-199707000-00003.

Kangasniemi, M. (2010). Equality as a central concept of nursing ethics: A systematic literature review. Scandinavian Journal of Caring, 24, 824–832. https://doi.org/10.111/j.147-6712.2010.00781.x.

Kasdovasili, E-I., & Theofilou, P. (2016). How nurses experience their profession and their relationship with the patients? A qualitative analysis. International Journal of Caring Sciences, 9(2), 534–541.

Khalil, D.D. (2009). Nurses' attitude towards "difficult" and "good" patients in eight public hospitals. *International Journal of Nursing Practice, 15*(5), 437–443. doi: 10.1111/j.1440–172X.2009.01771.x.

Koekkoek, B., van Meijel, B., Tiemens, B., Schene, A., & Hutschemaekers, G. (2011). What makes community psychiatric nurses label non-psychotic chronic patients as "difficult": Patient, professional, treatment and social variables. *Social Psychiatry and Psychiatric Epidemiology, 46*(10), 1045–1053. doi: 10.1007/s00127–010–0264–5.

Koloroutis, M. (Ed.). (2004). *Relationship-based care.* Creative Health Care Management.

Manos, P.J., & Braun, J. (2006). *Care of the difficult patient: A nurse's guide.* Routledge.

Marcum, J.A. (2015). Caring for patients during challenging clinical encounters. *Journal of Evaluation in Clinical Practice, 21*, 404–409. doi: 10.111/jep.12312.

Maupin, C.R. (1995). The potential for noncaring when dealing with difficult patients: Strategies for moral decision making. *Journal of Cardiovascular Nursing, 9*(3), 11–22.

Michaelsen, J.J. (2012). Emotional distance to so-called difficult patients. *Scandinavian Journal of Caring Sciences, 26*(1), 90–97. doi: 10.1111/j.1471–6712.2011.00908.x.

Michaelsen, J.J. (2020). The 'difficult patient' phenomenon in home nursing and 'self-inflicted' illness. *Scandinavian Journal of Caring Sciences.* Advance online publication. doi: 10.1111/scs.12890.

Olson, R., Bidewell, J., Dune, T., & Lessey, N. (2016). Developing cultural competence through self-reflection in interprofessional education: Findings from an Australian university. *Journal of Interprofessional Care, 30*(3), 347–354. http://dx.doi.org/10.3109/13561820.2016.1144583.

Pennsylvania Code. *§ 21.18. Standards of nursing conduct:1 b (7).* http://www.pacodeandbulletin.gov/Display/pacode?file=/secure/pacode/data/049/chapter21/s21.18.html&d=reduce.

Pennsylvania Department of State. *Professional Nursing Law, The Act of May 22, 1951, P.L. 317, No. 69 Cl. 63.* https://www.dos.pa.gov/ProfessionalLicensing/BoardsCommissions/Nursing/Documents/Applications%20and%20Forms/Professional%20Nurse%20Law.pdf.

Potter, P.A., Perry, A.G., Hall, A., & Stockert, P.A. (2017). *Fundamentals of nursing* (9th ed.). Mosby Elsevier.

Project Implicit. (2011). *Overview.* https://implicit.harvard.edu/implicit/takeatest.html.

Russell, S., Daly, J., Hughes, E., & Hoog, C.O. (2003). Nurses and 'difficult' patients: Negotiating non-compliance. *Journal of Advanced Nursing, 43*(3), 281–287. doi: 10.1046/j.1365–2648.2003.02711.x.

Sitzman, K., & Watson, J. (2014). The first caritas process. In K. Sitzman, & J. Watson, *Caring science, mindful practice: Implementing Watson's human caring theory* (pp. 41–52). Springer Publishing.

Stockwell, F. (1972). *The unpopular patient.* RCN Publications.

Tobiano, G., Marshall, A., Bucknall, T., & Chaboyer, W. (2016). Activities patients and nurses undertake to promote patient participation. *Journal of Nursing Scholarship, 48*(4), 362–370.

Ujhely, G. (1967). *The nurse and her "problem" patients.* Springer Publishing.

United States Department of Health and Human Services, National Institute of Mental Health. (n.d.). *Center for Epidemiologic Studies Depression Scale.* http://www.chcr.brown.edu/pcoc/cesdscale.pdf.

Watson Caring Science Institute. (2010). *Core concepts of Jean Watson's theory of human caring/caring science.* https://www.watsoncaringscience.org/files/PDF/watsons-theory-of-human-caring-core-concepts-and-evolution-to-caritas-processes-handout.pdf.

Wolf, Z.R., Brennan, R., Ferchau, L., Magee, M., Miller-Samuel, S., Nicolay, L., Paschal, D., Ring, J., & Sweeney, A. (1997). Creating and implementing guidelines on caring for difficult patients: A research utilization project. *MEDSURG Nursing, 6*(3), 137–144.

Wolf, Z.R., & Robinson-Smith, G. (2007). Strategies used by clinical nurse specialists to care for "difficult" clinician-patient situations: A descriptive study. *Cinical Nurse Specialist, 21*(2), 74–84.

Multiple-Choice Questions

1. **Which factors lead to the labeling of a patient as difficult? Select all that apply.**
   A. Behavior
   B. Compliance
   C. Living conditions
   D. Health status
   E. Attitudes

2. **What is an effect of a strained nurse-patient relationship?**
   A. Lack of trust
   B. Open communication
   C. Adherence to medication regimen
   D. Reduced hospitalizations

3. **What is one intervention that could improve the nurse-patient relationship?**
    A. Closed communication
    B. Self-reflection
    C. Authoritative tone
    D. Implicit bias

4. **What is the best action the nurse could take to improve relationships with patients of diverse backgrounds?**
    A. Ask the family to interpret for the patient
    B. Give the patient materials in their native language
    C. Encourage the patient to ask questions
    D. Self-reflect on own biases and stereotypes

CHAPTER 6

Neglect and Negligence
of Patients

Denise Nagle Bailey, EdD, RN,
MEd, MSN, CSN, FCPP

Objectives

    1. Describe factors underlying incidents of neglect and negligence that harm patients.

    2. Examine behavioral triggers for incidents of neglect and negligence of patients by health care professionals.

    3. Analyze examples of neglect and negligence in clinical settings.

    4. Compare strategies and interventions used to mitigate neglect and negligence of patients.

Critical Incident

A 93-year-old, wheelchair-bound woman was a resident in a long-term assisted care facility. The patient spent several happy years as an active member of the retirement community until her health status began to steadily decline, requiring her family to place her in a unit with an increased level of care. The patient became increasingly dependent on staff to assist her with routine Activities of Daily Living (ADLs).

The patient was pleasant, upbeat, non-demanding, and did not complain, even though she suffered daily with chronic, severe pain from rheumatoid arthritis. She was unable to raise her arms or move her legs more than an inch or two, a result of progressive arthritis-related deformities. As a retired registered nurse (RN), she hesitated to ask for assistance from nurses and staff, because she remembered how hectic it was for her as she once cared for patients. The patient's hesitance to ask for help was also predicated by her desire to be viewed as a good patient. Nursing staff often passed by her room, stopping by only to administer scheduled medications and to assist with ADLs requiring bathing, diaper changes, and transfers in and out of bed or chair.

Adequate staffing was problematic, particularly on weekends and holidays. Nurses and nursing assistants were often observed as hurried and quick to leave her room by both the patient and family members. If the patient pressed her call bell, it was for a justifiable reason; however, because of the patient's kind demeanor and non-complaining nature, she was often the last resident to receive a bath, obtain a diaper change, or eat breakfast. It was not uncommon for her to be wheeled out to an empty dining room at 11:00 or 11:30 a.m. for breakfast, relegated to eating in total isolation. Often the patient was wheeled back to the dining room for lunch an hour or less after eating breakfast. This delayed dining schedule ultimately resulted in her weight loss and decreased interaction with other residents and care staff and participation in scheduled activities.

One Saturday morning, a nurse and several attendants entered the patient's room after she experienced an episode of fecal incontinence. After staff completed a diaper change and the patient was placed back in her wheelchair, she requested a PRN pain medication since the nurse was already in the room. The nurse handed the patient her call bell, commenting that it was to be used only in a situation where she felt she was dying.

The patient became progressively more withdrawn and depressed, admitting to family that she feared to ask nurses for anything, even diaper changes and pain medication. She frequently sat in a wet or soiled diaper for extended periods of time. The patient was admitted to a hospital three times within a short period of time for severe urinary tract infections (UTIs), once with methicillin-resistant Staphylococcus aureus (MRSA). Ultimately, the patient died in the hospital from an acute UTI and sepsis.

Background

Similar and more serious cases of neglect surface in the literature and in anecdotes shared among family members and friends about their loved one admitted to long-term care settings. The nursing staff's negative behavior matches one of the constructs in Halldorsdottir's (1991) description of a continuum and typology of caring and uncaring. Such behavior can be explained as life-restraining or biostatic mode is uncaring; the patient perceives the nurse as indifferent, insensitive, and detached. The nurse-patient relationship is compromised in the clinical situation of neglect.

Unfortunately, elder mistreatment may not be reported and can be ignored (McAlpine, 2008). Elder mistreatment is typically carried out by persons with a continuing relationship with older persons, for example, caregivers in long-term care facilities who are trusted. Caregivers are responsible to meet the needs of persons under their care; regrettably, they might mistreat residents or, conversely, need to care for victims of mistreatment. When patients are neglected or care is negligent, caregivers' duty has been violated. When vulnerable persons are mistreated in health care facilities, the violation is termed institutional mistreatment (Halphen & Dyer 2019).

This chapter does not reflect self-neglect, another potential threat to patients' safety and well-being. The critical incident detailed in this chapter describes but one example of patient neglect resulting from prolonged wait times for diaper changes, pressure injuries of the buttocks, depression, withdrawal, and a perceived sense of fear and desperation expressed by the individual being cared for. The resident died as a result of an acute UTI and sepsis. Of related interest is a qualitative study on a diverse, community-based, stratified random sample ($N = 90$) of patients who contacted health care providers about at least one symptom of UTIs and participated in semi-structured interviews and focus groups (Welch et al., 2012). Adherence to recommendations, symptom relief, and satisfaction with care were examined. Almost 50 percent experienced no symptom relief following no treatment, no diagnostic tests, and either nonadherence to a treatment or ineffective treatment. No symptom relief was linked to not having received a treatment recommendation. However, some participants that had treatments noted that symptoms did not improve. Other participants perceived that providers considered their symptoms as not serious compared to their other health conditions or as a normal part of aging. They also perceived that some providers determined that adults' symptoms did not warrant treatment. Participants liked their providers and were overall satisfied with care in the primary-care context of the broader provider-patient relationship. However, for this community-based sample, providers needed to expand their approaches to meet patients' needs.

Residents of long-term care settings suffer from UTIs. UTIs represent the most common infection site for long-term care residents and the cause of bacteremia (Richards & Stuart, 2018). Risk factors are "urinary catheters, benign prostatic hypertrophy and prostatitis in men, atrophic vaginitis and estrogen deficiency in women, diabetes, neurogenic bladder, dementia, dehydration, and function impairment" (Richards & Stuart, 2018, para. 11). It is dangerous to consider UTIs as part of normal aging or so common in older persons residing in long-term care institutions that serious harm is not viewed as an outcome. Residents may not be able to clearly articulate their symptoms due to cognitive changes. Nursing staff must then be vigilant, assess signs and symptoms of UTIs, and request nurse practitioner or physician assessment so that diagnosis and treatment follow. Given that not all treatments are effective, nursing staff need to continue to assess residents' conditions. Not to do so suggests negligence. Whether care is provided in primary care or long-term care settings, it is the responsibility of care providers to consistently monitor and consider more holistic views of the care needs of their patients, consistent with Welsh et al.'s (2012) findings.

Definitions: Neglect and Negligence

Neglect is a form of mistreatment carried out by an individual who is entrusted with the care of another human being resulting in the lack of attention toward that individual through disregard, disrespect, or carelessness in meeting the other's needs. Exact language used to define neglect varies from jurisdiction to jurisdiction (National Adult Protective Services Association [NAPSA], 2019). Commonly reported types of negligence shared by adult protective services agencies include:

- **Physical neglect** includes failing to attend to a person's medical, hygiene, nutrition, and dietary needs, such as dispensing medications, changing bandages, bathing, grooming, dressing, or failure to provide ample food to maintain health.
- **Emotional neglect** includes causing emotional pain, distress, or anguish by ignoring, belittling, or infantilizing the needs of adults. This includes neglecting or discounting the emotional well-being of others, as well as actions to isolate adults from visits or contact by family and friends.
- **Abandonment** involves deserting the caregiving needs of an individual while neglecting to arrange sufficient care and support for the duration of the absence.
- **Financial neglect** involves disregarding a person's financial obligations such as failing to pay rent or mortgage, medical insurance or invoices, utility and garbage bills, property taxes or assessments.

- **Self-neglect** involves seniors or adults with disabilities who fail to meet their own essential physical, psychological, or social needs, which threaten their health, safety and well-being. This includes failure to provide adequate food, clothing, shelter, and health care for one's own needs [NAPSA, 2019, p. 1].

Negligence and neglect of patients are not just a growing issue of concern exclusive to the United States. In England and Wales, patient protection from ill-treatment and willful (intentional) neglect has been supported by the passage of more stringent laws that now attempt to shield patients from acts of omission in cases of ill treatment and willful neglect (Griffiths, 2015). The creation of new offenses related to these acts allow for the prosecution of care workers and care providers. The number of prosecutions for ill treatment and willful neglect by nurses has risen considerably since the release of two reports, the Francis Report in England (2013) and the Andrews Report in Wales (2014), that underscored incidents of poor patient care that resulted in deaths of patients.

The British Parliament removed the restrictions concerning when a health care worker can be prosecuted for ill treatment and willful neglect, through the passage of the Criminal Justice and Courts Act of 2015. The Act applies to care providers, including organizations that provide health care to children and adults. Included are general practitioner (GP) practices, hospital and community trusts, health boards, and Clinical Commissioning Groups (CGCs). According to Griffith (2015), a care provider commits a breach of duty under the Criminal Justice Act 2015 when:

- A care worker ill-treats or willfully neglects an individual.
- The care provider's activities are managed or organized in a way that amounts to a gross breach of their duty of care.
- In the absence of the breach, the ill treatment or willful neglect would not have occurred or would have been less likely to occur [p. 1].

Therefore, to be found guilty of a violation (Griffiths, 2015), the judicial authority needs to conclude that a care provider committed a gross breach of the duty of care for a patient. Here, the health care organization "will have had to have fallen far below the standard normally expected of it in the discharge of its duty of care" (p. 1).

When considering what acts constitute ill treatment and willful neglect, under recent changes to the British Criminal Justice and Courts Act of 2015, areas of uncertainty are not expressly defined. Police and prosecutors are dependent upon the facts and circumstances of each situation, in addition to applying the conclusions of cases previously determined by the courts. Furthermore, as new incidents are identified and reviewed, it is important to recognize that these laws are not meant to penalize health care workers, impede the clinical judgment of professionals, or deter health care organizations from making decisions where genuine accidents and errors result. Neglect, ill treatment, and willful neglect were defined by Griffith (2015) in the following manner:

> **Neglect:** would occur where a cardiac nurse failed to do what they would do in the care and treatment of a person. This has been held to include falsifying records, failing to give medications, and failing to provide cardiopulmonary resuscitation (CPR).
> **Ill treatment:** includes any behavior that a court would reasonably consider to be abusive.
> **Willful neglect:** would occur when a cardiac nurse failed to do what they would be expected to do in the care and treatment of a person. This has been held to include falsifying records, failing to give medications, and failing to provide cardiopulmonary resuscitation (CPR). To be convicted of the offense, the neglect must be willful.

Terminology to describe this uncaring behavior helps to focus on varying levels of undue harm, even death to vulnerable patients. Furthermore, the negligence and neglect unearthed in England and Wales gave rise to a global concern, thus highlighting the serious and harmful outcomes that surface when nurses and health care staff fail to provide appropriate care to vulnerable patients across all settings of practice. These settings cross borders and continue around the world.

In the United States, the Social Security Act (SSA; 2018) defined abuse pertaining to adults to be "the knowing infliction of physical or psychological harm or knowing deprivation of goods or services that are necessary to meet essential needs or to avoid physical or psychological harm" (SSA, Sec.2011. [42 U.S.C. 1397j] Subtitle 1). Subtitle 16 (A) of the SSA noted neglect to be "the failure of a caregiver or fiduciary to provide the goods or services that are necessary to maintain the health or safety of an elder." State-based legislation has also been enacted to protect vulnerable persons.

In contrast, the Pennsylvania General Assembly enacted the Older Adults Protective Services Act (1987). The Act defines neglect (Chapter 1) in the following manner:

> Neglect. The failure to provide for oneself or the failure of a caretaker to provide goods or services essential to avoid a clear and serious threat to physical or mental health. No older adult who does not consent to the provision of protective services shall be found to be neglected solely on the grounds of environmental factors which are beyond the control of the older adult or the caretaker, such as inadequate housing, furnishings, income, clothing, or medical care.

Additionally, the Older Adults Protective Services Act mandates that suspected abuse by employees, such as withholding of services, must be reported orally to the agency administrator and followed by a written report. Details are provided in the legislation.

Table 8 below identifies and summarizes another set of categories on neglect that appear in selected literature and provides definitions and examples of different types of neglect.

Table 8. Types of Neglect

Type	Definition	Example
Physical neglect	Includes failing to attend to a person's medical, hygiene, nutrition and dietary needs	Neglecting dispensing medications, changing bandages, bathing, grooming, dressing, or failure to provide ample food to maintain health
Emotional neglect	Includes causing emotional pain, distress or anguish by ignoring, belittling, or infantilizing the needs of adults	Neglecting or discounting the emotional well-being of others, as well as actions to isolate adults from visits or contact by family and friends
Abandonment	Involves deserting the caregiving needs of an individual while neglecting to arrange sufficient care and support for the duration of the absence	Nurse leaves unit without informing supervisor or charge nurse and ensuring the safety and welfare of assigned patients

Type	Definition	Example
Financial neglect	Involves disregarding a person's financial obligations	Failing to pay rent or mortgage, medical insurance, invoices, utility and garbage bills, property taxes or assessments
Self-neglect	Involves seniors or adults with disabilities who fail to meet their own essential physical, psychological or social needs, which threaten their health, safety and well-being	Includes failure to provide adequate food, clothing, shelter, and health care for one's own needs

Adapted from: National Adult Protective Services Association (2019). *What is neglect*? napsa.now.org.

In contrast, medical negligence includes:

any tort or breach of contract based on health care or professional services rendered, or which should have been rendered, by a health care provider to a patient. The standard of skill and care required of every health care provider in rendering professional services or health care to a patient shall be that degree of skill and care ordinarily employed in the same or similar field of medicine as defendant, and the use of reasonable care and diligence [18 Del. C. 6801(7)].

Medical negligence, as detailed in the Delaware statute, speaks clearly to a refusal or failure of those responsible to provide food, shelter, health care, or protection for a vulnerable individual or group of individuals (Davidson, 2004; Ziminski & Phillips, 2011).

The Pennsylvania Supreme Court defines medical malpractice as "the unwarranted departure from generally accepted standards of medical practice resulting in injury to a patient, including all liability-producing conduct arising from the rendition of professional medical services" (*Toogood v Rogal,* 824 A2d 1140, 1145 [Pa. 2003]). Medical negligence is one of the elements of malpractice, commencing when a health care provider has acted below the standard of care in which other similarly situated professionals would act, injuring a patient as a result (18 Del. C. 6801[7]).

Malpractice may be interpreted as broader than negligence; malpractice incorporates:

negligence, intentional misconduct, breaches of contract guaranteeing a specific therapeutic result, divulgence of confidential information, unauthorized postmortem procedures, failures to prevent injuries to certain nonpatients, and defamation [Weld & Bibb, 2009, p. 4].

A definition of negligence is the "failure to use such care as a reasonably prudent and careful person would use under similar circumstances" (Joint Commission, n.d.). Negligence also involves a refusal or failure to fulfill any part of a person's obligations to a patient and can be either intentional or unintentional on the part of the one providing care. Additionally, a care provider's failure to maintain a patient's personal hygiene or failure to provide physical aids, including dentures, glasses, canes, and walkers fall under the category of negligence and neglect (Rosen et al., 2018).

Literature

Reader and Gillespie (2013) conducted the first systematic review of literature located on the nature, frequency, and causes of patient neglect in health care institutions.

The authors researched the body of literature, which is still poorly understood, in this heightened area of public concern across Europe and North America. Their research is the first to differentiate patient neglect as a distinct entity removed from issues of patient safety topics, including medical error.

A variety of databases (PubMed, Science Direct, and Medline) were searched to identify research studies investigating patient neglect (Reader & Gillespie, 2013). Ten articles and four government reports met author criteria for inclusion, each containing primary data relating to the occurrence or causes of neglect in patients. Qualitative and quantitative extraction of data captured: (1) the definition of neglect; (2) the behaviors that were connected to neglect; (3) frequency of neglect; and (4) causes of neglect.

Results (Reader & Gillespie, 2013) revealed two types of patient neglect. First identified is procedural neglect, which focuses on the failures of health care staff to achieve "objective standards of care" (p. 1). The second type of neglect pertains to caring neglect, which was identified as staff behaviors that convey to patients and other observers the impression that staff do not care. Perceived frequency of behaviors considered neglectful were determined to be dependent on the observer. Health care staff were less likely to report neglect than patients and family members; however, nurses reported negligent acts of other nurses more frequently than on their own behaviors. Causes of patient neglect were often attributed to institutional or organizational factors (e.g., high workloads constraining the behaviors of health care staff, and burnout), and the patient-caregiver relationship.

Reader and Gillespie's (2013) systematic review of literature on patient neglect in health care institutions led to the authors' development of a conceptual model to assist in identifying and understanding two specific types of neglect occurring in the institutional setting. *Procedural neglect* refers to care that falls short of the nurse or health care professional meeting objective standards that are observable. Regulations and protocols fall within this category. Examples include failure of a nurse to clean a patient after an episode of incontinence or failure to feed and/or provide water to an incapacitated patient. Procedural neglect involves a violation of an institutional standard or procedure and does not include the perceptions of patients and family. Behaviors of staff can be measured objectively.

Caring neglect includes behaviors that fall into a category that typically falls below the radar, because these behaviors are not directed by specific procedures or objectified using metrics. The behaviors are, however, integral to the quality of patient care and are considered very important to family members (e.g., ignoring a request for patient glasses, dismissing a request to return to bed after sitting in a wheelchair for an extended period). The essential difference here is that procedural neglect is evaluated from an institutional perspective, while caring neglect is evaluated from a patient perspective. The researchers (Reader & Gillespie, 2013) commented that it is crucial for health care professionals to understand that the manifestation of caring neglect may ultimately lead to procedural neglect. Patient outcomes could be improved through the vigilance of nurses, supervisors, and administrators to assess the clinical setting for signs of caring neglect and take steps to mitigate any incidents immediately.

Reader and Gillespie's Conceptual Model of Patient Neglect (2013) can be further explained as additional components of the model are identified and integrated into the model. Antecedents to patient neglect include distal cause factors (underlying problems, e.g., poor management; organizational culture) and proximal causal factors (aspects of the working environment, e.g., high workloads; staff shortages). These sub-constructs directly contribute to patient neglect and its two constructs, procedural neglect (care behavior falling short of objectives and standards of good care) and caring neglect (care belief that leads to the perception that staff is uncaring). Outcomes include: (1) widespread physical and emotional harm that are a result of a systematic presence of procedural and caring neglect; (2) localized physical and emotional patient harm; and (3) emotional patient harm (e.g., harm to a single patient or event as a result of procedural and caring neglect).

Recommendations for analyzing patient neglect (Reader & Gillespie, 2013) included incorporating a social psychology–based conceptual model of patient neglect (explained above) into the institutional setting to detail the nature and occurrence of patient neglect. According to the researchers, adapting the model into institutional settings would assist in the clarification of:

- differences between patients and health care staff in how they perceive neglect
- the association with patient neglect and health outcomes
- the relative importance of system and organizational factors in causing neglect
- the design of interventions and health policy to reduce patient neglect [p. 1].

To evaluate programs or strategies aimed at preventing or reducing abuse in persons 60 years and over, Baker et al. (2016) conducted a systematic review. They asserted that abuse of older persons was not often reported. Elder abuse included physical, psychological, or sexual abuse, neglect, and/or financial exploitation. The researchers addressed education on elder abuse, programs to reduce factors affecting abuse, policies, legislation, programs to detect the rate of abuse, programs for victims of elder abuse, and programs to rehabilitate perpetrators. They appraised seven studies for method, intervention type, setting, target audience, and intervention components and intensity. They analyzed studies in which patients or caregivers were abusers and who were harmed by persons they knew well, such as a relative or friend, or by a professional caregiver. Results were inconclusive, limited due to the quality of studies.

Harm was associated with limited training, inadequate supervision, and resource challenges. Older persons were distressed by abusive situations (Baker et al., 2016). Furthermore, the outcomes of abuse, including neglect, might result in premature resident mortality. Both educational programs and programs to reduce factors that might decrease elder abuse were described. The researchers suggested that trained groups of caregivers may have lower rates of abusive behavior. More research is needed to recognize the potential for elder abuse, to increase caregivers' awareness and attitudes toward abuse, to increase detection of abuse, and to improve knowledge and skill among health care professionals and to direct care providers when providing care to patients. The researchers mentioned that the impact of educational programs for caregivers on reducing abuse events was beginning to be recognized in studies.

Kolanowski et al. (2017) conducted a scoping review on behavioral and psychological symptoms of dementia (BPSD). They aimed to identify patient, caregiver, and environmental determinants of five BPSD: aggression, agitation, apathy, depression, and psychosis. They noted that BPSD was linked with declining function, risk for physical abuse, poor quality of life, caregiver burden, and one-third of the cost of dementia-related care. The researchers used the theoretical framework of Kales et al. (2015) to orient their question. The chief constructs of Kales et al.'s framework, depicted as a cycle, are: Neurogeneration associated with dementia→Increased vulnerability to stressors→Behavioral and psychological symptoms of dementia (BPSD)→Patient factors→Caregiver factors→Environmental factors. Citations included samples of adults 55 years or older, with dementia and BPSD, residing in any setting, and a dementia diagnosis using a standard, valid approach. A research librarian managed the search process. A total of 692 articles were eligible for methodological review and appraisal of quality and risk of bias. Random selection of articles resulted in 168 receiving full review; 56 high quality/low-bias articles were summarized in the narrative report.

Aggression was a persistent behavior and, if left untreated, increased caregiver burden and promoted a cycle of reoccurring aggression (Kolanowski et al., 2017). Determinants of agitation were younger age, male gender, type of dementia, dementia severity, premorbid personality traits, presence of pain, and boredom. An intervention balancing arousal states and individualized sensory stimulation reduced agitation in older adults with dementia. Also, appropriate amounts of sensory stimulation and music reduced agitation. Communication episodes between caregiver and care recipient were also associated with less agitation. Apathy was related to severe cognitive impairment in dementia. Additionally, specific cognitive abilities were linked with depressive symptoms. The researchers asserted the need of health and human service professionals and other caregivers to recognize that BPSD might be triggered by modifiable environmental factors. Perhaps assisting nursing staff who provide basic nursing interventions to persons with dementia and other residents could benefit from periodic educational sessions. The complexity of causes and management of BPSD discussed in in-service programs might help nursing staff to be open to using tailored approaches for patients whose behavior manifests aggression, agitation, apathy, and psychotic symptoms. Reducing these symptoms as a result of tailored interventions may result in less alarming episodes and reduced caregiver burden.

Rosen et al.'s (2018) research into elder abuse and neglect in the emergency department (ED) revealed that neglect and negligence of patients was common and "may have serious medical and social consequences but are infrequently identified" (p. 1). The authors espoused that an ED visit represented a unique opportunity for health care providers to identify potential abuse and initiate intervention; however, these occasions are usually missed. ED providers should be concerned about elder abuse and neglect and are urged to document their findings in detail. ED interventions for confirmed or suspected elder abuse or neglect include treatment of acute medical problems, trauma, and psychological issues; safeguarding patient safety; and reporting incidents to the authorities. These protocols and interventions can be applied across all clinical settings and to all health care professionals.

Case Examples

New York City officials (Hartocollis, 2009) determined that neglect and a subsequent cover-up by hospital staff was the cause of death for a Jamaican immigrant woman who sought treatment at a city-run, psychiatric emergency room in Brooklyn. Investigators concluded that hospital staff failed to render basic medical care to the patient who had a psychiatric history. After the patient died on the floor of the waiting room while awaiting treatment, staff attempted to cover up their negligence.

A formal report followed the case investigation, indicating a systematic failure to provide appropriate and timely care to the patient (Hartocollis, 2009). Death was attributed to a blood clot, causing the patient collapse on the waiting room floor, while staff did nothing to assist her. Additionally, the report revealed that patients in the waiting room were not routinely observed for suicidal behavior and were frequently subdued with drugs and restraints. Staff were also cognizant that patients were being abused by other patients as they awaited care.

According to the investigative report (Hartocollis, 2009), continuity of care was absent over four medical shifts. The victim was never examined, even though a physician ordered an electrocardiogram and blood work that were never done. Additionally, the charge nurse made three false entries in the medical record, stating that 45 minutes prior to the patient expiring, she observed the patient to be in normal condition, which was ultimately proven to be false.

This sentinel event prompted the hospital to launch a series of institutional reforms, along with a court mandated $2-million settlement to the family. The 58-page report released by the Department of Justice determined that the charge nurse falsified her testimony when the victim was in full view of other patients in the waiting room (Hartocollis, 2009).

Another case involving nursing staff negligence (Brent, 2018) ultimately led to the death of a 71-year-old man. He was transferred from an acute care facility to a rehabilitation center after undergoing bypass surgery and developing subsequent complications from colonized MRSA. The patient's status improved during hospitalization, although he required the placement of a feeding tube for nutrition. He was transferred after 81 days of acute care to the rehabilitation facility. His status improved initially during the first 25 days of treatment, with documented improvement in strength and mobility. The patient also developed a good relationship with staff. After this initial period of care, the patient's condition deteriorated quickly and he was transported from the rehabilitation facility to an emergency department (ED), where he died less than 24 hours later. Multi-stage organ failure and sepsis were causes of death listed on the death certificate.

A liability lawsuit (Brent, 2018) was subsequently filed against the rehabilitation center by the patient's family. The lawsuit alleged that the patient developed two, stage three (necrotic) pressure injuries when at the facility, a result of substandard perineal care and failure to reposition him throughout the day. The patient did not receive adequate nourishment nor ordered medications, and had no monitoring of temperature or intake and output while on diuretics. It was also determined that there was insufficient documentation and fabrication of the medical record, along with failure to clean the patient's room.

The trial court ruled in favor of the family, focusing on the rehabilitation center and nursing staff's negligence, which were determined to be the cause of death (Brent, 2018). Issues involving the nurses' failure to provide an overall standard of care to the patient (i.e., failure to monitor and properly chart intake and output of a patient who was ordered Lasix [diuretic drug], dehydrated, and poorly nourished) added to the legitimacy of the case. The patient was sent to the ED, where no mention of the pressure injuries appeared on the accompanying medical record from the rehabilitation facility. Family members also stated that the patient was left lying in his feces after ringing the call bell, with no response from staff.

On appeal by the nursing home, the appellate court held that the evidence and inferences made at the trial level fully supported the jury's verdict in favor of the patient's family (*HCRA of Texas, Inc. d/b/a Heartland Health Center-Bedford v. Margarie Fay Johnston et. al.*, No. 2–03–321-CV Court of Appeals of Texas, Fort Worth, November 3, 2005). Brent (2018) noted that the court determined that, although the skin lesions were not mentioned in the rehabilitation center's record, it did not negate their existence. More so, it was established that a considerable degree of deliberate indifference was evident in the staff at the rehabilitation facility regarding patient rights. The staff did not demonstrate awareness or acknowledgment of the patient's severe risk for serious harm.

Other members of the health care delivery team (i.e., administrators and physicians) also failed to provide appropriate supervision of staff and failed to intervene on behalf of the patient. Brent (2018) suggested that the director of nursing and the nursing staff, who were involved in the care of the patient, would most likely face disciplinary action by the state board of nursing, with unprofessional conduct cited as the basis for such action.

Malpractice actions against nurses are not normally reported unless the matter is addressed by the respective state's appellate court. However, inappropriate behavior or actions by nurses are often addressed through the state licensing agency's administrative review process. By way of example, In the Matter of Permanent Registered Nurse License Number 833714 Issued to BETTY KENT KNIGHT, Respondent, Before the Texas Board of Nursing, March 10, 2020, the Nursing Board revoked Knight's license for failure to perform and/or document certain required patient treatments. The Nursing Board concluded that Knight, while employed as a registered nurse at a dialysis center in Lufkin, Texas, failed to administer ordered medications, failed to perform certain line dressing changes, failed to assess post-treatment assessments, and failed to document these various procedures. The Nursing Board concluded that Knight's negligent actions were likely to injure the patients and concluded the permanent revocation of Knight's RN license was appropriate.

Institutional Culture: Care Challenges

In all health care settings, including long-term care facilities, the aforementioned exemplars demonstrate the importance for professional nurses to follow a strict standard of patient care in daily practice consistent with their duty to care and to avoid serious allegations of negligence, neglect, and patient harm. Recommendations to nurses working in challenging institutional care settings should focus upon efforts to create a professional work culture that ensures the provision of optimum patient care and outcomes. Recommendations (Brent, 2018) for improving clinical practice and considerations follow:

- Provide patient care that is ordered, meets your standards of practice and overall standards of care, and what is required by your legal and ethical duties.
- When a patient or family member rings or asks for help, respond as quickly as possible.
- Document all care provided accurately and completely.
- Never fabricate or falsify a patient's medical record.
- Testimony from staff members and physicians who care for a patient may easily support a finding of negligence that leads to a patient's death.
- If a director of nursing ensures that your nursing staff is providing the care required for all patients.

- Regularly review the *Code of Ethics for Nurses with Interpretive Statements* and incorporate the Code into your everyday practice [Brent, 2018, p. 1].

National initiatives are available to track patient and resident mistreatment, and it is the responsibility and mandate of health care institutions to report harmful incidents. For example, state long-term care ombudsman programs (LTCOP) are mandated by federal law to report data on abuse to the National Ombudsman Reporting System (National Long-Term Care Ombudsman Resource Center [NORS], n.d.). Facilities may underreport data. Along with various types of abuse, gross neglect is defined thusly:

> Gross neglect: Failure to protect a resident from harm or the failure to meet needs for essential medical care, nutrition, hydration, hygiene, clothing, basic activities of daily living or shelter, which results in a serious risk of compromised health and/or safety, relative to age, health status, and cultural norms [NORS Complaint Codes and Definitions, 2019, para. 5].

Sadly, long-term care institutions have been cited for abuse violations. By 2008, NORS accrued about 269,000 complaints. Percentages connected to elder mistreatment included:

Failure to respond to request for assistance (6.9 percent)
Injury of unknown origin, falls, improper handling (3.2 percent)
Staff attitudes related to dignity or respect (4.4 percent)
Symptoms unattended (2.6percent)
Personal property lost, stolen, used by others, destroyed, withheld (2.2 percent)
Staff unresponsive, unavailable (2 percent)
Physical abuse (1.8 percent)
Resident-to-resident abuse (1.3 percent)
Verbal/mental abuse (1.4 percent)
Gross (i.e., willful) neglect (0.9 percent) [Halphen & Dyer, 2019, para. 4].

Tracking these data helps federal and state agencies to monitor patients' and residents' risk of harm and threatened safety.

Signs, Symptoms, and Assessment of Negligence and Neglect

Signs and symptoms of negligence and neglect have been repeatedly linked to untreated health issues when nurses fail to satisfy basic patient needs and safety requirements (Bailey, 2017; Ziminski & Phillips, 2011). Untreated health issues, malnutrition, unsanitary living conditions (including hospitals and other institutional settings), dehydration, inadequate protection of patient safety, and failure to maintain hygiene are all markers of neglect and negligence that place patients at great risk. Indecent exposure (i.e., failure to adequately clothe a patient) is also an indicator of negligence (Rosen et al., 2018).

The more overt signs and symptoms of negligence (e.g., pressure injuries resulting from failure to turn patients; severe excoriation of the perineum from a patient sitting in feces) are easier to identify and mitigate than those that are more clandestine (e.g., lack of nutritional support and water; isolation; psychological abuse). Geriatric patients residing in long-term care facilities are placed at particular risk of suffering the consequences of negligence and neglect by virtue of their marginalized health status and increased vulnerability (Bailey, 2017; Hess, 2011; Iannuzzi, 2015).

Vulnerability (Bailey & Dougherty, 2013) includes health disparities in populations that are often a result of poor resources or increased exposure to risk. Vulnerable groups, especially the poor, the elderly, the sick and dying, and those with mental illness, are just a few of the marginalized groups of individuals known to have high incidences of morbidity, mortality, and premature death. It is important for nurses to factor in vulnerability and risk in the populations they care for and in the settings in which care is delivered.

When conducting physical assessments of patients in any clinical setting, it is crucial for nurses and health care professionals to incorporate an evaluation to rule out negligence and neglect, based on patient risk factors and behavioral indicators, and promptly take appropriate measures to eliminate intentional or unintentional acts of suffering.

As patient advocates, nurses are responsible to pursue their suspicions of neglect and negligence. To further assess negligence and other types of mistreatment, nurses should interview patients or residents alone so they can answer directly about abuse, neglect, or exploitation. They might ask the following questions to assess patients' or residents' risk:

1. Has anyone at home ever hurt you?
2. Has anyone ever touched you without your consent?
3. Has anyone taken anything that was yours without asking?
4. Has anyone ever scolded or threatened you?
5. Have you signed any documents that you didn't understand?
6. Are you afraid of anyone at home?
7. Are you alone a lot of the time?
8. Has anyone failed to help you take care of yourself when you needed help?

[Halphen & Dyer, 2019, para. 7]

Another opportunity to assess nurses' suspicions of patient mistreatment is the administration of the Brief Abuse Screen for the Elderly (BASE) (Reis & Nahmiash, 1998). The BASE is a clinician, self-administered instrument to evaluate abuse of older patients. Four items are included. Item formats are scaled *Yes, No* and 1 = *No, not at all*; 2 = *No, only slightly, doubtful*; 3 = *Possibly, somewhat*; 4 = *Probably, quite likely*; and 5 = *Yes, definitely*. Comments are invited and a checklist is provided for type of abuse (physical; psychosocial; financial; neglect [includes passive and active]). The instrument can be self-administered by trained nurses, nurse practitioners, and nurse managers to document their concerns of elder mistreatment. Reporting suspicions of patient or resident harm is the next step.

Ethical and Legal Implications

Ethical and legal implications of patient care, for nurses and health care professionals, require strict adherence to the same standards of best practices, regardless of whether nurses are practicing in hospitals, long-term care agencies, outpatient settings, or other locations. Provision of health care services requires strict adherence to laws promulgated for the general public (Bailey, 2017; Ziminski & Phillips, 2011). Clearly, there is no justification for negligence, neglect, or abuse by health care professionals.

The ANA's *Code of Ethics for Nurses with Interpretive Statements* (2015) serves as an important guide for nurses as they deliver care and carry out nursing responsibilities. Nurses must adhere to the Code as they carry out their nursing responsibilities and do so by providing quality patient care and honoring the ethical obligations set forth by the profession. Furthermore, adhering to and incorporating the four ethical principles (respect for autonomy, nonmaleficence, beneficence, and distributive justice) into daily nursing practice (Stanhope & Lancaster, 2014) are central to decreasing the incidence of negligence and neglect in the clinical setting across any areas of practice.

The ANA Code of Ethics (2015) upheld the fundamental principles of the dignity, value, and individuality of all persons regardless of economic situation, personal characteristics, or health problems. This declarative statement serves as the cornerstone for all nursing practice where nurses are duty-bound to care for people compassionately and respectfully. Part of the ethical code for nurses that is incontrovertible is predicated on protecting patients from harm and abuse, thus reducing the incidence of harmful or injurious acts to those cared for (ANA, 2015). This ethical doctrine articulated by the ANA supports appropriate measures and practices to safeguard vulnerable clients, through integration of these measures into daily practice by all nurses. The ANA (2015) continued to identify respect for persons as a core ethical principle that includes the right to autonomy, which is considered an essential element of nursing practice.

All health professionals are duty-bound in adhering to specific obligations established by their specific discipline and scope of practice. The obligations are interpreted by a set of principles grounded in bioethics. This approach to understanding ethics within a nursing context is referred to as principlism, in which four important principles are included: respect for autonomy, nonmaleficence, beneficence, and distributive justice (Stanhope & Lancaster, 2014). Application of the deontological ethics decision process is critical for nurses to incorporate into daily practice and can serve as a useful tool to mitigate incidents of negligence and neglect. The process comprises four steps:

1. Determine the moral rules (e.g., tell the truth) that serve as standards by which individuals can perform their moral obligations.

2. Examine personal motives for proposed actions to ensure that they are based on good intentions in accord with moral rules.

3. Determine whether the proposed actions can be generalized so that all persons in similar situations are treated similarly.

4. Select the action that treats persons as ends in themselves and never as mere means to the ends of others [Stanhope & Lancaster, 2014, p. 56].

Nurses working in hospitals, other institutional settings, and homes need to develop a keen awareness for state and local laws and institutional policies intended to protect patients from undue harm. Albeit not all facilities have specific policies in place for staff to follow; therefore, it is crucial for nurses to take a proactive stance to serve as advocates in the development of task forces to draft, implement, and operationalize these working documents within the institutional milieu. This strategy could assist in reducing harmful injustices to vulnerable patients as nurses increase their awareness in identifying and in reporting negligent acts.

A corollary to these measures includes affording all nurses (staff nurses, nurse managers, administrators, and nursing assistants) an opportunity to access topic-related educational materials for professional development. These essential tools could assist nurses in daily practice and be useful as they begin conversations with risk managers, social workers, and other members of the interprofessional health care team on the topics of neglect and negligence (Hess, 2011; Pehale, 2010). Personal accountability is also a crucial factor for all nurses to consider in the protection of patients from acts of negligence, neglect, and abuse (Hess).

The daily professional life of the nurse entails multiple patient interactions that are placed within a myriad of cultural and social contexts (Wolf, 2014). During an initial interaction with a patient, it is important to mention that nurses meet individuals who need care for the first time and most often are strangers. Wolf articulated that "nurses typically answer the call to care by greeting their patients." Their greeting begins a relationship initiated during a meeting that as interaction begins to develop, a connection between the nurse and patient unfolds.

It is imperative that nurses pay particular attention to the ethical principle of beneficence when considering patients' vulnerability. The principle requires that nurses do good and prevent undue harm to patients. Although nurses are limited by time, place, and talent in the "amount of good that can be done" (Stanhope & Lancaster, p. 639), nurses have an obligation to carry out actions that do not place "an undue burden" on the provider of care (p. 639). Nurses and other health care professionals have a clear obligation to honor the principle of beneficence in patient care.

Summary

Nurses are obligated by their profession to identify and report all acts of abuse. However, nurses should report acts of negligence and neglect and, when in doubt, discuss suspected cases of patient harm with nurse managers or administrators (Hess, 2011). Ethical principles (respect for autonomy, nonmaleficence, beneficence, and distributive justice) serve as a moral compass to guide nurses as they encounter more subtle but harmful acts against patients.

Nurses must be equally aware of specific indicators, interventions, and reporting mechanisms required by law and individual state nurse practice acts enacted to reduce the incidence of neglect and negligence and thwart harmful acts against patients. Developing a foundational understanding and appreciation for theoretical elements and principles related to negligence and neglect warrants dissemination of pertinent information to all nurses and interprofessional team members to decrease negative patient outcomes (Hess, 2011). Empowering staff through continuing education and pursuing a proactive stance to educate vulnerable and at-risk patients (including the general public) about the signs and symptoms of negligence and neglect can "avert [these] more subtle forms of abuse and prevent even more serious events among fragile populations" (Bailey, 2017, p. 8).

Negligence, particularly related to the aging population, is commonplace across many areas of practice in institutional settings and elsewhere; however, identification of negligence is more obscure than more visible injuries and nurses are not mandated by law to report such cases compared to abuse where reporting requirements exist (Hess, 2011). Unfortunately, negligence and abuse comprise harmful acts that collectively present more serious medical and social consequences as they relate to the assessment of patients in EDs or other settings of professional practice (Rosen et al., 2018). ED assessment, and similarly, assessment of patients across all other practice settings, should include observing the patient-caregiver interaction, obtaining a comprehensive medical history, and including a head-to-toe physical examination. Formal screening protocols may also be useful.

Providers concerned about elder abuse or neglect need to document pertinent findings in detail. Interventions for suspected or confirmed elder abuse or neglect include evidence-based treatment of acute medical, traumatic, and psychological problems so that patient safety is promoted. It is also important for nurses to report to administrators for immediate action any findings of neglect when any employee is seen inflicting harm or to authorities or agencies dealing with elder abuse and neglect outside of the institutional milieu (Hess, 2011; NAPSA, 2019; Rosen et al., 2018).

Other strategies that would decrease negligence and neglect in vulnerable patients look to nurses and patient care technologists (PCTs [or nursing assistants or nurses' aides]) or nursing assistants as they deliver bedside care, since they spend more face-to-face contact with patients, caregivers, and other family members than other members of the health care delivery team. Nurses and PCTs are in a unique position to observe interactions between patients and their caregivers that may raise red flags requiring further investigation. Additionally, nurses and PCTs provide basic hygiene to geriatric patients, including diaper changes. Careful assessment during routine care may further assist in the identification of otherwise missed physical findings that are suspicious and need further investigation by supervisory staff and administrators (Rosen et al., 2018).

Criminal justice systems are taking a more serious look at allegations of negligence and neglect of patients by nurses and health care workers around the globe. New laws to alleviate these harmful acts toward patients are being enacted and, as a result, are being reported in the literature. Conducting background checks on applicants seeking employment is another measure that can be used to identify nurses and staff members who have prior criminal records. Therefore, to ensure patient safety, improve health outcomes and circumvent harmful acts toward patients, Griffith (2015) stated that it is critical for those entrusted with the care of vulnerable clients to "demonstrate that they have discharged their duty of care to their patients by acting with probity, applying the standards of care required by the law and professional regulator[s], and ensuring their records accurately reflect their involvement with patients" (p. 2).

Risk managers, quality improvement leaders, and administrators of long-term care nurses typically understand legislation for long-term care settings (Rose, 2018). They monitor complaints, generated from reasonable suspicions, that abuse may have occurred. They next prepare reports even when evidence in inconclusive. Institutional leaders encourage employees to use incident reporting systems. However, employees may fear retaliation when acting as whistleblowers.

Negligence and neglect of patients by nursing staff can be reconceptualized as missed nursing care. However, most of the studies on missed nursing care have been implemented in acute care settings (Kalisch et al., 2013). Kalisch (2006) brought attention to missed or incomplete nursing care and described its many aspects: neglected ambulation turning, feeding, patient education, discharge planning, emotional support, hygiene, fluid balance documentation, and surveillance.

Of concern is that patient neglect may often represent failure to perform basic nursing care. Missed nursing care often is basic nursing care. However, basic nursing care lacks research evidence (Cleary-Holdforth, 2019; Zwakhalen et al., 2018). Although research on missed nursing care is increasing and studies on negligent nursing care are continuing, more attention is needed on programs addressing missed nursing care, such as teamwork development among health care providers (Joint Commission, 2005). Training interventions used are simulation, crew resource management, and other approaches. Checklists, goal sheets, and case analysis are some of the tools used to improve teamwork. An example of a self-managed work team approach of nurse aide staff members was described by Yeatts et al. (2004) in Texas nursing homes. The study's initial aims were reducing turnover and absenteeism, improving resident satisfaction, and increasing employee empowerment. Administrator participation and commitment to the success of the team were essential as were manager supports and weekly meetings. Continuing attention to team-based participative-management strategies are needed, such as described in this example. Organizations need to continue to increase interdisciplinary training.

Resources are available to assist administrators in long-term care institutions and other health care agencies to increase the knowledge of the health care team and to alert them to information on elder abuse and neglect. For example, the Center of Excellence on Elder Abuse & Neglect, University of California, Irvine, School of Medicine (2019) has a website to promote excellence in care. Information organized by professional discipline is available, and includes health care professions, judicial, law enforcement, legal, and other links.

Strategies

See Table 9 for strategies to prevent neglect and negligence of patients.

Table 9. Strategies to Prevent Neglect and Negligence of Patients

Strategies to Effect Change	Evidence-Based Citations
Provide periodic training program about awareness and attitudes toward abuse, detection of abuse, and skills to prevent patient escalation	Baker et al. (2016) Kolanowski et al. (2017)
Provide sensory stimulation, including music, to reduce agitation in older adults with dementia	Kolanowski et al. (2017)
Respond as quickly as possible when a patient or family member rings a bell or asks for help	Brent (2018)
Daily inspect (head-to-toe) all parts of patients' bodies	Bailey (2017) Hess (2011) Iannuzzi (2015)
Privately pose questions to patients and residents about abuse, neglect, or exploitation	Halphen & Dyer (2019)
Report suspicions of abuse or neglect to administrators and agencies for immediate action	Hess (2011) NAPSA (2019)

Conclusion

This chapter investigated neglect and negligence in clinical settings and analyzed how uncaring acts of nurses and other health care staff negatively impact patient outcomes. Review of the literature also corroborated the pervasiveness of negligence and neglect in society as represented by vulnerable individuals living in the community who are cared for by health care professionals, families, and friends.

Hope (2018) discussed negligence within the context of professional nursing and noted that the impact of negligence within the profession has markedly increased, particularly as nursing continues to evolve as a "specialized and independent occupation" (p. 1). Acts of negligence and neglect tend to be more obscure and are more difficult to identify than more overt forms of abuse. Identification, reporting, and reduction of abusive acts are called for in the prevention of more serious harm caused by nurses who cross into this harmful realm of practice.

Nursing as a caring and time-honored profession can fall short of providing optimum care when nurses fail to incorporate ethical and moral principles into daily practice. Historically, the roots of the nursing profession have been predicated upon upholding and adhering to the ethical principles and tenets set forth in the Nightingale Pledge created by Lystra Gretter in 1893 (Stanhope & Lancaster, 2014). The Nightingale Pledge and its statement of ethics and principles serves as a celebrated reminder for all professional nurses, not only in the United States but across the globe, to do no harm to those entrusted in their care.

Discussion Questions

1. What is meant by negligence and neglect? Describe how these safety threats lead to poor patient care.

2. Describe behaviors of nurses and staff members that may indicate negligence and neglect of patients.

3. Discuss the ethical obligations of nurses for patients in daily practice, considering how adhering to ethical standards improves patient outcomes.

4. Analyze the differing viewpoints that health care staff and patients may have regarding neglect.

5. Examine the serious nature of legal sanctions in the literature in relation to how acts of negligence and neglect impact nurse practice.

AUTHOR SELECTIONS

Freeman, I.C., & Hennen, C. (2017). *Creating an Abuse Prevention Culture in Residential Long-term Care Vital Practices to Support Enhance Legal Compliance* [PowerPoint]. https://theconsumervoice.org/uploads/files/events/Consumer_Voice_2017_Abuse_Prevention.PowerPoint.pdf.

Mazzola, D. (2010). *I'm a person too* [Poem]. Family Friend Poems. https://www.familyfriendpoems.com/poem/im-a-person-too.

REFERENCES

American Nurses Association. (2015). Code of ethics for nurses with interpretive statements. https://www.nursingworld.org/practice-policy/nursing-excellence/ethics/code-of-ethics-for-nurses/.

Angel, S., & Vatne, S. (2017). Vulnerability in patients and nurses and the mutual vulnerability in the patient-nurse relationship. Journal of Clinical Nursing, 26(9–10), 1428–1437. doi:10.1111/jocn.13583.

Bailey, D.N. (2017). Abuse, negligence, and missed nursing care: Nursing considerations. PADONA Journal, 29(1), 6–12.

Bailey, D.N., & Dougherty, A. (2013). A nurse-led wellness program for migrant backstretch workers. Nursing Forum, 49(1), 1–9.

Baker, P.R., Francis, D.P., Hairi, N.N., Othman, S., & Choo, W.Y. (2016). Interventions for preventing abuse of older people. *Cochrane Database of Systematic Reviews*, Issue 8. Article CD010321. doi: 10.1002/1465 1858.CD010321.pub2.

Brent, N.J. (2018, March 1). *Nursing staff's professional negligence causes death of a patient: Avoiding liability bulletin, ethics, nursing, patient care*. CPH & Associates. https://www.cphins.com/nursing-staffs-professional-negligence-causes-death-of-patient/.

Center of Excellence on Elder Abuse & Neglect, University of California, Irving, School of Medicine. (n.d.). *Information by Professional Discipline*. http://www.centeronelderabuse.org/Information_By_Professional_Discipline.asp.

Chen, P., McKenna, C., Kutlik, A.M., & Frisina, P.G. (2013). Interdisciplinary communication in inpatient rehabilitation facility: Evidence of under-documentation of spatial neglect after stroke. *Disability and Rehabilitation, 35*(12), 1033–1038. doi: 10.3109/09638288.2012.717585.

Cleary-Holdforth, J. (2019). Missed nursing care: A symptom of missing evidence. *Worldview on Evidence-Based Nursing, 16*(2), 88–91.

Griffith, R. (2015). Patient protection from ill-treatment and willful neglect. British Journal of Nursing, 24(11). https://doi.org/10.12968/bjon.201.24.11.600.

Halldorsdottir, S. (1991). Five basic modes of being with another. In D. Gaut, & M.M. Leininger (Eds.), *Caring: The compassionate healer* (pp. 37–49). National League for Nursing Press.

Halphen, J.M., & Dyer, C.B. (2019, July). Elder mistreatment: Abuse, neglect, and financial exploitation. *UpToDate.* https://www.uptodate.com/contents/elder-mistreatment-abuse-neglect-and-financial-exploitation?search=elder%20mistreatment&source=search_result&selectedTitle=1~16&usage_type=default&display_rank=1.

Hartocollis, A. (2009, June 20). City finds neglect and cover-up in patients' death. *The New York Times.* http://nytimes.com/2009/06/20nyregion/20hospital.html?pagewanted=print.

Hess, S. (2011). The role of health care providers in recognizing and reporting elder abuse. *Journal of Gerontological Nursing, 37,* 28–34.

Hope, I. (2018, January 23). Nursing negligence and its impact in the nursing profession. *RN Speak.* https://www.rnspeak.com/nursing-negligence-and-its-impact-in-the-nursing-profession/

Iannuzzi, K. (2015). *Nursing home elder abuse and neglect: A preliminary guide for risk prevention and patient advocacy* [Unpublished Capstone Project, Utica College].

Joint Commission. (2002). *Negligence definition.* https://www.google.com/search?q=joint+commission+definition+negligence&rlz=1C1EJFA_enUS791US791&oq=joint+commission+definition+negligence&aqs=chrome.0.69i59l2j0.9882j0j4&sourceid=chrome&ie=UTF-8.

Joint Commission. (2005). *Health care at the crossroads: Strategies for improving the medical liability system and preventing patient injury.* https://www.jointcommission.org/-/media/deprecated-unorganized/imported-assets/tjc/system-folders/topics-library/medical_liabilitypdf.pdf?db=web&hash=B7E4D12D38C7A469FCEE06073E5D2C64.

Kalisch, B.J. (2006). Missed nursing care: A qualitative study. *Journal of Nursing Care Quality, 21,* 306–313. https://doi.org/10.1097/00001786-200610000-00006.

Kalisch, B.J., Xie, B., & Ronis, D.L. (2013). Train-the-trainer to increase nursing teamwork and decrease missed nursing care in acute care patient units. *Nursing Research, 62*(6), 405–413. doi: 10.1097/NNR.0b013e3182a7a15d.

Kolanowski, A., Boltz, M., Galik, E., Gitlin, L.N., Kales, H.C., Resnick, B., Van Haitsma, S.S., Knehans, A., Sutterlin, J.E., Sefcik, J.S., Wen, L., Petrovsky, D.V., Massimo, L., Gilmore-Bykovsky, A., MacAndrew, M., Brewster, G., Nalls, V., Jao, Y-L., J. & Scerpella, D. (2017). Determinants of behavioral and psychological symptoms of dementia: A scoping review of the evidence. *Nursing Outlook, 65,* 515–529. http://dx.doi.org/10.1016/j.outlook.2017.06.006.

McAlpine, C.H. (2008). Elder abuse and neglect. *Age and Ageing, 27,* 132–133. doi: 10.1093/ageing/afr008.

National Adult Protective Services Association. (2019). *What is neglect?* https://www.napsa-now.org/get-informed/what-is-neglect/.

National Long-Term Care Ombudsman Resource Center. (n.d.). National Ombudsman Reporting System (NORS). https://ltcombudsman.org/omb_support/nors.

National Long-Term Care Ombudsman Resource Center. (2019, October 1). *National Ombudsman Reporting System (NORS) Complaint Codes and Definitions.* https://ltcombudsman.org/uploads/files/support/NORS_Codes_and_Definitions.pdf.

Penhale, B. (2010). Responding and intervening in elder abuse and neglect. *Ageing International, 35,* 235–252. doi: 10.1007/s12126-010-9065-0.

Pennsylvania Older Adults Protective Services Act, 35 P.S. § 10225.101 et. seq. (1987).

Reader, T.W., & Gillespie, A. (2013). Patient neglect in healthcare institutions: A systematic review and conceptual model. *BMC Health Services Research, 13,* 156. doi: 10.1186/1472-6963-13-156.

Reis, M., & Nahmiash, D. (1998). Validation of the indicators of abuse (IOA) screen. *Gerontologist, 38*(4), 471–480. https://medicine.uiowa.edu/familymedicine/sites/medicine.uiowa.edu.familymedicine/files/wysiwyg_uploads/BASE_0.pdf.

Richards, M.J., & Stuart, R.L. (2018). Causes of infections in long-term care facilities: An overview. *UpToDate.* https://www.uptodate.com/contents/causes-of-infection-in-long-term-care-facilities-an-overview?search=uti%20long%20term%20care&source=search_result&selectedTitle=1~150&usage_type=default&display_rank=1.

Rose, V.L. (2018). Preventing abuse, neglect, and exploitation of residents in nursing homes. *Annals of Long-Term Care, 26*(3), 11–14. doi: 10.25270/altc.2018.06.00034.

Rosen, T., Stern, M.E., Elman, A., & Mulcare, M.R. (2018). Identifying and initiating intervention for elder abuse and neglect in the emergency department. *Clinics in Geriatric Medicine, 34*(3), 435–451. doi: 10.1016/j.cger.2018.04.00.

Social Security Act of 1935, 49 Stat. 620. [As Amended Through P.L. 115–123, Enacted February 09, 2018]. Subtitle B-Elder Justice. Sec. 2011. [42 U.S.C 1397j] Definitions.

Stanhope, M., & Lancaster, J. (2014). *Foundations of nursing in the community: Community oriented practice* (4th ed.). Mosby Elsevier.

Texas Board of Nursing, Eligibility and Disciplinary Committee. (2020, March 10). *Order of the Board. In the Matter of Permanent Registered Nurse License Number 833714 Issued to BETTY KENT KNIGHT, Respondent. Notice of Disciplinary Action 7/20.* https://www.bon.texas.gov/discipline_and_complaints_ disciplinary_action_072020.asp.

University of California Irvine, School of Medicine, Center of Excellence on Elder Abuse & Neglect. (2019). *Information by professional discipline.* http://www.centeronelderabuse.org/Information_By_ Professional_Discipline.asp.

Welch, L.C., Botelho, E.M., Joseph, J.J., & Tennstedt, S.L. (2012). A qualitative inquiry of patient-reported outcomes. *Nursing Research, 61*(4), 283–290. doi: 10.1097/NNR.0b013e318251d8f6.

Weld, K.K., & Bibb S.C.G. (2009). Concept analysis: Malpractice and modern-day nursing practice. *Nursing Forum, 44*(1), 2–9.

Wolf, Z.R. (2014). *Exploring rituals in nursing, Joining art and science.* Springer Publishing.

Yeatts, D.E.., Cready, C., Ray, B., DeWitt, A., & Queen, C. (2004). Self-managed work teams in nursing homes: Implementing and empowering nurse aide teams. *Gerontologist, 44*(2), 256–261.

Ziminski, C.E., & Phillips, L.R. (2011). The nursing role in reporting elder abuse: Specific examples and interventions. *Journal of Gerontological Nursing, 37*(11), **19–23.** https://doi.org/10.3928/00989134-20111010-01.

Zwakhalen, S.M., Hamers, J.P., Metzelthin, S.F., Ettema, R., Heinen, M., de Man-Van Ginkel, J.M., Vermeulen, H., Huisman-de Waal, G., & Schuurmans, M.J. (2018). Basic nursing care: The most provided, the least evidence based–A discussion paper. *Journal of Clinical Nursing, 27,* 2496–2505. doi: 10.1111/jocn.14296.

MULTIPLE-CHOICE QUESTIONS

1. **Which of the following descriptions is used for negligence?**

    A. Failing to attend to a person's health care needs: medical, hygienic, and nutritional

    B. Deserting the caregiving needs of an individual

    C. Causing emotional pain, distress, or anguish by belittling the needs of adults

    D. Refusal/failure to provide food, shelter, health care, or protection for vulnerable persons

2. **Which of the following are signs and symptoms of negligence and neglect?**

    A. Loss of weight and confusion

    B. Failure to maintain hygiene and dehydration

    C. Losing physical aids (e.g., dentures, canes) and replacing them

    D. Complaints of being cold and adjusting clothing and temperature

3. **Which of the following causes have been attributed to patient neglect in health care institutions, according to Reader and Gillespie?**

    A. Patient-caregiver relationship

    B. Marginal health states

    C. Complex care needs

    D. Failure to report problems

4. **Which of the following approaches should nurses take to address patient neglect or negligence?**

    A. Follow professional standards of care

    B. Know state and local laws

    C. Discuss problems with care teams

    D. Report all acts of negligence and neglect

CHAPTER 7

Physical Abuse of Patients

Zane Robinson Wolf, PhD, RN,
CNE, FCPP, ANEF, FAAN

Objectives

1. Describe factors given as causal explanations of physical abuse incidents that harm patients.
2. Examine behavioral patterns that might signal imminent incidents of physical abuse of patients.
3. Analyze examples of violence and abuse in different clinical settings.
4. Compare caring-based interventions and strategies aimed at eliminating physical abuse of patients.

Critical Incident

An 80-year-old man resided in an assisted living facility where most of his direct care was provided by nursing assistants. He had significant pain and vomited after being assaulted by a nursing assistant. For a total of two days, none of the staff noticed that the resident had bruises on his neck and chest. The resident received no pain medication. He died and his body was transported to a funeral home. The funeral director subsequently reported suspicions of abuse: a very large bruise on the man's body. A postmortem examination revealed evidence of assault: broken ribs, a punctured lung, and internal bleeding. The nursing assistant who was the perpetrator was charged with criminal homicide, aggravated assault, and neglect of care. She was convicted of third-degree murder, aggravated assault, and neglect of a care-dependent person. Two registered nurses and another nursing assistant were arraigned and pled guilty to neglect of a care-dependent person. The nurses failed to supervise and monitor the staff (Brent & Adams, Assoc., 2008).

Rosen et al. (2020) conducted a case control prospective study. They contended that health care providers did not often recognize elder abuse as a common threat to patients' well-being. The researchers examined successfully prosecuted physical abuse cases from an urban district attorney's office. Physical abuse victims 60 years of age and older with falls were matched with older persons having unintentional falls. Physical abuse victims had more bruising and maxillofacial, dental, and neck injuries than counterparts. The researchers noted that there were clinically identifiably injuries in abused persons.

Nurses and other health care providers might review older persons' injuries on entry to emergency units and on admission to hospitals and long-term care agencies to distinguish intentional versus unintentional injuries. They also need to periodically inspect the skin of vulnerable persons across the lifespan.

Background

The incident described above represents an extreme example of a crime that ended with the death of a resident. It brings attention to the need to examine the problem of physical abuse committed by nursing staff. Other examples of nurses who have physically abused patients are published. One involved a nurse who placed a medication in a restrained patient's mouth and covered her mouth with a cloth ("Nurse who verbally abused," 2014). A second example took place when a vagrant needed to be moved to another emergency unit location. A nurse pushed the patient into the corridor and poured the patient's urine onto his feet and shoes (Castledine, 2001). Patients had previously complained about the nurse's behavior. The nurse was convicted of physical abuse; incidents included different assaults on three patients that included slapping, kicking, or dragging a patient by the neck. Staff reported the behavior; however, prior to that, some staff had resigned their positions at the hospital due to the nurse's behavior and aggression directed toward them. Finally, this senior staff nurse lost his license due to incidents of repeated physical abuse (Castledine, 2003). His behavior finally caught the attention of supervisors and the state board of nursing.

Physical abuse is defined as intentional action by health care providers resulting in bodily injury to persons in their care. It is an intentional act of violence, including kicking, pinching, punching, shoving, and unwanted physical restraint (Barber, 2007). Persons frequently physically abused are individuals with disabilities, older persons, and pregnant women.

Physical abuse by employees is an acknowledged, serious problem in health care settings (Barber, 2007). Physical abuse is mediated by cultural norms and is an international phenomenon (Barber, 2007). It is more than employee misconduct. It may go unnoticed by health care staff, including supervisors and administrators of health care agencies. Frontline staff may not report violence due to fear of recrimination from staff with whom they work.

The primary aim of all health care providers is to relieve suffering. Therefore, when nursing staff harm patients by physical means they fail to provide caring interventions. Their actions are in direct conflict with the nursing goal of promoting the health and well-being of those cared for. Nursing staff that abuse patients fail to do what they morally should do: honor the person for whom they are responsible. The ethical principle of do no harm is violated when nurses and staff they supervise harm vulnerable patients or residents.

Institutional Culture: Care Challenges

However, it may be difficult to separate nursing care that is abusive from nursing care that poorly adapts to patients' or residents' needs (Skovdahl et al., 2003). For example, the need to bathe patients versus the pain caused by the activity confronts direct care providers (Wierucka & Goodridge, 1996). The challenge for health care providers and their leaders is to reflect on the nature of the harm identified and attempt to identify the intent of an employee in a nursing situation. Consistent with the Joint Commission's (TJC's, 2018) perspective noted in a *Sentinel Event Alert*, a culture of trust established in a health care institution helps employees report instances deemed hazardous to patient safety. Intention not to harm (beneficence) or to harm (maleficence) is central when analyzing the care provided.

Prior to an employee reporting an incident of physical abuse, leaders need to establish a culture of safety and to encourage reporting of hazardous situations as a performance expectation of employees. They must promote the psychological safety of staff in reporting (TJC, 2018). Equating an employee's intentional, harmful behavior with a hazardous condition requires an institutional reconceptualization of typical error-prone situations, such as medication errors, to include persons judged hazardous who harm patients or residents. They are obvious risks to patients' health and well-being. A system-wide safety net with an incident reporting system is essential. So, too, is leaders' recognition of potential threats to whistleblowers.

The context of a health care facility could affect staff behavior. Cultural and social environments might implicitly support aggressive staff behavior against patients or residents. Instead of blaming staff, the behavior of individuals being cared for who act out are blamed for incurring staff's negative responses. Attributing or justifying the cause of physical harm and inflicting pain to patients or residents to the social or health care context (Hirst, 2002) cannot continue. There is no place for intentional acts of physical violence against patients or residents.

Literature

The literature review on physical abuse of patients by staff revealed three examples of patients who have been abused. Various databases were accessed. Physical abuse against older persons, pregnant women, and psychiatric patients are examples that are explored next.

Older Persons

The vulnerability of older persons was examined in a literature review on elder abuse, and focused on injury, mistreatment, or neglect (Wierucka & Goodridge, 1996). The prevalence of elder abuse was reported at 40 per 1,000 in a survey. Acts of abuse were committed across different health care settings. The authors speculated that counts might be conservative estimates. Survey findings and other studies showed that staff witnessed abuse incidents. Whether they reported them or not was in question. The authors noted that facilities with more beds may have less abuse. They suggested that standardization of services to meet the needs of average patients could result in staff inflexibility, despite demands of residents requiring more complex care. Periodic educational offerings need to target the indicators and prevention of older person neglect.

The authors suggested that understanding resident expressions of frustration and language difficulties between staff and residents requires staff to intensify their efforts to identify residents' needs (Wierucka & Goodridge, 1996). Dependent, frail residents and aggressive individuals could be more at risk for abuse. They implied that residents of long-term care facilities, still connected to their communities and neighborhoods, contributed to a supportive institutional environment. They emphasized that nursing assistants' low pay, an indicator of value, was further complicated by the care burden of residents of long-term care facilities. Aspects of the care burden are resident aggression, discrimination, emotional exhaustion or burnout, risk for assault, and staff's need for education and support.

Wierucka and Goodridge (1996) recommended the establishment of positive relationships between registered nurses and nursing assistants as an abuse-reduction strategy. They advocated respect for nursing assistants and promotion of self-esteem through education on clinical and leadership concepts. Examples included conflict management, characteristics of abuse and abusing situations, and reporting mechanisms. Also, nursing administrators' monitoring of staff-resident ratios, acuity level, and tasks could recognize the contributions of nursing assistants and trigger recognition and promotion of their excellent performance. Overt appreciation of the value of their work, tangible support from administrators, and involvement in care planning might foster caring interventions and hopefully eliminate resident abuse.

Nursing assistants' stressors in the workplace were examined through self-reports of their conflict, aggression, and burnout (Goodridge et al., 1996). The study's rationale was the incidence of elder abuse and mistreatment in health care institutions. Because nursing assistants provide most of the direct care to residents of personal care homes and long-term care facilities, they experience multiple stressors resulting from some of the demands of basic nursing care. The physical and psychological needs of residents require nursing assistants to provide intensive physical and emotional care.

The researchers (Goodridge et al., 1996) speculated that conflict, aggression, and burnout might be associated with elder abuse and mistreatment. For example, disturbing resident behaviors and racial and ethnic cultural differences add to the stress experienced by nursing assistants. Staff experience mistreatment from residents, including physical abuse. Furthermore, nursing assistant burnout and resident aggression could predict psychological abuse of residents. They perceive no institutional support, according to the researchers, and burnout may result in decreased quality and quantity of nursing care.

Nursing assistants ($N = 126$) completed a questionnaire on resident conflict, aggression toward nursing assistants by residents, and burnout prior to participation in a staff education program on abuse prevention and the Staff-Burnout Scale for Health Professionals (Goodridge et al., 1996). Participants were stable employees and not likely to quit working in the next six months. Most felt close or very close to residents and that their job performance was good or very good. Over 75 percent rated the care at the facility as good or very good. Most had enough time to complete their work. Burnout scores were comparable to other health care providers. Physical and verbal abuse, feeling unappreciated, and conflict between nursing and other nursing assistants were the greatest stressors. Also, workload, shift work, racial intolerance, physical demands of the job, and empathy for resident suffering and diminished quality of life were also stressors. Frequent types of conflicts consisted of residents' unwillingness to dress, wanting to go outside the facility, client complaints, and personal hygiene struggles. Seventy percent of nursing assistants experienced physical aggression (pushed, grabbed, shoved, pinched, kicked, bitten) from residents. They were spat at, had their hair pulled and buttocks and breasts touched, and were punched. Psychological aggression was slightly more common than physical assaults. Most incident reports involved cognitively impaired residents during staff assistance with self-care. Some occurred during incontinence care. Few nursing assistants reported abuse by residents, perhaps due to frequent events. They would appreciate assistance with the abuse; they also preferred education on communication and physical management of residents with dementia, depression, and aggressive behavior. It is difficult to predict nursing assistants' reactions to psychological or physical abuse carried out by residents against staff.

Elder abuse was defined in the context of long-term care settings as commonly used by a group of registered nurses (Hirst, 2002). An ethnoscience approach helped to understand the language of the members of this cultural group. A taxonomy was constructed on the phenomenon of elder abuse using participants' answers to questions as datapoints. Participants were interviewed first on perceptions of abuse and then with responses to terms in the first interviews, sorted into subcategories and behavioral clusters. Frequencies shaped the taxonomy of resident abuse and validated the analytic categories. The visual schema included category, subcategory, and behavioral cluster labels. The environmental context, described as content bound and context free, was presented. The context-bound situation indicated that participants were influenced by it. Context-free acts of abuse took place regardless of circumstance.

Characteristics of abuse included the perception to hurt, acts of omission or commission, the context of care, intentional or unintentional, and behavioral clusters (Hirst, 2002). In the model of resident abuse, the context-free act/behavior (or always wrong) was committed and intentional, and seen in offensive language (emotional, such as swearing), physical acts (corporal and emotional, punishment, such as slapping), material acts (emotional, taking away control, such as stealing), failure to meet physical needs (corporal and emotional, such as not taking to the toilet), failure to meet psychosocial needs (emotional, inappropriate language, such as using "granny/grandpa"). Resident abuse, a relational experience, was non supportive; perpetrators did not promote older residents' well-being.

Skovdahl et al. (2003) studied the interactions between persons with dementia and aggressive behavior. They compared caregivers having problems dealing with aggressive behavior and those who did not. The communication issues that persons with dementia demonstrated required that caregivers make decisions about care to serve the best interests of residents and to provide good care. The process of showering was videotaped on two units to compare the difference expressed by staff in being satisfied and capable with resident aggressiveness or with feeling overwhelmed by caring for persons with dementia exhibiting aggression. One patient on each unit, described as aggressive, was videotaped as nursing staff cared for the patient during morning care. Analysis of the texts based on the six video recordings followed a phenomenological hermeneutic method.

Being involved and developing a positive interaction was described as resident and caregiver sequences unfolded (Skovdahl et al., 2003). For the unit satisfied with care (*power unit*), the resident's needs and experiences were attended to as she was listened to and respected. She used her own abilities and cooperated with care activities. Most of the time a caregiver worked alone. As aggressive behaviors were expressed, the staff gave her more information to help her understand the situation. The caregivers repeated information in different ways, and encouraged her to voluntarily participate in care, as compared to being forced to participate. The caregivers were calm and systematic. They set limits and explained what they thought was necessary. When the resident was physically aggressive, they moved the resident's hands away. A caregiver was flexible and empathetic, for example, when the resident complained of being cold.

In contrast, another resident was confined to routines and negative interactions by the staff that expressed being overwhelmed with aggressive behavior, in the *power over* unit (Skovdahl et al., 2003). The caregivers worked together, often two or three of them. The resident wanted to make her own decision about when to take a shower. She interpreted the shower as being seen as a dirty person. The caregivers ignored the resident and showered her even as she became physically and verbally abusive. Caregivers ignored the resident's protests and used their power to hold her arms and legs. She physically attacked them and expressed that she was important while the caregivers were scum. Of note is that the first unit had received education on care of persons with dementia who were aggressive. Education for caregivers and opportunities for reflection and alternate activities as compared to rigid routines were advocated, so that *power over* did not produce more *power over* actions. The researchers submitted that how caregivers provide care is preferable to just completing the essential task of showering residents.

Elderspeak, a type of patronizing communication used with older adults, has been both supported and critiqued when used in hospitals and nursing homes by care providers (Grimm et al., 2015). According to the researchers, contextual cues that stimulate elderspeak, perhaps based on assumptions, are cognitive impairment, physical incompetence, and old age. Certified nursing assistants ($N = 26$) were asked during semi-structured interviews about situations in which elderspeak was used, reasons why it was used, situations in which it was appropriate and less appropriate, residents' reactions to elderspeak, and what residents might think about it. Themes as reasons for elderspeak use were making the resident feel comfortable, making the caregiver seem friendlier to residents, helping the resident better understand verbal communication, and getting the resident to cooperate. Elderspeak was used by nursing assistants to help residents to do something or cooperate and with residents with dementias. Elderspeak was less appropriate when residents were angry and not cognitively impaired.

Nursing assistants saw the inappropriateness and degrading aspects to elderspeak, and its utility in caregiver situations (Grimm et al., 2015). The researchers shared a concern that elderspeak might result in resistance to care with cognitively impaired persons, such as agitation and aggression. Due to differences in the findings on this topic, more research is called for.

In a systematic review of literature on abuse of older adults (Baker et al., 2016), studies published in 2015 and 2016 and selected from 19 databases were appraised in which elder abuse prevention programs were implemented. Older persons were abused in various settings: home, institutions, and community. The researchers framed elder abuse as a global problem affecting millions with economic costs and poorer health, injuries, and premature death as abuse outcomes. Lack of training, supervision, and resources were suggested as causal.

Seven studies with a total of 1,924 participants and 740 other persons were represented (Baker et al., 2016). Many studies had a high risk of bias. A low quality of evidence was identified for most. The researchers questioned programs aimed at increasing knowledge of staff and decreasing abusive behavior. Programs on victims who were abused may have resulted in increased older persons' reports of abuse events. Of interest were the instruments used in studies, for example, Caregiver Psychological Abuse

Behavior Scale, Hospital Anxiety and Depression Scale, Hartford Physical Abuse Subscale, and Modified Version of the Conflict Tactic Scale. Programs were focused on attitude change, education, effective communication, and stress and conflict management. Activities displayed in a logic model on interventions or programs for preventing elder abuse included: education, reduction of factors influencing elder abuse, policies for elder abuse, legislation on elder abuse, increased detection rates of elder abuse, victims of abuse, and rehabilitation programs for elder abuse perpetrators. Outcomes were targeted at improving quality of care and living conditions, so that barriers to quality care could be avoided in situations of potential abuse, and improvements of long-term care realized. The impact of programmatic interventions was avoidance of potential elder abuse, lower rates of elder abuse in communities and in institutions and reduced recurrent elderly abuse. The researchers used the framework of primary, secondary, and tertiary intervention to assess program effectiveness. They provided a matrix that organized studies by these levels and by participants.

Baker et al. (2016) recommended that randomized controlled trials be conducted on interventions to prevent and reduce elder abuse. The effect of program plans in interventional studies in which evidence-based protocols were administered with fidelity could stand out as prototypes for long-term care institutions.

Common Definition and Applications for Psychiatric Patients

The next exemplar of physical abuse is seen in the care of patients admitted to facilities for psychiatric are. Physical restraints have been used to reduce aggressive behaviors of older persons in long-term care, psychiatric, and hospital settings (Steinert et al., 2010) and have been characterized as abusive interventions. Application of such restraints is common across the world. Consequently, a Delphi study (Bleijlevens et al., 2016) was conducted to induce a consistent definition of physical restraints, in the hope of using it in comparative descriptive design research. Gerontological experts who were identified in the literature from 14 countries, having produced research and clinical applications in the literature, participated in a three-round study. The first round emailed survey included 34 definitions and obtained 40 participants; the second, 47; and the third, 47. The consensus process resulted in the following definition of physical restraints: "Any action or procedure that prevents a person's free body movement to a position of choice and/or normal access to his/her body by the use of any method, attached or adjacent to a person's body that he/she cannot control or remove easily" (Bleijlevens et al., 2016, p. 2309). The definition can easily be applied to patients in psychiatric facilities.

In contrast, seclusion is defined as "a control measure that consists of confining an individual to a location for a specific period of time and from which the person may not leave freely" (Goulet et al., 2017, p. 212). Seclusion is commonly used for patients with psychiatric disorders. Literature on restraints and seclusion often addresses both and examines the effect of "restricting individuals' freedom of movement, physical activity, or normal access to the body" (Negroni, 2017, p. 100).

Most likely attentive to concerns that restraint and seclusion of persons with psychiatric disorders has stimulated, the American Psychiatric Nursing Association (2014) developed and revised a position paper emphasizing safety and standards on the use of restraint and seclusion for individuals receiving psychiatric services and their caregivers. The paper advocated protection from needless trauma associated with seclusion and restraint use, professional growth and learning on safety, support of autonomy and personal control, use of quality care and risk-reduction standards, evidence-based practice to support interventions for behavioral emergencies, and cultural development on minimal seclusion and restraint use and ultimate elimination. Fundamental principles were identified on the individual's right to be treated with respect and dignity and never to use seclusion or restraint for coercion. Also advocated were alternative approaches to preventing behavioral emergencies, leadership involvement on staffing levels and staff education, oversight of seclusion and restraint use in organizational performance improvement efforts, and support of less intrusive, preventive, evidence-based interventions for behavioral emergencies.

Restraint and seclusion (R/S) have been commonly used by health care providers in many countries to control patient aggression, including prevention of self-harm. These interventions have been interpreted as violence by providers against patients. An international effort was described (LeBel et al., 2014) in efforts to put forth an evidence-based model of preventing and reducing conflict, violence and factors contributing to what now are termed coercive methods. Funding was obtained in the United States in support of curriculum development on R/S use in inpatient settings. A Six Core Strategies Model was developed based on a prevention-oriented, trauma-informed care framework. Core strategies were: "(a) active leadership toward organizational change; (b) using data to inform practice; (c) developing the workforce; (d) using R/S prevention tools; (e) actively including consumers and advocates in the care setting; and (f) rigorously debriefing R/S events after they occur" (LeBel et al., 2014, p. 24).

Incentive grants were awarded in the U.S. with the result that participating facilities reported reduction in restraint and seclusion use (LeBel et al., 2014). The number of clients restrained or in seclusion also decreased. Reports from different states and facilities demonstrated dramatic reductions in use and duration. Other results noted were reduced medication use, consumer injuries, staff injuries, and worker compensation usage. Cultural changes, changes in practice, and alternative modalities were emphasized in several states, with trauma-informed care and consumer inclusion notable. The rollout of the Six Core Strategies framework in Finland provided methods and approaches worth replicating. For example, monthly violence and seclusion data and progress were shared with staff, and counseling and crisis management principles were emphasized. New South Wales, Australia, and North West United Kingdom also engaged in restraint and seclusion reduction. Data were used in all examples to document the outcomes in countries cited. Sustaining changes and preventing drift away from the Six Core Categories model were concerns of the authors who recommended the influence of dedicated leaders.

In contrast, a systematic review (Jalil & Dickens, 2017) was conducted on mental health nurses' experience of anger and anger's relationship with their attitudes and clinical practice. The researchers noted that mental health nurses need to self-regulate their emotional states, since negative emotions can affect patients' emotional regulation. They focused on anger, as a subjective state or trait, as potentially influenced or reinforced by social factors. They narrowed the review to examine if exposure to clinical practice, such as patient aggression, was associated with nursing staff anger. They appraised 12 studies, most of which consisted of cross-sectional surveys. Participant ($N = 1,471$) roles varied. Anger of mental health nurses was lower in one study than anger norms in nonclinical settings. Patients' aggressive behavior evoked anger most commonly. Aggression interrupted routine nursing tasks, resulting in the great anger. Nurses' angry responses could be motivated by increased administrative and clinical burdens of managing aggressive incidents.

Staff perceptions of anger and aggression were associated with patient self-harming and incidents of patient containment, such as physical restraints and/or seclusion for aggression (Jalil & Dickens, 2017). Also, perception of patients' anger was associated with staff approval of restraint use. Staff anger was also related to humiliating, personally directed, and verbally aggressive behavior of patients. Nurses' anger control related to job motivation; lack of control was linked to the reverse. The researchers proposed that nurses' anger could affect therapeutic relationships with patients. Nurses needed support to assist them to cope with patient aggression. The connection between aggression against staff leading to patients being placed in physical restraints and/or seclusion was worth investigating. If mental health nurses' anger in response to patient aggression resulted in physical restraint application (coercive containment method), staff physical abuse might follow or could be perceived as such by patients.

Abuse in health care has affected at-risk groups: children, persons with learning disabilities, older people, and individuals with histories of other types of abuse. To address health care abuse, a drama pedagogical model was implemented (Wijma et al., 2016) as a piloted staff intervention for those staff that perceived they failed during encounters with patients who consequently felt abused and suffered. The framework for the intervention included the elements of an environmental climate and clinical setting model in which abuse was indirectly enabled; dynamics prevalent in society were additional influences. Abuse prevention in health care was described as the responsibility of staff and managers. Abuse, culture, and structure were parts of the intervention model. According to the researchers, erosion of moral responsibility and fragmentation of services distorted the moral resources of staff and could lead to inhumane deeds. The researchers added the need to strengthen staff's moral resources to the intervention model that focused the intervention.

Additionally, the results of some surveys confirmed a lifetime prevalence of abuse in health care, according to researchers (Wijma et al., 2016). Qualitative studies also showed that patients felt powerless and ignored, and conversely staff defined abuse in health care as an ethical failure or ethical lapse yet did not take on their responsibility. Staff were defensive and dismissed abusive incidents; they suppressed incidents or forgot them and consequently did not learn from them. Rather than focusing on eliminating bad behavior, the researchers focused on good behavior and ways to expand on it. These results added to the framework that oriented a workshop.

Forum Play (FP), a Swedish modification of the Theater of the Oppressed, an approach used against social injustices, was the platform for the intervention (Wijma et al., 2016). The intervention was aimed at increasing individuals' ability to be liberated from oppression. FP uses improvisational role play, opportunities for reflection, and values-clarification methods. The researchers provided details for the FP workshop; activities were aimed at eliminating negative consequences of old behavior, testing of new behavior, and evaluation of whether the new behavior achieved desired consequences. Presumptions of the old behavior were analyzed.

The researchers conducted 16 workshops, led by drama instructors, at an obstetrical/gynecological clinic in Sweden (Wijma et al., 2016). All staff remembered abuse incidents in which they acted as bystanders or perpetrators of abuse; their actions did not agree with their moral framework. Results of the intervention revealed increased empathy of staff during post-intervention interviews. Justifications, explanations, and trivializations of abuse in health care incidents decreased for the staff. The silence surrounding abuses in health care was replaced by awareness and increased daily conversations among staff. Staff reported increased ability to act consistent with their moral beliefs. Abuse in health care transitioned from being an individual to a group problem; the abuse in health care problem became a shared one. Shame about the negative outcomes of abuse for patients was connected to a change toward actions consistent with their moral compass. Staff were more courageous about acting regarding abuse present in health care situations.

The researchers constructed two figures depicting what happens when nothing is done in abusive situations and what happens when staff learn to act in abusive situations (Wijma et al., 2016). A figure depicted the regret feedback loop. Regret was felt when staff were uneasy about an abusive situation and suppressed or forgot it. The researchers suggested that regret was based in the feeling that the staff had participated in something morally wrong. Regret may lead to efforts to correct abuse and for learning to take place from awareness of patients' suffering. Role playing clinical scenarios in which patient abuse occurs might assist health care providers to identify triggers and responsibilities for preventing abusive situations. Workshops that encourage staff to reflect on and modify behaviors and clinical environments could be used in different health care settings for different patient situations.

Restraint application has also resulted in patient injury (Duxbury, 2015). The author argued against restraining patients and listed minor and major physical injuries linked to physical restraints. Examples are coma, fractures, lacerations, choking, incontinence, physical asphyxia, and death. She cited cases in the United Kingdom and the United States; physically restraining adults and children resulted in death by asphyxia. Restraint as a clinical intervention, part of a menu of coercive measures including seclusion, could also show cultural and social bias and exist in a non-therapeutic culture. Coercive measures are also used to stop patients' attempts to leave a facility, to control conflict over medications, and to set boundaries. Clinical records may lack a description of an aggressive situation. Duxbury recommended education, training, and supervision. The idea that restraint is therapeutic was questioned.

Duxbury (2015) questioned whether restraint application was used as a last resort. In addition to violence, restraint application justifications were verbal aggression, agitation, property damage, and staff denying requests. The need to maintain control of past patient behavior influenced nurses' decisions to restrain. Patient factors also included danger, stress, diagnosis, medication administration, and injury to self or others. Insufficient number or inexperienced staff and reduction of physical injury to involved persons and patient safety were also reasons to restrain. In contrast, nurses also wanted to avoid restraining patients. There were conflicts between the need to restrain and using a controversial intervention and one they disliked.

Leadership, cultural changes across organizations, and elimination of negative interactional styles, authoritarian behavior, and poor communication skills were identified as factors that might prevent restraint episodes (Duxbury, 2015). Duxbury recommended a trauma informed care philosophy, rather than restraining that might result in trauma, injury, or death. Orientation and ongoing staff development were proposed;

topics might include therapeutic safety and boundaries, therapeutic relationship characteristics, de-escalation techniques, patient participation and empowerment, and strength-focus care planning. The non-therapeutic, unnecessary, and life-threatening effects of restraint application were emphasized.

Aggressive and violent acts often take place in psychiatric inpatient settings, at times injuring staff (Duxbury, 2015). Duxbury explored aggression and violence and examined the common practice of applying physical restraints, sometimes called a restrictive practice or restrictive intervention. She described restraints as common interventions in the United Kingdom for inpatients requiring psychiatric care, applied when patients' exhibit aggressive and violent behavior. Restraints may control aggressive behavior and can be a response to physical violence against staff by patients. Relatives and others have physically assaulted staff.

Many institutions have reduced restraint use, and trauma informed care has emerged as an alternative approach to violence and aggressive behavior (Duxbury, 2015). Restraints involve force and restrict patients' movement. As a last resort, restraints can cause psychological and physical trauma. Duxbury challenged staff defenses to promote alternate interventions.

In the next study, the complexities of psychiatric nursing care are examined. The authors provided a perspective on the influences of how the cultures of a country and health care providers may be in conflict. In Japan, psychiatric nurses were concerned about patient situations seen as problems in providing ethical care to patients needing psychiatric services (Toda et al., 2015). Paternalism, patient autonomy, dignity, safety, interference with patient care, and education for family members due to enforced confidentiality were some of the conflicts that oriented the study. Patient advocacy, described as protection of patients' rights and benefits, was a challenge for psychiatric nurses when caring for these vulnerable patients. The study explored experienced psychiatric nurses' ($N = 21$) clinical judgment for patient advocacy (CJPA) on the necessity to intervene as patient advocates. Situational components influenced their advocacy as did ethical, cultural, and social factors. Textual versions of semi-structured interviews, focused by case examples, were analyzed in situational contexts and clinical judgment was examined. Cases varied; they consisted of patients and the following factors: families, community residents, community-based supporters, health care professionals, isolation/physical restraints, receiving medical care at other departments, medical treatments, and refusals of treatment.

Nurses were aware of disregard of or impediments to patients' rights (Toda et al., 2015). Major problems in psychiatric nurses' CJPAs were: conflicts with surrounding people impeding patients' rights to life and safety (13 cases), health care professionals' policies impeding patients' self-determination (11 cases); own violent behaviors impeding appropriate treatment and welfare services (7 cases); own or families' recognition impeding patients' self-actualization, inadequate medical treatment or nursing care impeding patients' liberty (7 cases); and kin's heartless conduct impeding patients' property rights (1 case) (Toda et al., 2015, p. 769). CJPA categories consisted of protecting patients from: inappropriate actions of families and community residents; inappropriate actions of health care and welfare professionals; and patients' futures. Principles of human dignity, self-determination, autonomy (freedom), and protection of patients' property were some determinants of the reasons and ways nurses intervened in the cases. The nurses' moral sense and Japanese norms also influenced CJPAs. Patients' violent acts and statements threatened health care professionals' safety. Nurses tried to act consistently with patient rights, their own safety, and that of other health care professionals. Patients did not express their needs and tended to seek harmony. Psychiatric nurses acted for the well-being of patients without patients expressing requests or demands. This study illustrates the complexities of psychiatric patient care from the perspective of Japanese psychiatric nurses, the challenges of having personal moral codes and ethical principles that contrast with Japanese norms, and the difficulties of making clinical judgments on how to intervene as advocates for patients.

Victimization and adverse experiences in psychiatric institutions were described in a quantitative retrospective study (Santos Mesquita & Costa Maia, 2016). Among established forms of victimization were physical assault, sexual assault, threats, and verbal abuse. However, the researchers added adverse experiences that could occur within psychiatric institutions. A semi-structured interview preceded patient participation. Portuguese psychiatric patients ($N = 95$) in four psychiatric institutions participated, using the Experiences in Psychiatric Institution Inventory, including items (5-point scale) on occurrence of psychiatric experiences and witnessed experiences. Other negative experiences were also elicited. Total Experiences of Self varied between 0 and 7 ($M = 1.75$). Total Witnessed Experience varied between 0 and 7 ($M = 1.7$). Summed Self and Witnessed or Total Global Experiences varied from 0 to 14 ($M = 2.92$). Being close to frightening or violent patients (37.9 percent) was the most disturbing experience. Watching other patients suffer physical violence represented 19.9 percent of respondents, and 14.7 percent indicated use of excessive force. Twenty-nine (30.5 percent) of patients reported 0 Total Experiences of Self; 1 Total Experiences of Self resulted in 22 (23.2 percent). An array of negative experiences was reported, for example, envy from other patients, being restrained, being humiliated, and being punished. Seven patients noted that the worst experience was being hospitalized against their will.

Obstetrical Nursing

Abusive nursing care has been reported in countries in which working conditions are very difficult and patients are very poor. During nursing care situations, nurses may humiliate, verbally coerce, and physically harm patients (Jewkes et al., 1998). In one situation, the cruelty of nurses described in local news prompted an exploration of South African obstetrical care. The study's findings (Jewkes et al., 1998) led to understanding the nature of the abuse patients experienced and why nurses treated patients in abusive ways.

The researchers provided a historical context for nursing in South Africa (Jewkes et al., 1998). In the late 19th century, white women established nurse education programs. Africans attended nursing schools starting in the 1920s. Nursing education was racially segregated. Few Africans entered nursing schools until after World War II. Nurses and midwives included most of educated African women and were elite in their societies. The status of nurse education helped to distance African nurses from their communities, far from native life. Nurses were taught to be subordinate to physicians and other authority figures that controlled patients' lives. Apartheid affected such nurses. Official racial discrimination ended in the 1990s; however, nurses still worked in difficult conditions. Work and home situations were very difficult and included domestic and other forms of violence in their society.

Framed by this context, Jewkes et al. (1998) conducted an ethnographic study on obstetrical public health services in Western Cape Province, South Africa. An antenatal clinic was the chief setting; another clinic was also studied. Informants were midwives, enrolled nurses, family planning advisors, and general workers. Observations, individual interviews, and focus group discussions were held. Perceptions of the work environment and problems in it were explored with staff. Other informants were pregnant women 17 to 40 years of age; 90 interviews were conducted. Only one interview took place in the clinic; the remainder were in women's homes. Most findings focused on the clinic in which abuses occurred often.

Most of the patients were interviewed throughout their pregnancy and after delivery (Jewkes et al., 1998). Patients at the first clinic reported being shouted at, beaten, neglected, and told they were stupid; midwives were not kind, not caring, and were rude and inhuman. Patients were afraid of midwives and were criticized by midwives if they did not schedule appointments for labor services unless they came to the clinic at 3:00 a.m. The area was dangerous for travel. Midwives were abusive during labor and slapped patients.

Booking the deliveries early was the way in which the midwives controlled their work (Jewkes et al., 1998). Their workday ended at lunch, even though they were scheduled to work until 4:30 p.m. Alternatively, the nursing staff claimed that patients abused them; they thought patients were ignorant and did not respect their position as nurses or their knowledge.

Another clinic setting was seen by patients as more positive, yet midwives there were reported by women to be verbally abusive (Jewkes et al., 1998). Staff at both clinics did not think that patients benefited from education they provided. Staff indicated that patients resisted being taught. Nursing staff across the nursing hierarchy or at different levels or grades considered patients illiterate and irresponsible. Coercion of patients was sanctioned as was the perception that patients were inferior persons. International factors, offered as explanations of neglect and abuse of patients, include structural elements, such as shortages, staffing levels, salaries, and conditions of service. Nonjudgmental, caring, interpersonal relationships were offered as a potential solution and a change from what is considered acceptable patient/staff interactions to more supportive relationships. The struggle in the international nursing community for power and middle-class status was offered as an explanation for why nurses abused and neglected patients. A critical examination of abuse, debate, and leader involvement in changes in nurse-patient relationships were recommended. Similarly, explorations of patient autonomy and dominant professional nursing perspectives needed to be carefully examined. This study is an exemplar that illustrates how status issues might provide a context for patient abuse.

Summary

The literature presented provides evidence of physical abuse of patients using three clinical situations with patients. Citations also revealed that nurses and others have been attempting to find causes of physically abusive behavior and strategies to eliminate it. Also needed is an examination of patients' sense of security when hospitalized for psychiatric problems (Santos Mesquita & Costa Maia, 2016). What is needed are robust strategies that are combined into protocols that can be tested in clinical trials and more studies that elicit patients' experience of caregivers across institutions and primary care settings.

Additionally, education of staff in these three clinical settings might provide opportunities for self-reflection and self-awareness and knowledge of alternate strategies to manage difficult clinical situations in which abuse might result. Behavior change could result as clinicians reconsider past practices and replace them, so that ultimately abuse is eliminated, other strategies for caring for patients are enacted, and cultural norms reset, regardless of type of setting.

Strategies

Table 10 includes strategies that could be implemented to assist nurses to change situations and modify provider behaviors in which physical abuse occurs.

Table 10. Strategies to Change Health Care Provider Behaviors Aimed at Preventing Physical Abuse of Patients

Strategies to Effect Change	Caring Theory-Based Citation
Education on dementia behaviors and interventions; increased interaction with nursing assistants to promote revised model of engagement; mutual vulnerability of nursing assistants and long-term care residents; listening to stories of nursing assistants	Giovannoni (2019) King & Barry (2019) Vitali (2019) Wagner (2019)
Support groups for nursing assistants	King & Barry (2019) Turkel & Ray (2013) Wagner (2019)
Education on interventions to eliminate restraint and seclusion	Vitali (2019)
Dissemination of information on status issues and cultural patterns for nurses caring for laboring patients; workshops for nurses on caring and uncaring behaviors	King & Barry (2019) Turkel & Ray (2013) Wagner (2019)

Strategies reinforce the need to educate nursing staff on how to address difficult patient situations and to stop physically abusing patients. Cultural and status issues also need to be examined, so that nursing staff gain insight about their perspectives. The patient situations that nursing assistants experience at work are challenging; they need to be supported by administrators and taught methods to deal with conflict with patients whose level of cognition and aggressive behavior could result in abuse of their caregivers.

Conclusion

Physical abuse is a contradiction to the essential ethical principal framing health care providers' work: do no harm. Although the incidence of physical abuse has been known to many health care providers and carefully examined, additional attention needs to be paid to eliminating it. Difficult patient situations in which clinicians' safety is threatened may be anticipated throughout health care settings as part of the job. However, opportunities for the creation of evidence-based protocols are many and will guide nurses' and other clinicians' actions.

Discussion Questions

1. How do you plan to respond to situations in which you witness physical abuse?

2. What is the difference between units in which *power over* behaviors are enacted by staff and *power units* in which residents listen to and respect patients? (Skovdahl et al., 2003)

3. Why are restraint and seclusion practices, as used in patient care, explained as coercive behaviors?

4. What are alternative strategies to the use of restraint and seclusion for patients?

5. Why do status issues among providers, for example between patients and nurses, persist, resulting in harm to patients?

AUTHOR SELECTION

Conde, S. (2003). Unsung heroes. In *Debutante in Cowboy Boots* [Poem] (pp. 22–23). Whimsy.

REFERENCES

American Psychiatric Nurses Association. (2014). *Position Statement: The Use of Seclusion and Restraint.* https://www.apna.org/files/public/Seclusion_&_Restraint_Position_Paper.pdf.

Baker, P.R., Francis, D.P., Hairi, N.H., Othman, S., & Choo, W.Y. (2016). Interventions for preventing abuse in the elderly. *Cochrane Database of Systematic Reviews.* https://www.cochrane.org/CD010321/PUBHLTH_interventions-preventing-abuse-older-people.

Barber, C.F. (2007). Abuse by care professionals. Part 1: An introduction. *British Journal of Nursing, 16*(15), 938–940.

Barber, C.F. (2007). Abuse by care professionals. Part 2: A behavioural assessment. *British Journal of Nursing, 16*(16), 1023–1025.

Bleijlevens, M.H., Wagner, L.M., Capezuti, E., & Hamers, P.H. (2016). Physical restraints: Consensus of a research definition using a modified Delphi technique. *Journal of American Geriatric Society, 64,* 2307–2310. doi: 10.1111/jgs.14435.

Brent & Adams Associates. (2008, July 21). Elder abuse symposium honors victim of nursing home neglect. https://www.brentadams.com/news/elder-abuse-symposium-honors-victim-of-nursing-home-neglect-20080721.cfm.

Castledine, G. (2001). A&E nurse who physically and racially abused patients. *British Journal of Nursing, 10*(8), 490.

Castledine, G. (2003). Senior staff nurse who physically abused clients in a home. *British Journal of Nursing, 12*(14), 837.

Castledine, G. (2005). Nurse who physically abused patients. *British Journal of Nursing, 14*(12), 633.

Conde, S. (2003). *Debutante in cowboy boots.* Whimsy.

Duxbury, J.A. (2015). The Ellen Skellern Lecture 2014: Physical restraint: In defense of the indefensible? *Journal of Psychiatric and Mental Health Nursing, 22,* 92–101.

Giovannoni, J. (2019). Holding sacred space for loving-kindness and equanimity for self/other. In W. Rosa, S. Horton-Deutsch, & J. Watson, *A handbook for caring science: Expanding the paradigm* (pp. 355–371). Springer Publishing.

Goodridge, D.M., Johnston, P., & Thomson, M. (1996). Conflict and aggression as stressors in the work environment of nursing assistants: Implications for institutional elder abuse. *Journal of Elder Abuse & Neglect, 8*(1), 49–67.

Goulet, M-H., Larue, C., & Lemieux, A.J. (2017). A pilot study of "post-seclusion and/or restraint review" intervention with patients and staff in a mental health setting. *Perspectives on Psychiatric Care, 4*, 212–220.

Grimm, T.M., Buchanan, J., & Afflerbach, S. (2015). Understanding elderspeak from the perspective of certified nursing assistants. *Journal of Gerontological Nursing, 41*(11), 42–49.

Hirst, S.P. (2002). Defining resident abuse within the culture of long-term care institutions. *Clinical Nursing Research, 11*(3), 267–284.

Jalil, R., & Dickens, G.L. (2017). Systematic review of studies of mental health nurses' experience of anger and of its relationships with their attitudes and practice. *Journal of Psychiatric and Mental Health Nursing, 25*, 201–213. https://doi.org/10.1111/jpm.12450.

Jewkes, R., Abrahams, N., & Myo, Z. (1998). Why do nurses abuse patients? Reflections from South African obstetric services. *Social Science and Medicine, 47*(11), 1781–1795.

Joint Commission. (2018, December 11). Developing a reporting culture: Learning from close calls and hazardous conditions. *Sentinel Event Alert, 60*, 1–8.

King, B.M., & Barry, C.D. (2019). Mutual vulnerability: Creating healing environments that nurture wholeness and well-being. In W. Rosa, S. Horton-Deutsch, & J. Watson, *A handbook for caring science: Expanding the paradigm* (pp. 373–384). Springer Publishing.

LeBel, J.L., Duxbury, J.A., Putkonen, A., Sprague, T., Rae, C., & Sharpe, J. (2014). Multinational experiences in reducing and preventing the use of restraint and seclusion. *Journal of Psychosocial and Mental Health Nursing, 52*(11), 22–29.

"Nurse who verbally abused." (2014). Nurse who verbally abused clients banned from practice by NMC. *Learning Disability Practice, 18*(6), 6. doi: 10.7748/ldp.18.6.6.s4.

Rosen, T., LoFaso, V.M., Bloemen, E.M.; Clark, S., McCarthy, T.J., Reisig, C.; Gogia, K., Elman, A., Markarian, A., Flomenbaum, N.E., Sharma, R., & Lachs, M.S. (2020). Identifying injury patterns associated with physical elder abuse: Analysis of legally adjudicated cases. Annals of Emergency Medicine, 76(3), 266–276. https://www.doi,org/10.1016/j.annemergmed.2020.03.020.

Santos Mesquita, C., & Costa Maia, A. (2016). When the safe place does not protect: Reports of victimization and adverse experiences in psychiatric institutions. *Scandinavian Journal of Caring Science, 30*, 741–748. doi: 10.1111/scs.12300.

Skovdahl, K., Kihlgren, A.L., & Kihlgren, M. (2003). Dementia and aggressiveness: Video recorded morning care from different units. *Journal of Clinical Nursing, 12*, 888–898.

Steinert, T., Lepping, P., Bernhardsgrütter, R., Conca, A., Hatling, T., Janssen, W.,…Whittington, R. (2010) Incidence of seclusion and restraint in psychiatric hospitals: A literature review and survey of international trends. *Social Psychiatry and Psychiatric Epidemiology, 45*, 889–897.

Toda, Y., Sakamoto, M., Tagaya, A., Takahashi, M., & Davis, A.J. (2015). Patient advocacy: Japanese psychiatric nurses recognizing necessity for intervention. *Nursing Ethics, 22*(7), 765–777. doi: 10.1177/0969733014547971.

Turkel, M.C., & Ray, M.A. (2013). Creating a caring practice environment through self-renewal. In M.C. Smith, M.C. Turkel, & Z.R. Wolf (Eds.), *Caring in nursing classics: An essential resource* (pp. 407–413). Springer Publishing.

Vitali, N. (2019). Teaching from the heart. In W. Rosa, S. Horton-Deutsch, & J. Watson, *A handbook for caring science: Expanding the paradigm* (pp. 225–241). Springer Publishing.

Wagner, A.L. (2019). Narrative healing. In W. Rosa, S. Horton-Deutsch, & J. Watson, *A handbook for caring science: Expanding the paradigm* (pp. 587–597). Springer Publishing.

Wierucka, D., & Goodridge, D. (1996). Vulnerable in a safe place: Institutional elder abuse. *Canadian Journal of Nursing Administration, 9*(3), 82–104.

Wijma, B., Zbikowski, A., & Brüggermann, A.J. (2016). Silence, shame and abuse in health care: Theoretical development on basis of an intervention project among staff. *BMC Medical Education, 16*, 75. doi: 10.1186/s12909-016-0595-3.

Multiple-Choice Questions

1. How is physical abuse of patients inflicted by health care providers differentiated from neglect?

    A. Unintentional harm resulting in bodily injury

    B. Intentional harm resulting in bodily injury

    C. Intentionally avoiding difficult patients

    D. Necessary actions performed for patients

  2. Which of the follow characteristics of institutional cultures helps employees to report hazards to patients that might harm them?
    A. Trust
    B. Autonomy
    C. Persistence
    D. Justification

  3. Which of the following patient characteristics might position them to be at increased risk of abuse?
    A. Needing complex physical care and having dementia
    B. Being dependent, frail, and aggressive
    C. Being acutely ill and acting very needy
    D. Acting culturally different from providers

  4. Which of the following patient behaviors alerts nurses to the possibility of physical abuse by nursing assistants working in homecare setting?
    A. Require a great deal of physical care
    B. Complain about care received
    C. Swear about physical care received
    D. Mistreat nursing assistants

CHAPTER 8

Bullying by Nurses

Jeannine Uribe, PhD, RN

Objectives

1. Examine the issue of bullying of nurses by other nurses at the levels of peer, administrator, classroom, and clinical faculty.
2. Discuss evidence-based literature related to decreasing the incidence of bullying in all settings.
3. Differentiate types of bullying.
4. Explain solutions to bullying as applied in health care and educational institutions.

Critical Incident

The nurse earned her associate degree and next enrolled in a BSN completion program. She had worked as a nursing assistant when completing the associate degree. As a registered nurse, she was employed in a variety of jobs, including per diem in cardiovascular surgical, surgical, and medical units during vacations and holidays of the BSN program. Her travels afforded experiences in nursing homes and home care settings.

The nurse decided to practice on a labor and delivery/postpartum unit and took a nursing review course and an obstetrical nursing course, both approximately three weeks long. She felt comfortable entering an obstetrical unit. She also pursued a master's degree in public health nursing to eventually practice nursing as a maternal child nurse in the community.

The new nurse's preceptor on the obstetrical unit shared jokes told by the nursing staff about what they thought the newcomer would be like. Several thought she was older and more experienced and were surprised by her youth and eight years of nursing experience. Many nurses on the floor did not have their BSN degree and had only worked in that hospital since graduation. No nurse on the unit was planning on more education. On the first day of work, the newcomer felt on display and scrutinized. Although everyone greeted her, they warned her she had a lot to learn.

During three months of orientation with her preceptor on day shift, the orientee struggled to establish a routine. However, the preceptor often asked her to provide care to other patients or to do tasks in addition to assigned patients. Often when assigned a new task, she received incomplete information; one or two steps were missing from instructions. Next the preceptor berated her for missing steps. She was also shouted at and humiliated by a physician for not obtaining a patient's complete surgical case history; the preceptor was unavailable.

The new nurse learned to ask other nurses for help and to read the policy manual for additional information. When assigned to the second shift, the new nurse was told by the regular nurses how they managed the postpartum floor. If patients had requests, they were required to walk to the nurses' station. When one of the newcomer's patients asked for a hot cup of tea, she was told not to deliver it, that patients had get it themselves. The shift nurses did not mention that walking could be therapeutic for the new mothers, but the mothers would never stop asking the nurses for assistance.

After her orientation/evaluation period ended, the nurse chose the late shift and was welcomed and felt understood by more experienced nurses. She learned that the night shift nurses chose the shift to avoid the negativity of cliques on other shifts.

The nurse experienced bullying, which was covert and concealed at times. Antagonism, gossiping, criticizing, undermining, withholding information, and cliquish behavior were experienced. All are listed in the literature as examples of bullying behavior.

The new nurse unknowingly had joined a well-established unit but was not accepted by the nursing staff. She was expected to provide professional work, measured by unit nurses' standards, had insufficient time to adjust to the new role, and was without assistance to ease her transition. The preceptor did not organize the orientation and withheld information, thus putting patients in danger. Corrections by the preceptor were callous and unkind and delivered in front of staff. The newcomer was judged by the level of care she provided; the other nurses did not give the same type of care and did not welcome new ideas. By changing shifts, the new nurse had limited learning opportunities. Ultimately, she stayed one year despite loving the patients.

Background

Bullying is a part of civilization and has been documented historically and studied in elementary and high schools, in businesses, and in journalism; it is evident in American politics. Daniel (2010) stated that incivility in politics dates back to the formation of the United States' democracy. Bullying is not new to the profession of nursing.

Florence Nightingale was bullied by the military establishment during the Crimean War for her determination to change conditions she related to sanitation. She fought to improve the conditions for soldiers but was denied supplies. Nightingale was told that her work needed to be completed by the physicians (Cook, 1913; Fee & Garaofalo, 2010). In another instance, an 1883 article from the *British Medical Journal* showed nurse superintendents were being bullied by physicians who wanted to control the training, hiring, and firing of nurses. Surprisingly for the times, the nurses stood up to the "rude bullying of the ungentlemanly men" who had been given charge of the institution (St. John's House, 1883, p. 1037). They banded together and left the place to form their own group and to manage their own trained nursing care.

Nurses in the United States also suffered from bullying. An American nurse leader, Isabel Stewart, wrote in a 1922 article, "Perhaps we have been a little inclined to pay too much attention to the reactionary autocrat and to the blustering and bullying type of elder brother" referring to the medical profession (Stewart, 1922, p. 423). Their aim was to prevent the women from starting their profession and to keep them under male, medical domination. The bullying extended outside of the hospitals, where physicians and state legislators argued against nursing leaders' right to govern nursing schools and the registration of nurses; nurses did not have the brains to carry out the work (Graduate Nurses Association Convention, 1903). The nurses also reported reading disparaging remarks in editorials of newspapers, taking action against their ideas beyond the professional realm and into the public arena. The dominance or bullying of men over women, especially in the health care arena between male, privileged doctors and their *assistant* nurses, was a norm of behavior in the late 19th and early 20th centuries and to a lesser degree continues today.

It is remarkable, however, that nurses bully other nurses at all levels from students to managers and administrators. Bullying between nurses began in the past with strict and punitive instructors and superintendents and continues to be an existing problem in nursing. Gillespie et al. (2017) mentioned nurse bullying connected to identification of nurses as an oppressed group. Oppressed people turn their power struggles inward toward each other rather than toward the system. Of concern is that the provision of patient care, nurse retention in the workplaces and relationships with colleagues are negatively affected when nurses are bullied. Therefore, bullying must be eliminated. This chapter examines the effect of bullying for nurses in educational and practice settings and among peers and leaders at work.

Literature

Research on bullying in nursing programs consists of continued attempts to conceptualize bullying actions; different terms are used for bullying behaviors in nursing literature. The American Nurses Association (ANA, 2015) position paper defined incivility, bullying, and workplace violence but did not clearly differentiate among each of the three concepts. *Incivility* is observed in rude, discourteous actions, gossip, spreading rumors, and refusal to assist a coworker. *Bullying* is similar and includes power differentials; *workplace violence* includes physical actions against another (ANA, 2015). Because of the similarity among experiences for threatened health care providers, bullying and violence share common issues.

Mobbing is a term describing repeated, emotional abuse by a group acting against an individual (Karsavuran & Kaya, 2017). Katrinli et al. (2010) referred to *horizontal peer bullying* as harm caused by a coworker who does not have power or authority over the other but is done for self-serving reasons of advancement because of a competitive environment. Dellasega (2009) used the term *relational aggression* to refer to a variety of subtle, indirect, and emotional behaviors by nurses. Adams and Maykut (2015) described bullying as *uncaring*.

The negative behaviors associated with bullying are linked to manners by which nurses relate to one another, such as the *resentful nurse*, the *backstabbing nurse*, and the *green-with-envy nurse*. Each type has specific behaviors shown as nurses act out against other nurses (Dellasega, 2009, p. 55). The ANA's Position Paper called such types of actions *incivility* and described bullying as "rude and discourteous actions, of gossiping and spreading rumors, and of refusing to assist a coworker" (ANA, 2015, p. 2). Wing et al. (2015) termed *incivility* a milder hostility, thus separating it from bullying. However, the gray areas of aggressive relational actions have the same effect and make nurses feel vulnerable. Another term, *workplace violence,* occurs in health care settings and may be perpetrated by a nurse as well as other health care providers. This term typically refers to violence against a nurse from a patient, a family member, or a visitor (AJN Reports, 2016).

Microaggression is a term used by Brown (2019) to describe bullying demonstrated by verbal snubs, insults, and other hostile actions delivered subtly and which may surface from implicit bias. Brown (2019) reported that women were more sensitive to identifying bias and negative comments than male peers. Social norms in American society reinforce the feminine use of relational, subtle aggression, expressed as microaggression, because of the cultural customs of boys being taught to be independent while girls are taught that emotional relationships are the way to interrelate. Girls are encouraged to gain control over others by having dominance in the relationship gained by carrying out nonphysical and veiled actions used as strategies to gain this interpersonal power (Simmons, 2002).

Across the United States, there is an increasing number of incidents of workplace bullying. As a result, a group of activists in California in 2001 formed the Healthy Workplace Campaign to protect workers as well as employers from a stressful environment related to bullying. The organization declared that antidiscrimination laws did not cover issues of bullying at work. Organizational leaders wrote the Healthy Workplace Bill to encourage states to promote policies to increase the number of employers who take action to encourage reporting and investigation into workplace bullying (Healthy Workplace Campaign, 2019).

Discrimination is another term comparable to workplace bullying; both involve aggression in the workplace and an environment of intimidation. The U.S. Equal Employment Opportunity Commission (EEOC) established that minor offensive conduct will not meet standards of being illegal. However, employees experiencing hostile behaviors that result in loss of employment or wages, or behavior that any reasonable person can recognize as harassment will be followed up by the Equal Employment Opportunity Commission (EEOC, 2018). Witnesses to this type of offensive behavior may also make a claim against the employer (EEOC, 2018). Earnshaw et al. (2018) conducted a systematic review of elementary and secondary school bullying. They found that victims had experienced discrimination due to having socially devalued characteristics related to sexual orientation, ethnicity, disability, and body size.

The Occupational Safety and Health Administration (OSHA), a federal government institution under the Department of Labor, recently posted recommendations and regulations specifically related to violence and bullying in the workplace. OSHA declared that it is a duty of an employer to provide a safe work environment free from risk of injury and death to employees (OSHA, n.d.). OSHA administrators started to acquire data specifically linked to health care and social service workplace incidents of bullying (OSHA Workplace Violence Proposed Rule, 2016). From that data, OSHA created a 60-page booklet on preventing and dealing with workplace violence in hospitals, residential treatment settings, community clinics, homes, and non-residential mental health settings (U.S. Department of Labor, 2016). General duty clauses of OSHA standards were added to protect employees from workplace violence and retaliation for reporting workplace bullying and violence (OSHA, 2016).

Bullying in Nursing Education

Nursing, with its specific uniform, work rituals, and specialized language and value system, has been described as having its own culture (Wolf, 1988). Compared to other cultures, in the community of nurses there are established social rules for dynamic interactions. Suominen et al. (1997) pointed out that nurses struggle globally with gender and power issues, using rituals to present a standard of care in the face of human suffering. Socialization into the culture of nursing ought to occur in the schools with nursing faculty taking the initiative to introduce students to the professional and civil behaviors of the profession. The university setting, typically a considerate and amicable atmosphere with policies and regulations keeping students and faculty on their best behavior, allows faculty time to observe nursing students, discuss issues with them, and present as a role model to demonstrate professional interactions in the nursing profession.

Bullying in the nursing education setting has been reported as instigated against students by students and faculty and extends into hospital environments during clinical learning experiences. Several studies have determined that students feel bullied in clinical agencies by professors, clinical instructors, and staff nurses working on units of clinical institutions. Minton and Birks (2019) studied student nurses in the clinical setting. Students voiced many complaints of bullying, harassment, and incivility during their clinical days. Birks et al. (2018) surveyed students who reported extensive complaints of sexual, racial, physical, and verbal abuse toward them and identified a variety of institutional staff as originators of the abuse. Students' response to abuse included physical manifestations, emotional distress, and loss of confidence in their abilities to be a nurse (Minton & Birks, 2019). Students felt disrespected by faculty and staff because they were of low status in the nursing hierarchy. Student nurses in clinical settings may feel aggression directed toward them while learning professional skills under a clinical instructor or a floor nurse. Negative clinical experiences can decrease students' confidence level and may have long lasting effects on their professional development (Buonaguro, 2020). Burkely (2018) cited the ANA's Code of Ethics as the source for prompting hospital administrators and nursing faculty to have a zero-tolerance policy of staff bullying of students during clinical experiences.

Nurse executives and managers responded to a survey regarding issues related to student bullying in hospital environments and linked high acuity and a general lack of preparation of the students and discord between hospital and academic institutional goals as creating issues on nursing units (Clark et al., 2011). Nurse leaders wanted students to have additional education in areas of effective communication, conflict resolution, and critical-thinking skills to improve decision making to decrease student stress levels (Clark et al., 2011). Cultivating professional collegiality through establishing communication and codes of conduct between hospital and academic institutions may help to advance expectations and goals for meeting both hospital and student needs (Clark et al., 2011).

Peer Bullying in the Workplace

Nurses are the most trusted profession in the United States (Brusie, 2020), yet some new nurses might disagree when describing experiences with their work colleagues. Nurses have been accused of *eating their young*, the phase that illustrates the power differential between experienced nurses and their intolerance of newcomers. Experienced nurses may take aggressive steps to push new nurses around, scold them, or punish them by withholding information. Newly hired nurses are also at risk for bullying because they may be oriented to the hospital and the unit's policies, procedures, and regulations, through online education modules. This cognitive method of educating new nurses to the unit does not accomplish familiarizing them with the culture they are entering. Staff solidarity and tight cohesion may develop as new nurses learn the ethos of a unit, as they attempt to join the group, or are left isolated. Nurses who are bullied will not ask coworkers for help, fearing rejection and comments about their nursing skills. The environment of intimidation can lead to patient care errors because neophytes are not comfortable asking domineering coworkers about patient problems (ANA, 2015).

Newly graduated nurses need time to adjust their abilities to the needs of a full-time position; however, bullying can result from staff judging neophytes as incompetent or inept. Preceptors are very important for orienting new staff and protecting them from unjust comments and power struggles. Hawley and Williford's (2015) research studied primary and secondary school bullying programs. They examined theories related to bullying and recommended an examination of power structures in an academic organization. Key figures have power and influence and can guide a culture change during orientation. Preceptors who are influential can be selected to orient newcomers, especially if they have status and are willing to support orientees during a stress-free orientation period.

Peer-to-peer bullying can include a group culture that demands allegiance to their norms of nursing care; although the element of the power differential is missing, the group determines the culture of the unit. Conflict on nursing units can be witnessed because of differences in professional experience, age, personality, and communication style (DiMeglio et al., 2005). Differences in the ethos between the shifts the nurses work can also create tension and result in bullying (DiMeglio et al., 2005).

A critical outcome affected by bullying in hospitals is patient care quality. Patients and family members can sense bullying and may voice feelings of discomfort to the nurse victim or to the unit manager. Observing tension between nurses, nurses and ancillary staff, or between nurses and physicians raises concern for the family members and whether loved ones will receive appropriate care (Laschinger, 2014). A report released by Press Ganey (2017), the organization responsible for surveying patient experiences, shows that nurse managers influence patient and nurse outcomes, which are affected by the manager's authority over the workplace environment under the leader's control (Press Ganey, 2017).

It is natural that anyone entering a profession after college graduation will experience the stress of adapting to a new position. This is especially true of recent nursing graduates who may never have experienced providing patient care for a full 12-hour shift and who enter the workplace with anxiety and feelings of inadequacy about nursing skills (Duchscher, 2009). Nurses who are bullied may experience somatic symptoms that affect their work performance. McKenna et al. (2003) studied first year nurses who were bullied, and some reported they experienced symptoms including headaches, fatigue, low self-esteem, loss of appetite resulting in weight loss and feelings of post-traumatic stress disorder (McKenna et al., 2003). Victims of bullying are affected in the provision of their work and resigning their position, which often leads to leaving the profession (Wilson & Diedrich, 2011). Johnson and Rea (2009) found links to nurses leaving their job and the profession when bullied.

Losing an employee is expensive to the hospital system, and managers who are aware of this result of bullying need to work on changing the culture and social context of their units through a variety of actions. These actions include building resilience in their nursing staff, which requires management's commitment to encouraging self-care and stress management (Halfer & Benedetto, 2020). Research shows that managers are responsible for the workplace environment and need to have specific conversations with staff about what constitutes bullying and how to prevent it (Major et al., 2013).

The Joint Commission (TJC, 2016) published a paper addressing health care bullying, reporting that intensive care units, emergency departments, and behavioral health units were those with the highest rates of bullying. However, the report did not describe who were victims and who were bullies (TJC, 2016). Leaving the job, burnout, and higher rates of absenteeism resulted from incidents of bullying, increasing the costs to the hospital, as well as affecting the well-being of staff who remained on the job (TJC, 2016). Other areas in hospitals were affected and were bringing bullying to light. The Association of periOperative Registered Nurses (AORN) acted in 2009 to form the Council on Surgical and Perioperative Safety to improve patient safety through decreasing workplace violence, realizing its devastating effects on all involved (Kirchner, 2009).

Studies have indicated that hospital policies must have clear definitions of bullying and delineation on actions to take if bullying occurs. Johnson et al. (2015) found through discourse analysis that anti-bullying policies may not contain the word *bullying*, and that managers' role may not be clearly described. Sabri et al. (2015) noted that nurses need training on bullying policies to understand definitions and actions associated with it so they can identify and report problematic situations. Nurses need to work in an environment where they feel safe to report bullying; this means that all stakeholders agree that bullying is unacceptable at that institution. All must support the necessity of reporting bullying and creating pathways of reporting bullying in the agency.

Creating a structural environment of empowerment, one that supports learning, organizational goals, and flexibility, helps new nurses through the orientation process. Support for the neophytes includes monitoring their need for resources, such as education to expand nursing knowledge and clinical skills and mental and emotional support as they join the profession (Wing et al., 2015).

Báez-León et al. (2016) introduced a model on intention to help and helping behaviors related to witnessing bullying in health care institutions. The model's concepts, based on literature, were proposed to predict intention to help and helping behavior when bystanders witness bullying. The concepts include guilt and tension (arousal), group identity (facilitates witness identification with victim), support to peer's initiative (to intervene), and absence of fear of retaliation (reflects cost/benefit analysis of helping victim). These concepts represent mobilizers of helping behavior. The researchers recommended that organizations develop policies to foster health care providers' support of bullied clinicians. Employees of health care institutions need to increase their understanding of how to act when witnessing difficult, unprofessional situations involving nurses and other colleagues (Báez-León et al., 2016).

Managers and Bullying

Nurse managers are responsible for nursing staff assigned to their units and for satisfaction with the clinical environment. Managers set the unit culture and the tone. Skarbek et al. (2015) conducted a phenomenological study of nurse managers who witnessed bullying and their interventions. All nurse managers agreed they would not tolerate bullying, would offer support to the victim, and would address it directly on the unit to create a respectful and healthy work environment. This is an expected response of nurse managers in control of their administrative skills. However, there is a greater problem for staff nurses when managers are bullies.

Power differentials are established elements of the problem of bullying. For example, Causon (2007) surveyed managers who described intimidation by other managers and between managers. Most common examples were verbal attacks, lack of invitations to meetings, and the abuse of power. Also, when managers do not recognize their actions as bullying, a larger problem is created that may leave the nurse without recourse. Suppressing responses to bullying events allows the problem to continue and may eventually affect more staff.

Intimidation and issues of bullying may be hidden or public, leading to questions about why nurses may not intervene and assist nurses under attack. Hawley and Williford (2015) mentioned the bystander effect described in research literature. Experiments showed that people continued to walk by without aiding a person in need. If a person helps that individual, then others may stop to assist. Often no one wants to be the first to become involved with the person needing assistance. Learning bystander theory might help staff nurses reevaluate inaction and be the first to help the victim (Hawley & Williford, 2015).

Nursing research could determine if the bystander effect occurs in hospitals when health care workers witness bullying. Sessions on actions to support bullied nurses and other staff might encourage colleagues to develop strategies and supportive relationships, so that when witnessing bullying episodes, they stand for victims and deescalate situations rather than waiting for others to help.

Nursing care should be performed in a caring environment. However, when nurses work with managers who bully, the delivery of quality patient care can decrease due to nurse distress. Jiang et al. (2017) found that bullying by managers inhibits employee responses to problems, their internal motivation, and creativity in solving patient issues. Nurses may hesitate to respond to client needs or problems because they fear criticism and intimidation from managers or from other health care workers in authoritative positions. Fear and hesitation could ultimately have a negative impact on patient outcomes.

Workplace violence is a global issue, and many factors influence the type of violence nurses experience. The International Council of Nurses (ICN) has been working with the World Health Organization (WHO) to create publications and policies to prevent health care workplace violence. Violence against health care workers, including physical and verbal harassment, is instigated by patients, families, and fellow health workers. WHO encourages prevention through analysis of risk in the environment, culturally sensitive understanding, and properly managed and trained staff that need respite from the pressures of work overload (International Labour Office, ICN, & WHO, 2002). Although not bullying, aspects of workplace violence can be interpreted as bullying.

It is difficult to understand why an individual is chosen to be a victim of bullying, and causes have been suggested. Victimization from bullying may be linked to childhood experiences of abuse and may contribute to the vulnerability of nurses who experience violence in hospitals. Sabri et al. (2015) studied hospital nurses and compared a variety of variables to see their effect on the nurses' experience of workplace violence (WPV).

Ethnic and racial differences in WPV among racial groups were noted. The researchers recommended developing assessment tools and policies to protect nurses and assess vulnerabilities to WPV, such as past childhood abuse and intimate partner violence (Sabri et al., 2015). Studies of adverse childhood experiences (ACEs) also have been linked to risk of poor health. Research is underway that may contribute to nurse managers' and nursing faculty's understanding of victimization and workplace violence (Monnat & Chandler, 2015).

Alternatively, nurse managers, directors, and executives were surveyed for their experiences with bullying, and 60 percent reported seeing or experiencing incidents of bullying in their institutions (Hampton, 2020). Some managers were pressured to bully providers to achieve institutional and unit goals; consequently, managers also experienced bullying from their direct reports (Hampton et al., 2019). Hampton and Rayens (2019) identified a protective factor, psychological empowerment (PE), was used by nursing leaders who were bullied. PE is defined as having a mental state of feeling in control of the work to get done and the self-belief of having the ability to get the job done. Managers with high PE scores felt less intimidation and less desire to leave their job because of bullying in the workplace (Hampton & Rayens, 2019). Further examination of how PE develops in managers might be beneficial to prepare future nursing leaders for success.

Studies have documented managers' bullying of staff. Johnson and Rea (2009) concluded that managers bullied experienced staff nurses. Staff nurses reported that bullying can occur at any point in a nurse's career (Johnson & Rea, 2000). Gallant-Roman (2008) suggested that nurse managers must support zero-tolerance policies against bullying; however, this creates a challenge when the nurse manager is the bully.

Since 1983, the Magnet Recognition Program has placed an increased amount of control of the hospital workplace into the hands of nurses. The list of 14 qualities that draw nurses to a hospital in search of excellence is explained by the American Nurses Credentialing Center (ANCC) (Lippincott Solutions, 2016). ANCC criteria encourage administrators to build a healthy, safe, stimulating workplace by giving nurse leaders and nurses the ability to use evidence-based practice, transformational leadership, system improvements, outcome measures, and other tools. Magnet hospital nurses are encouraged to strive for excellence. Janzekovich (2016) studied horizontal violence prevalence at Magnet and non–Magnet hospitals. She found nurses in Magnet status hospitals were almost equal in their reporting of having been bullied during the week of the study. She noted that bullying was slightly more prevalent in Magnet hospitals than in non–Magnet hospitals and explained this result as managers being under tremendous pressure to accomplish the focus points to achieve and maintain Magnet status (Janzekovich, 2016).

Solutions to Creating a Healthy Academic and Work Environment

Bullying is a documented and researched issue for nursing in academic and health care settings. Critical to creating a healthy academic and workplace environment is a change of culture in places nurses learn and work. Acknowledging bullying's presence and knowing it creates a hostile atmosphere affecting staff, students, and patients mean changing the culture of the institution with support from the highest level of administration to the newest employees.

Only a small percentage of nurses are bullies and bullied, but one incident of bullying can affect many in the work environment. When one staff member bullies another on the team, others are affected, and aspects of patient care can suffer. Student learning is affected, and staff camaraderie lessens. Nurses, including administrators, managers, nursing staff, and students, need to change the culture and environment of health care institutions from one of bullying to one of caring teamwork.

Create Change in Nurses

First, nurses and other staff need to recognize when bullying is occurring. This is difficult because the bullying is often hidden (McKenna et al., 2003). Nurses may not know what to do if bullying occurs. Gillespie et al. (2017) developed a program for nursing students to complete over three years of their nursing studies. Web-based activities and classroom discussions helped students learn definitions of bullying, observe recorded simulations of bullying, and discuss in teams how to respond to bullying situations (Gillespie et al., 2017). Portions of the Health Resources and Services Administration (HRSA) online program, stopbullying.gov, also presents a web-based program as a long-term solution to educate communities on how to stop bullying. This program could be adapted and applied to nursing situations. Bullying also incorporates aggression with the presence of a power differential between the bully and the victim (HRSA, 2016).

Additional efforts are needed on how nurses can work individually on strengthening factors that have been identified as placing them at higher risk to become victims of bullying. For example, the contributions of each of the nursing staff to the team might start a change in the unit culture. Dellasega (2009) underscored the importance of self-reflection to understand how others view oneself, unit colleague relationships, and positive or negative attitudes about the work environment. Nurses could develop self-reflection skills to examine work relationships and practices. Cultivating caring behaviors and compassion, two critical elements of healing-focused nursing care, can be enhanced through self-reflection (Adams & Maykut, 2015). Nurses can reflect on their role in bullying situations that occur on units and work to change the culture.

Anti-bullying programs have been developed to reduce or eliminate bullying behavior, for example, conflict resolution. But the HRSA program (2016), stopbullying. gov, which provides training modules to help schools stop bullying behavior, does not recommend this strategy as it is difficult to confront a bully even in mediated situations. Another program, the BE NICE Champion program, developed by a taskforce of nurses in an East Coast hospital, educated staff nurses on all shifts about bullying by giving them the opportunity to watch scenarios and role-play situations of intimidation (Keller et al., 2016). The four tenets the program encouraged were: stand by, support, speak up, and sequester the victim if needed (Keller et al., 2016). The program was successful. Several nurses reported they assisted in de-escalating bullying situations. At the end of the program, nurse managers were responsible to intervene in future cases of bullying and to eliminate uncivil behavior (Keller et al., 2016).

Create Change in Managers

Press Ganey released a report in 2017 on the importance of the work environment for producing positive outcomes for patients and nurses. Findings indicated that when nurses were in a positive work environment, they experienced less burnout, continued to work at the hospital, and were generally satisfied with work (Press Ganey, 2017). In a study of more than 170,000 nurses, the Press Ganey report noted that the nurse manager's role in different nursing units influenced nurse-nurse interactions and nurse-physician relationships when bullying occurred. Five other factors—autonomy, professional development, participation in quality improvement activities, safe handling and mobility practices, and appropriate staffing levels—also related to the nurse manager's influence on the work environment (Press Ganey, 2017).

According to the report (Press Ganey, 2017), nurse managers benefit from preparation for their role through education on leadership positions. Education on role functions could reduce bullying situations. Nurse executives and nurse managers needed to examine personal autonomy and capacity to direct unit environments through hiring, staffing levels, interprofessional interactions and building a cohesive culture (Press Ganey, 2017). Empathetic nurse managers who created a nurturing workplace environment with efficient processes decreased workplace stress and encouraged camaraderie and autonomy, all of which may help improve quality patient outcomes (Press Ganey, 2017).

Members of the health professions and academics should focus on prevention of bullying. However, managers are responsible for workplace culture and establish rules for handling behavior that demeans, threatens, or offends nurses and students. Zero tolerance for bullying of coworkers and students is important to establish an inviting atmosphere where people want to work in short- and long-term settings. Knowledge of a culture in which bullying flourishes could result in decreased candidate applications for employment. When students experience bullying in clinical environments, they may decide against future employment in that organization, based on treatment and witnessed events (Burkley, 2018).

Programs have provided a framework relating to the affective domain of learning as applied to clinical environments. Meires (2018) recommended the framework of emotional intelligence and learning to delay anger and modulate temper in self and other staff members (Meires, 2018). Meires recognized bullying and incivility in the workplace as a burst of emotion with many causes that can be dealt with if staff stop to question threatening actions and recognize the bullying reaction for what it represents. An unacknowledged issue concerning bullying is that coworkers often fail to recognize when colleagues are being bullied.

Zero tolerance has been proposed by researchers and nurse educators to demonstrate responsibility for maintaining a safe workplace and a commitment to safety for nurses (Burkley, 2018; Gallant-Roman, 2008). Castronovo et al. (2016) envisioned a system of incentivizing a hospital to address issues of bullying by surveying staff for incidents and viewpoints of bullying experienced in the institution. The researchers (2016) proposed surveying employees on bullying and publishing score reports for each institution. This could allow patients and potential employees to view the hospital's score and decide to apply for a position or to avoid the institution (Castronovo et al., 2016). Surveys are available to measure bullying. They presented their recommendations to federal agencies, noting bullying's administrative burden and administrators' indecision about which department would administer the measures (Castronovo et al., 2016).

It is difficult for health care leaders to persuade staff to report workplace violence. Findorff et al. (2005) noted that serious bullying events can be remembered, but when bullying was not considered serious, it might not be accurately recollected in a survey. Participants in studies may fear retaliation, especially if bullies are their bosses. With no or little reporting, managers may not identify a bullying problem in their institution (Findorff et al., 2005). Safe reporting mechanisms for bullying need to be implemented based on suggestions of staff and managers.

Much of the literature addresses solving the bullying problem between bully and victim. Future research on the sociocultural aspects of bullying in nursing is needed. Maunder and Crafter (2018) suggested a sociocultural assessment, in consideration of the context where the bullying occurs. Their approach uses a multilayered examination including the system, the community culture, and those in charge of creating the environment where bullying occurs. A multi-causal model, including the sociocultural environment of academic, clinical, and individual behavior that allows bullying behavior to continue (Monks et al., 2009), might also structure studies.

Emotional intelligence (EI), when applied to lateral violence, requires training and a desire to champion this method. Training is needed because confronting another nurse about bullying creates anxiety and stress. Jones and Argentino (2010) studied EI and anxiety associated with confrontation. They found that nurses having difficulty maintaining their emotions showed high anxiety scores when confronting other nurses about inappropriate behavior such as bullying. Analysis of narrative responses revealed that nurses did not have rules to guide them for maintaining appropriate behavior and felt anxious about having to confront another nurse.

Strategies

The following table includes strategies to decrease bullying as supported by evidence-based citations.

Table 11. Strategies to Decrease Bullying

Strategies to Effect Change	Evidence-Based Citations
Provide clinical and emotional support delivered by experienced nurses. Create an empowering workplace through collaboration and collegial relationships.	Wing et al. (2015)
Present annual web-based program for junior and senior nursing students to actively learn responses to workplace bullying through reflection and role play.	Gillespie et al. (2017)
Use HCAHPS model of surveying to incentivize hospital management to deal with issues.	Castronovo et al. (2016)
Teach nurses a method of questioning their emotions (develop EI) to control their responses during times of conflict.	Meires (2018)
Investigate bullying with a multi-layered model to examine the environment and individual behaviors of bullying.	Monks et al. (2009)
Implement NIOSH program Workplace Violence Prevention for Nurses Program.	Centers for Disease Control and Prevention (n.d.)

Much of the literature on bullying focuses on the victim and the bully rather than on the system that sets up the situation for bullying. Adams's (2015) book, *Workplace*

Mental Health: Manual for Nurse Managers, is a manual of guidelines for managers related to the stressful hospital setting. She offers perspective on system issues that create the space for bullying. Further examination of the system and the hierarchy in hospitals may reflect why bullying affects nurses. Research shows that managers do not recognize nurses' good work; they are unable to control their work, how decisions are made, and the challenges of systemic factors that are changeable (Adams, 2015; Dellasega, 2009; Huseman, 2009). Adams (2015) offered suggestions, such as policy changes, recognition of bullying, education of staff about civil behavior, and manager training to end bullying; however, these suggestions focused on the individual behavior instead of changes in the system.

The commonly held attitude that violence and bullying are norms in health care settings needs to change. Brous (2018) and Hoyle et al. (2018) conducted a qualitative study by reviewing newspaper accounts to evaluate how news stories described violence toward nurses. They found that acceptance of violence was a part of the role of nurse. The Massachusetts Nurses Association is fighting this notion of violence as a norm of the nursing profession and is seeking legislation to protect nurses (AJN Reports, 2016). Hoyle et al. (2018) noted that sensationalized press coverage prevented applicants to nursing programs from choosing nursing as a profession.

Groups of American nurses are encouraging increased legal protection for nurses. The American Journal of Nursing (2016) reported on actions taken across the United States, such as increasing the penalty for assaulting a nurse and developing in-house crisis teams that are called when violence escalates. OSHA needs to continue to push for federal standards and regulations of safety to protect health care workers (Pfeifer, 2017). Keller et al. (2016) encouraged nurses to support the Healthy Workplace Bill, a bill addressing workplace bullying and the creation of a peaceful workplace for all workers.

Conclusion

Training

Training on dealing with bullying and workplace violence is recommended for academic and clinical settings. Keller et al. (2016) promoted the BE NICE program, started by nurses to educate other nurses on how to respond to bullying through methods of de-escalation and by supporting peers through incidents of bullying. This program addresses the bystander theory by encouraging nurses to assist colleagues instead of not responding to bullying situations.

Training programs should identify the characteristics of bullying and offer ways to respond to it and to prevent it (AJN Reports, 2016; American Journal of Nursing, 2015; Brous, 2018; Brown et al., 2018; Sabri et al., 2015). Topics need to include self-care, stress management, resilience building, and coping mechanisms for use in the workplace (Duchscher, 2009; Halfer & Benedetto, 2020; McKenna et al., 2003). An example is the National Institute of Occupational Safety and Health's (NIOSH's) training on bullying. The program teaches methods to prevent and manage violence. In addition, NIOSH has an online web-based program on workplace violence to teach nurses how to identify warning signs of violence and how to communicate with a violent person to deescalate the situation. Nurses may need support after experiencing violent events; information on sources is also available in the course (Hartley et al., 2019).

Brown et al. (2018) developed a program called enABLE to prepare nurses for these dangerous encounters with threatening persons. After iterations, they present scripted simulation experiences to educate their staff on how to protect themselves and their patients and how to get help. Participants are taught escape methods and physical methods for subduing an aggressor. Staff are assessed for traumatic reactions during the scenarios and are also debriefed together to lessen stressful feelings (Brown et al., 2018).

Empowering Environment

Nurses must work in a culture where the norm is treating each other with respect (American Journal of Nursing, 2015; Hawley & Williford, 2015). The culture can develop when each nurse nurtures positive attitudes for connection, teamwork, and recognition for good work (Huseman, 2009; Meraviglia et al., 2009; Wing et al., 2015). Assessing the work environment for conditions that create stress and bullying is important as is making it safe for staff to report incidents (McKenna et al., 2003; Sabri et al., 2015). Shared governance (Olender et al., 2020) adds to nurses feeling empowered as does doing work that is creative and meaningful. Wing et al. (2015) used a change theory to examine that was meaningful to nurses. They found that when nurses were included in the goals of an organization and grew in their knowledge and expertise, they felt empowered by the environment. Offering support services for bullying experiences contributes to an empowered, safe environment (McKenna et al., 2003).

Management's Role

Managers' role includes creating a work environment that prevents bullying. Managers need to adopt a zero tolerance for bullying; all incidents of bullying must be recorded as an employee infraction (Brous, 2018). Examples of bullying behavior should be discussed with staff (Brous, 2018; Johnson et al., 2015; McKenna, 2003). Prompt intervention needs to be provided for victims of bullying and to be supported by managers (Dellasega, 2009). Managers need to identify interventions to be operationalized if bullying incidents occur. Details need to be specified in a policy manual. Orientation to the policies on bullying must be accessible for all staff members and available for annual review.

Legal Actions

Federal guidelines and programs are available to address bullying in clinical environments. Patients, families, and staff must recognize that bullying in the workplace is unacceptable. Allegations against individuals that bully may result when nurses and other clinicians are intimidated at work.

In sum, bullying is a complicated issue that shows the darker side of nursing. Nurses can take control, study the issue, and develop methods for preventing bullying, starting in nursing school and working in academia and clinical practice.

Discussion Questions

1. What is the process for a student to take if being bullied by a staff member at a clinical site?

2. Should a new graduate nurse take a job at a hospital where they were bullied as a student?

3. What political action can a nurse take to limit bullying in the workplace?

4. Which solution from Table 11 do you think is most comfortable for you to address if bullied?

5. What is the process a working nurse should take if bullied in the workplace by a physician or other health care worker in the institution?

AUTHOR SELECTION

Ó Tuama, P. *The facts of life* [Audio Poem]. On Being. https://onbeing.org/poetry/the-facts-of-life/.

REFERENCES

Adams, L. (2015). *Workplace mental health manual for nurse managers.* Springer Publishing.

Adams, L., & Maykut, C. (2015). Bullying: The antithesis of caring acknowledging the dark side of the nursing profession. *International Journal of Caring Sciences, 8*(3), 765–773.

AJN Reports. (2016). Violence against nurses in the workplace: Consolidated approaches are needed from employers, victims, and the political system. *American Journal of Nursing, 116,* 20–2.

American Nurses Association. (2015). *American Nurses Association Position Statement on Incivility, Bullying, and Workplace Violence.* https://www.nursingworld.org/~49d6e3/globalassets/practiceandpolicy/nursing-excellence/incivility-bullying-and-workplace-violence—ana-position-statement.pdf.

Báez-Léon, C., Moreno-Jiménez, B., & Aguirre-Camacho, A. (2016). Factors influencing intention to help and helping behaviour in witnesses of bullying in nursing settings. *Nursing Inquiry, 23*(4), 358–367. doi: 10.1111/nin.12149.

Birks, M., Budden, L.M., Biedermann, N., Park, T., & Chapman, Y. (2018). A 'rite of passage?' Bullying experiences of nursing students in Australia. *Collegian, 25*(1), 45–50.

Brous, E. (2018). Workplace violence: How it affects health care, which providers are most affected, and what management and staff can do about it. *American Journal of Nursing, 118*(10), 51–55.

Brown, R.G., Anderson, S., Brunt, B., Enos, T., Blough, K., & Kropp, D. (2018). Workplace violence training using simulation: A combination of classroom learning simulation and hands-on defense techniques improves preparedness. *American Journal of Nursing, 18*(10), 56–68.

Brown, T. (2019, November 19). Male clinicians miss microaggressions their female peers notice. *Medscape.* https://www.medscape.com/viewarticle/921527.

Brusie, C. (2020, January 7). Nurses ranked most honest profession 18 years in a row. *Nurse.org.* https://nurse.org/articles/nursing-ranked-most-honest-profession/.

Buonaguro, R. (2020). Bullying in nursing school? How students describe their reactions. *DEAN's Notes, 42*(2). http://web.a.ebscohost.com.dbproxy.lasalle.edu/ehost/detail/detail?vid=5&sid=4329d1dd-aacc-4e5e-836d-c6279d4d31ca%40sdc-v-sessmgr03&bdata=JnNpdGU9ZWhvc3QtbGl2ZSZzY29wZT1zaXRl#AN=147194707&db=ccm.

Burkely, J. (2018). Adopt zero tolerance for hospital staff bullying nursing students: Negative clinical experiences can have a formative influence on aspiring nurses. *American Journal of Nursing, 118*(5), 11.

Castronovo, M.A., Pullizzi, A., & Evans, S. (2016). Nurse bullying: A review and a proposed solution. *Nursing Outlook, 64,* 208–214.

Causon, J. (2007). Pressure is no excuse: A recent survey reveals the extent of bullying among public sector managers. *Nursing Standard, 21*(29), 64.

Centers for Disease Control and Prevention. (n.d.). *Occupational violence. Workplace violence prevention for nurses.* https://www.cdc.gov/niosh/topics/violence/training_nurses.html.

Clark, C.M., Olender, L., Cardoni, C., & Kenski, D. (2011). Fostering civility in nursing education and practice: Nurse leader perspectives. *Journal of Nursing Administration, 41,* 324–330.

Dellasega, C.A. (2009). Bullying among nurses: Relational aggression is one form of workplace bullying. What can nurses do about it? *American Journal of Nursing, 109*(1), 52–58.

DiMeglio, K., Padula, C.K., Piatek, C., Korber, S., Barrett, A., Ducharme, M., Lucas, S., Peirmont, N.,

Joyal, E., DeNicola, V., & Corry, K. (2005). Group cohesion and nurse satisfaction: Examination of a team-building approach. *Journal of Nursing Administration, 35*(3), 110–120.

Duchscher, J.E. (2009). Transition shock: The initial stage of role adaptation for newly graduated registered nurses. *Journal of Advanced Nursing, 65*(5), 1103–1113.

Earnshaw, V.A., Reisner, S.L. Menino, D.D., Poteat, V.P., Bogart, L.M., Barnes, T.N., & Schuster, M.A. (2018). Stigma-based bullying interventions: A systematic review. *Developmental Review, 48,* 178–200.

Fee, E., & Garaofalo, M.E. (2010). Florence Nightingale and Crimean War. *American Journal of Public Health, 100*(9), 1591.

Findorff, M.J., McGovern, P.M., Wall, M.M., & Gerberich, S.G. (2005). Reporting violence to a healthcare employer: A cross-sectional study. *AAOHN Journal, 53* (9), 399–406.

Gallant-Roman, M.A. (2008). Strategies and tools to reduce workplace violence. *AAOHN Journal, 56*(11), 449–454.

Gillespie, G.L., Grubb, P.L., Brown, K., Boesch, M.C., & Ulrich, D.L. (2017). "Nurses eat their young": A novel bullying educational program for student nurses. *Journal of Nursing Education and Practice, 7*(7), 11–21.

Graduate Nurses Association Convention. (1903, October 5). Minutes of the Convention of the Graduate Nurses Association of the State of Pennsylvania held October 5, 1903, in Pittsburgh, Pennsylvania. Roberta West Collection (MC 57 Box 1, Series 1, Folder 1). Barbara Bates Center for the Study of the History of Nursing, Philadelphia, Pennsylvania.

Halfer, D., & Benedetto, C. (2020). Evolution of a newly licensed RN transition-to-practice program: Theory and development supporting accreditation. *Journal of Nursing Administration, 50*(1). 28–33.

Hampton, D. (2020). The importance of resilience in helping leaders cope with psychological violence/workplace bullying. *Kentucky Nurse, 68*(1), 10. https://d3ms3kxrsap50t.cloudfront.net/uploads/publication/pdf/1997/Kentucky_Nurse_1_20.pdf.

Hampton, D., & Rayens, M.K. (2019). Impact of psychological empowerment on workplace bullying and intent to leave. *Journal of Nursing Administration, 49*(4), 179–185.

Hampton, D., Tharp-Barrie, K., & Rayens, M.K. (2019). Experience of nursing leaders with workplace bullying and how to best cope. *Journal of Nursing Management, 27,* 517–526.

Hartley, D., Ridenour, M., & Wassell, J. (2019). Workplace violence prevention for nurses: An online NIOSH course raises awareness of workplace violence and offers preventive strategies. *American Journal of Nursing, 119*(9), 19–20.

Hawley, P.H. & Williford, A. (2015). Articulating the theory of bullying intervention programs: Views from social psychology, social work, and organizational science. *Journal of Applied Developmental Psychology, 37,* 3–15.

Health Resources and Services Administration (HRSA). (2016). Bullying prevention and response training and continuing education online program. [PowerPoint]. https://www.stopbullying.gov/resources/training-center/bullying-prevention-training-course.

Healthy Workplace Campaign (2019). Healthy Workplace Bill. https://healthyworkplacebill.org.

Hoyle, L.P., Smith, E., Mahoney, C., & Kyle, R.G. (2018). Media depictions of unacceptable workplace violence toward nurses. *Policy, Politics and Nursing Practice, 19,* 57–71.

Huseman, R.C. (2009). The importance of positive culture in hospitals. *Journal of Nursing Administration, 39,* 60–63.

International Labour Office, International Council of Nurses and World Health Organization (2002). *Framework guidelines for addressing workplace violence in the health sector.* https://www.who.int/violence_injury_prevention/violence/interpersonal/en/WVguidelinesEN.pdf?ua=1&ua=1.

Janzekovich, C. (2016). Exploring the prevalence of horizontal violence in nursing between Magnet and non-Magnet hospitals. (Publication No. 2132). [Dissertation, Seton Hall University]. Seton Hall University Dissertations and Theses.

Jiang, W., Qinxuan, G., & Tank, T. (2017). Do victims of supervisor bullying suffer from poor creativity? Social cognitive and social comparison perspectives. *Journal of Business Ethics, 157*(2), 865–884.

Johnson, S., & Rea, R. (2009). Workplace bullying: Concerns for nurse leaders. *Journal of Nursing Administration, 39,* 84–90.

Johnson, S.L., Boutain, D.M., Tsai, J.H., & de Castro, A.B. (2015). Managerial and organizational discourse of workplace bullying. *Journal of Nursing Administration, 45*(9), 457–461.

Joint Commission. (2016, June). Bullying has no place in health care. *Quick Safety, 24.* https://www.jointcommission.org/resources/news-and-multimedia/newsletters/newsletters/quick-safety/quick-safety-issue-24-bullying-has-no-place-in-health-care/.

Jones, T.L., & Argentino, D. (2010). Nurse-to-nurse hostility, confrontational anxiety, and emotional intelligence: An integral, descriptive pilot. *Journal of PeriAnesthesia Nursing, 25*(4), 233–241.

Karsavuran, S., & Kaya, S. (2017). The relationship between burnout and mobbing among hospital managers. *Nursing Ethics, 24*(3), 337–348.

Katrinli, A., Atabay, G., Gunay, G., & Cangarli, B.G. (2010). Nurses' perceptions of individual and organizational political reasons for horizontal peer bullying. *Nursing Ethics, 17*(5), 614–627.

Keller, R., Budin, W.C., & Allie, T. (2016). A task force to address bullying: How nurses at one hospital implemented an antibullying program. *American Journal of Nursing, 116*(2), 52–58.

Kirchner, B. (2009). Safety: Addressing inappropriate behavior in the perioperative workplace. *AORN Journal, 90*(2), 177–180.

Laschinger, H.K. (2014). Impact of workplace mistreatment on patient safety risk and nurse-assessed patient outcomes. *Journal of Nursing Administration, 44*(5), 284–290.

Lippincott Solutions (2016). *History of Magnet Recognition Program.* http://lippincottsolutions.lww.com/blog.entry.html/2016/09/27/history_of_the_magne-PylM.html.

Major, K., Abderrahman, E., & Sweeney, J. (2013). "Crucial Conversations" in the workplace: Offering nurses a framework for discussing and resolving incidents of lateral violence. *American Journal of Nursing, 113* (4), 66–70.

Maunder, R.E. & Crafter, S. (2018). School bullying from a sociocultural perspective. *Aggression and Violent Behavior, 38,* 13–20.

McKenna, B.G., Smith, N.A., Poole S.J., & Coverdale, J.H. (2003). Horizontal violence: Experiences of registered nurses in their first year of practice. *Journal of Advanced Nursing, 42* (1), 90–96.

Meires, J. (2018). The essentials: Using emotional intelligence to curtail bullying in the workplace. *Urologic Nursing, 38*(3), 150–53.

Meraviglia, M., Grobe, S.J., Tabone, S., Wainwright, M., Shelton, S., Miner, H., & Jordan, C. (2009). Creating a positive work environment: Implementation of the nurse-friendly hospital criteria. Journal of Nursing Administration, 39, 64–70.

Minton, C., & Birks, M. (2019). "You can't escape it": Bullying experiences of New Zealand nursing students on clinical placement. *Nurse Education Today, 77,* 12–17.

Monks, C.P., Smith, P.K., Naylor, P., Barter, C., Ireland, J.L. & Coyne, I. (2009). Bullying in different contexts: Commonalities, differences and the role of the theory. *Aggression and Violent Behavior, 14,* 146–156.

Monnat, S.M., & Chandler, R.F. (2015). Long term physical health consequences of adverse childhood experiences. *Sociological Quarterly, 56*(4), 723–752.

Occupational Safety and Health Administration. (n.d.). OSHA Act of 1970 Introduction. https://www.osha.gov/laws-regs/oshact/section_1.

Occupational Safety and Health Administration. (2016). *Guidelines for preventing workplace violence for healthcare and social service workers.* OSHA 3148–06R 2016. https://www.osha.gov/Publications/osha3148.pdf.

Occupational Safety and Health Administration Prevention of Workplace Violence in Healthcare and Social Assistance, Proposed Rule, 81:88147–88167(2016). https://www.osha.gov/laws-regs/federalregister/2016-12-07.

Olender, L., Capitulo, K., & Nelson, J. (2020). The impact of interprofessional shared governance and a caring professional practice model on staff's self-report of caring, workplace engagement, and workplace empowerment over time. *Journal of Nursing Administration, 50,* 52–58.

Pfeifer, G.M. (2017). OSHA considers national standard to prevent healthcare workplace violence. *American Journal of Nursing, 116*(4), 15.

Press Ganey Associates. (2017, November 15). *Press Ganey Nursing Special Report: The influence of nurse manager leadership on patient and nurse outcomes and mediating effects of the nurse work environment.* https://www.pressganey.com/resources/white-papers/2017-nursing-special-report.

Sabri, B., St. Vil, N.M., Campbell, J.C., Fitzgerald, S., Kub, J., & Agnew J. (2015). Racial and ethnic differences in factors related to workplace violence victimization. *Western Journal of Nursing Research, 37*(2), 180–196.

Simmons, R. (2002). *Odd girl out: The hidden culture of aggression in girls.* Houghton Mifflin Harcourt Publishing.

Skarbek, A.J., Johnson, S., & Dawson C.W. (2015). A phenomenological study of nurse manager interventions related to workplace bullying. *Journal of Nursing Administration, 45*(10), 492–497.

Stewart, I.M. (1922). The evolution of nursing education. *American Journal of Nursing, 22* (6), 420–425.

Suominen, T., Kovasin, M., & Ketola, O. (1997). Nursing culture–some viewpoints. *Journal of Advanced Nursing, 25,* 186–190.

United States Equal Employment Opportunity Commission. (2020, January). *Harassment.* https://eeoc.gov/laws/types/harassment.cfm.

Wilson, B.L., & Diedrich, A. (2011). Bullies at work: The impact of horizontal hostility in the hospital setting and intent to leave. *Journal of Nursing Administration, 41*(11), 453–458.

Wing, T., Regan, S., & Laschinger, H.K. (2015). The influence of empowerment and incivility on the mental health of new graduate nurses. *Journal of Nursing Management, 23,* 632–643.

Wolf, Z.R. (1988). Nursing rituals. *Canadian Journal of Nursing Research Archive, 20,* 632–643.

MULTIPLE-CHOICE QUESTIONS

1. Which of the following bullying terms describes repeated, emotional abuse by a group against an individual?
    A. Horizontal peer
    B. Relational
    C. Microaggression
    D. Mobbing

2. When applied to bullying, which of the following phrases represents experienced nurses' intolerance for new nursing staff?
    A. Power differential
    B. Lack of cohesion
    C. Cultural dissonance
    D. Rite of passage

3. Which of the following health care personnel have the greatest responsibility for a healthy workplace environment?
    A. Each staff nurse
    B. Chief nurse administrator
    C. Nursing director
    D. Nurse manager

4. Which of the following strategies might assist a nurse witnessing an episode of bullying to stop an incident from escalating?
    A. Report the incident to the nurse manager
    B. Stand by a bullied coworker
    C. Act as a supportive preceptor
    D. Describe the bullying at a meeting

CHAPTER 9

Relational Incompetence

The Witnessing Nurse

Colleen Maykut, DNP, RN, FCAN

Objectives

1. Recognize that competence/incompetence is a nursing phenomenon.
2. Describe the meta-construct of relational incompetence.
3. Understand that witnessing and not intervening is an outcome of relational incompetence.
4. Articulate the paradigm shift required to rectify this dark side example from individual, organizational, and disciplinary perspectives.

Critical Incident

Mr. Jeffrey Ryan (37 years of age) of Pocologan, New Brunswick, Canada, died March 8, 2011, while serving a sentence for failing to adhere to his court conditions: refraining from driving a motorized vehicle due to a suspended driver's license. It was documented on admission (March 5, 2011) that Mr. Ryan had been taking opioids to address chronic pain from a gunshot wound to his abdomen. His plan of care did not include treatment for opioid use or strategies for managing withdrawal.

Nurses noted Mr. Ryan's increased agitation, physical tremors, nausea and vomiting, and a fall due to severe lightheadedness, all of which failed to activate transport to a local hospital. The nurse practitioner (NP) at the jail prescribed an antiemetic; he was placed in a specialized medical cell to be monitored. The patient was not checked in person by correctional officers every 15 minutes per correctional policy but was observed on screen. The nurses responsible for his care in the medical cell were not present. He was found dead the next morning. The investigation determined that no one had visited the cell to assess Mr. Ryan for over six hours.

In April 2019, the Nurses Association of New Brunswick's Discipline Committee found the NP's behavior reflected incompetence, professional misconduct, and disregard for the safety and welfare of patients. She was suspended. Also, Mr. Charles Murra, ombudsman, commented on the incompetence and inhumanity demonstrated by the professionals:

He wasn't just an inmate, an incarcerated person. He was also a person in our care ... he was dependent upon us for all the essentials of life and we failed in our primary duty to keep him healthy and safe.

Mr. Ryan's family is championing full disclosure of this incident to prevent gross incompetence from occurring to future inmates and their families (Donkin & Smith, 2019).

What is of concern is not the overall incompetence of the nurses involved, but the wrongdoing that occurred. Worth questioning is why nurses working in the jail failed to intervene when they witnessed incompetence in their peers. It is likely that all nurses at the jail were competent. The most knowledgeable, skilled, and interpersonally capable should have rectified their peers' negligent actions and behaviors.

The incident highlights failure to provide affirmation of a man's humanity and delivery of timely nursing care while Mr. Ryan was incarcerated in Canada's correctional system. Although others were involved in his case (correctional officers), nursing staff with advanced knowledge of mental health and addictions, health assessment, pharmaceuticals, and appropriate nursing care, and guided by ethics, should have intervened to prevent his unnecessary death.

The nurses involved in the incident failed to engage in relational practice, utilize their knowledge for body-mind-spirit care, and uphold the duty to care as described in their code of ethics. They became witnesses and failed to intervene in their peer's negligent professional practice, which resulted in their own relational incompetence (RI).

Individuals, including prisoners, who identify as high priority or marginalized populations often face neglect, stigma, and structural barriers to obtaining health care (Askola et al., 2017; Daibes et al., 2017) and a lack of funded programs. Programmatic funding limitations imply that marginalized people are invisible to funders, suggesting that their lives do not matter. A lack of funded health care programs may result in threatened health and inadequate services for vulnerable people and threatens their health and well-being. With inadequate or missing resources, such as health care programs, nurses and other members of the health care team find it difficult to establish caring connections with marginalized persons in need of health care interventions (Hyatt, 2017; Jones & Wright, 2017; Létourneau et al., 2017).

Since nurses are recognized health care professionals, their actions and beliefs must be guided by a code of ethics and standards of practice. The burden of incompetent practice, such as shown in the death of Mr. Ryan, lies with the prison employees and nurses who did not meet minimum standards of performance in the patient's situation. Conversely, little attention is typically paid to witnesses or bystanders during incompetent clinical situations as the persons who did not support, educate, and report peers who lacked the knowledge, skills, attributes, and attitudes reflective of professional practice.

Background

Relationships are foundational to the expression of nursing practice (Adams & Maykut, 2015; Benner, 2000; Létourneau et al., 2017; Roach, 2002). Nurses must have essential knowledge, skills, attitudes, and attributes to provide safe, competent, ethical, and compassionate care. Core relational abilities can also have a positive effect on patient outcomes (Meyer et al., 2009).

Undergraduate nursing education programs foster the acquisition of knowledge and clinical skills of nursing students. Clinical experiences with patients assist students to develop skill in communicating with patients (Expósito et al., 2018). However, additional education and practice are required to develop relational competence when interacting with patients and collaborating with members of the multidisciplinary health care team.

Faculty discuss numerous professional issues in nursing programs, and incompetent practice is one topic examined. However, understanding how to develop competencies to address the difficult problem of reporting witnessed professional incompetence with nurse colleagues and managers is an important ability and hopefully seldom needed. Compared to nursing students, new graduate nurses and experienced nurses may not have had the knowledge or experience in having difficult conversations with peers who demonstrate incompetence.

Safe, knowledgeable clinical practice requires registered nurses to be competent in creating and maintaining therapeutic connections and non-judgmental approaches to patient care (Askola et al., 2017; Daibes et al., 2017; Jones & Wright, 2017; Sutton et al., 2011; Tenkanen et al., 2011). In addition, nurses' authenticity, respect for patients and self, trust in self and others, and respect for human dignity are factors influencing nurses' commitment to establishing relationships with patients (Askola et al., 2017, 2018; Daibes et al., 2017; Gluyas, 2015; Jones & Wright, 2017; Létourneau et al., 2017) and collaborating with other members of the health care team.

Relational Competence and Incompetence

Relational competence, an interconnected set of relational values and attitudes that promote establishment and maintenance of positive relationships (Niederberger et al., 2013), is based on a theory built by psychological research. L'Abate et al. (2010) described relational competence and the abilities leading to developing positive relationships and whether skills can be developed through training (Niederberger et al., 2013). An important aspect of discussions on relational competence is knowing that individuals are aware that support is available if needed.

In contrast, a model on intention to help and helping behavior was developed by Báez-León et al. (2016) to explain the helping behavior of witnesses to bullying in nursing practice. The notion of vulnerability of bullied nurses can also be applied to incompetent nurses in this formulation, as both nurses might suffer from lateral violence. However, witnesses of nurse incompetence and bullying, who do nothing, perpetuate difficult situations (Báez-León et al. 2016) and promote relational incompetence.

The concepts in Báez-León et al.'s (2016) model were based on literature and include predictors of intention to help and helping behavior: guilt and tension (arousal), group identity (facilitates witness identification with victim), support to peer's initiative (to intervene), and absence of fear of retaliation (reflects cost/benefit analysis of helping victim). These concepts represent mobilizers of helping behavior. The researchers espoused prosocial interventions in support of victims and suggested that policies need to be developed to promote organizational responses and clinicians' understanding of how to act when difficult, unprofessional situations involving nurse colleagues (Báez-León et al., 2016) are witnessed.

The concept of relational incompetence (RI) is operationalized in examples of failed relationships among members of health care teams. One exemplar is the clinical situation observed when health care colleagues demonstrate incompetent practice behaviors and peers do not act. The peer observer, bystander, or witness is often tested to respond to this difficult situation and may not act.

RI is a dark side exemplar for nursing. The concept of RI is defined as an intentional act of failing to intervene in problematic health care situations to educate and support incompetent colleagues and not reporting their incompetent practice to managers. The RI concept is largely unexplored. A grasp of its characteristics is limited by the dearth of literature on the phenomenon.

RI is differentiated from relational competence. For example, when witnesses of emergency or serious events engage in helping behaviors, they demonstrate relational competence. If witnesses do not engage when colleagues need help, for example when incompetent, they are passive. They did not take the initiative to intervene. Choosing not to act in a situation demonstrating a peer nurses' incompetence illustrates RI.

Lack of awareness of RI factors and how to act in difficult situations, such as when observing the performance of a nurse colleague who is incompetent, can threaten patient safety. When incompetent behavior continues, patient safety is still at risk because peers did not intervene. Incompetent care persists without intervention. The good, caring nurse in the bystander position commits to colleagues in ways that liberate, support, and strengthen (Catlett & Lovan, 2011).

Since RI content may often be missing in courses of basic nursing education programs, the problem of incompetent health care providers might not be studied in depth and actions to resolve it are absent. Therefore, it is important to conceptualize RI, especially because ethical standards of nursing practice are compromised by the inactions of peer providers.

Ethical Implication

Witnessing incompetence in clinician behavior and failing to act signifies a moral disengagement from a peer (Brüggemann et al., 2019; Hyatt, 2017; Zhao & Xia, 2019). Inaction demonstrates a violation of autonomy, justice, beneficence, and nonmaleficence, principles which ground nursing's professional practice (American Nurses Association [ANA], 2015; Canadian Nurses Association [CNA], 2017; International Council of Nurses [ICN], 2012). Witnessing and identifying incompetent practice without confronting it suggests that peer bystanders may not be aware of what to do.

Not intervening could lead to identifying the bystander's behavior as relationally incompetent. This type of provider incompetence suggests that this exemplar of the dark side of nursing warrants attention. Nurses who have witnessed a colleague's incompetence do not own the total responsibility to offer support and compassion to them. Shaming and blaming a colleague who does not report incidents of incompetence, falls short of resolving the problem. Nurses can bring attention to managers and administrators by seeing incompetent clinical behaviors as a systems problem for health care institutions.

Witnessing, one aspect of RI, is based on the psychological experiments of Latané and Darley (1969), where subjects failed to assist others in need. An inverse effect was found in situations where as the number of bystanders or witnesses increased, the likelihood of intervening decreased. The researchers also described the increased crowd behavior of watching and not acting that was influenced by the seriousness of the situation.

The possibility of self-harm, a consequence of witnesses intervening, was a deterrent for coming to the aid of others, even when empathy and sympathy to their plight was self-reported (Báez-Léon et al., 2016; Latané & Darley, 1969). Although Latané and Darley's (1969) research is dated, understanding the contextual factors of human nature are applicable today. Latané and Darley's (1969) original study is replicated (Thomas et al., 2016). In addition, health care research has linked the concept of the bystander effect to patient safety (Brüggemann et al., 2019; Mcintosh, 2019), workplace culture (Báez-Léon et al., 2016), and climate safety (O'Donovan et al., 2019). These major issues require competent performance from both individuals and organizations.

Toxic workplace climates and ineffective leadership have led individuals to reject being accountable for their actions, neglect ethical performance, and displace their responsibility (Bandura, 2002; Hinrichs et al., 2012). Although diffusion of responsibility is comparable to displacement, in that the individual rejects their responsibility to act ethically, displacement is not for one specific individual, but shared equally among a group (Bandura, 2002; Hinrichs et al., 2012). Both concepts have been linked to incivility and bullying, workplace climate problems, and ineffective leadership. They show dehumanization as a disconnection from an individual's ethical foundation. Lack of responsibility also prevents the resolution of a situation in which peer incompetence is demonstrated. Therefore, the situation does not end and clinicians' failure to identify incompetent practice continues. Christensen's (2019) review suggested that nurses are at a critical risk when diffusing their individual knowledge to a lack of knowledge. However, the complexity of nursing practice is situated in structural hierarchies, power dynamics, and the pressure to conform; these factors affect behavior.

Literature

A summary of the theoretical and empirical literature provides content and context on RI and offers potential strategies from individual, organizational, and professional perspectives to mitigate the risk of RI. Competence is difficult to conceptualize as a singular concept and is a consequence of the complexity and variability in nurses' work (Aäri et al., 2008; Garside & Nhemachena, 2013). Therefore, incompetence is equally difficult to understand.

Roach (2013) explained her theory of *caring: the human mode of being*, a formulation framed by functional and ethical manifestations of caring. Among Roach's 6 Cs (compassion, competence, conscience, confidence, commitment, comportment) that represent actions of what nurses do when caring, is the concept of competence. Competence is defined "as the state of having the knowledge, judgment, skills, energy, experience, and motivation required to respond adequately to the demands of one's professional responsibilities" (p. 172). The concept of competence, according to Roach (2013), consists of some of the following descriptions: "Must know what the condition is about, how treated, and what is available to the patient; Know how to orchestrate each program and guide patient and family through it; and Importance of experience, understand this illness to be able to treat symptoms physical, emotional, and so on" (Roach, 2013, pp. 167–168). Caring competence is exemplified by compassion when nurses interact with others; it means that dominance is unacceptable and respect for the dignity and needs of patients and coworkers served is essential.

Utilizing Roach's (2002) definition of competence, an analysis of RI as a meta-construct with distinct expressions (*episteme* [knowledge], *techne* [actions], and *phronesis* [moral being]), might foster understanding its manifestations and stimulate a unified approach to address this challenging nursing problem. When RI is examined from a phronetic perspective, the answer to the question posed following the description of the critical incident—Why did all the nurses fail to intervene?—could be answered. These expressions are not mutually exclusive; they are integral to ensuring competent nursing practice.

Although individual incompetence was revealed in the exemplar, the witnessing of the peer nurses demands examination. Numerous examples from peer reviewed (Brüggemann et al., 2019; Wolf, 2012) and related literature (ANA, 2015; CNA & The University of Toronto Faculty of Nursing, 2004; Laing, 2013) support the multi-faceted complexity of individual incompetence in nursing practice and its consequences for society.

Individuals who are incompetent often lack awareness (Castledine, 2004; Dunning et al., 2003; Kruger & Dunning, 1999) of the necessary knowledge, skills, and values that can enable them to practice safely, competently, compassionately, and ethically. Instead of exploring individual incompetence, incompetence is addressed here as the fundamental responsibility of nurses, health care organizations, and educational institutions. As a group or team issue, RI is situated in a collective versus individual approach so that strategies are identified to decrease its effects.

Competence and Caring

Roach (2002) described the paradox of caring, suggesting it is more obvious when absent than when present. Her expressions of competence in nursing practice were guided by humans' ability to obtain the necessary awareness of the other (body-mind-spirit). According to Roach (2002), awareness was informed by multiple ways of knowing and was applied ethically by recognizing the uniqueness of each nursing care situation (Roach & Maykut, 2010). Competence becomes the expression of an individual's capacity to provide timely, relevant, and ethical nursing care. Alternatively, capacity refers to the nurse's present ability (a current snapshot of integration and application of multiple knowings). Capability conveys the nurse's highest attainable level of ability and is future oriented. The responsibility of the nurse is to engage in ongoing learning and competency that strengthens skill and fosters competent practice.

Competence, as a caring attribute, is framed by knowing of epistemology, anthropology, and ontology, as embodied awareness of what it means to be human and the necessary response to the other in relationship (Roach & Maykut, 2010). RI is reflected in a human response absent of authenticity, respect, dignity, and ethos, whether a result of an unintentional or intentional failure. The nurse as a caring person must intentionally integrate the 6Cs proposed by Roach (2002), including compassion, competence, conscience, confidence, commitment, and comportment, as an entangled, authentic expression of a professional response to the other, the person cared for (Roach & Maykut, 2010).

Competent practice is an expectation of professional nurses' performance. Registered nurse (RN) is a protected title, distinguishing and certifying an individual who graduates from an accredited learning institution, passes a licensing examination, and upholds the ethical values of the nursing profession (ANA, 2015; CNA, 2019; ICN, 2012). As members of the profession, individual nurses are held accountable for their practice by a state regulatory body, whose social contract with society is to uphold nursing practice standards that ensure practitioners are safe, ethical, compassionate, and competent in their interactions with others (ANA, 2014; CNA, 2019; National Council of State Boards of Nursing [NCSBN], 2019). Once employed, the individual RN has a responsibility to maintain the social contract through self-initiated programs of education to maintain competency (CNA, 2004; Whittaker et al., 2000), as reported periodically to regulatory bodies.

Health care organizations are also responsible for providing the necessary resources and support for nurses to enact the profession's social contract (Coventry et al., 2015; O'Donovan et al., 2019). Professional peers are also required to regulate nursing practice through upholding legal and ethical standards by activities that educate, support, and report nurses who fail to meet nursing's social contract.

Incompetence and Caring

Incompetence is ubiquitous in the profession of nursing due to contextual factors, ranging from individual capacity and capability (Adams & Maykut, 2015; Castledine, 2004; Cerrato, 1988; Gardner et al., 2008; Zhang et al., 2001) to organizational structures and human/non-human resource allocations (Coventry et al., 2015), and includes the role behaviors of professional peers (Báez-Léon et al., 2016; Cerrato, 1998). It is not surprising that nurses correctly or incorrectly assume that other nurses' performance is competent. This expectation is challenged when witnessing nurse behaviors that deviate from expected professional norms and are incompetent.

Individuals who are incompetent are ineffective and inefficient; they are unable to choose correct actions when responding to patient situations in which there is a demand for nursing care. The nurses lack the necessary awareness of inappropriate and dangerous responses they initiate; they are doubly burdened (Dunning et al., 2003; Kruger & Dunning, 1999). Lack of awareness of incompetent performance is problematic, as incompetent individuals may continue to overestimate their capacity to perform and are unable to achieve safe practice. Incompetence illustrates the inability to provide timely, relevant, and ethical nursing care.

Embodied awareness, necessary for the integration of relevant knowledge and competent action in a timely and effective manner, is influenced by a variety of factors. These include, but are not limited to: (1) internal (attributes, cognitive processing, and/or morality) (Castledine, 2004), (2) personal external (determinants of health) (Government of Canada, 2019), (3) professional nursing practice (acquisition of the necessary knowledge, skills, and attitudes) (ANA, 2015; CNA, 2017; ICN, 2012), and (4) environmental workplace factors (human and non-human resources) necessary to obtain and demonstrate competence (Cerrato, 1988; Coventry et al., 2015; Gardner et al., 2008; Hutchinson, 2016). Examples of factors as associated with embodied awareness reveal that there can be multiple expressions of competence-incompetence. A nurse may be incompetent in one situation due to limited resources and competent in the same situation a day later following an educational workshop.

Awareness of a nurse's personal limitations is crucial for identifying areas of incompetence and the necessary "knowing of" to lessen the risk of incompetence. However, it is naive to assume and expect that as members of a profession, nurses are exempt as individuals from the responsibility of critiquing actions, providing support, and upholding peers' practice by reporting those who do not demonstrate and maintain clinical competence

(Iacono, 2019; Wolf, 2019). Nurses need to be intentionally vigilant about their individual practice and that of peers so that RI is understood and confronted.

Analyzing Relational Incompetence

The importance of chains of knowledge (cognitive and psychomotor domains) and networks of understanding (affective domain), as framed by study of expertise (Hutchinson et al., 2016), is used to frame the analysis of incompetence from an *episteme*, *techne*, and *phronesis* perspective. Much literature focuses on *episteme* and *techne* as expressions of competence or incompetence (Dunning et al., 2003; Gardner et al., 2008; Kruger & Dunning, 1999; Zhang et al., 2001) in clinical practice. The paucity of literature exploring the influence of *phronesis* on incompetent professional practice provides an opportunity to acquire an awareness of the extent of RI.

Episteme (Knowledge)

This philosophical term encompasses knowing oneself, others, and the world (Benner, 2000). How nurses come to know and process information is through their cognitive capacity and capability on a continuum from basic recall as a minimum ability to evaluation as a higher-order skill (Hoque, 2016). Knowing includes acquisition, analysis, application, and transfer of the necessary knowledge to foster effective and efficient decision making (Graber et al., 2018; Hoque, 2016; Miller, 2010). Embedded in nurses' knowing are higher-order thinking skills, including but not limited to allocation and sustainable human and environmental resources, anticipation, mitigation of risk factors, communication within dyads and as a multidisciplinary team, understanding complexity and systems thinking, appropriate professional development to enhance performance, and progression from novice to expert, and using reflexivity to foster relational practice (Benner, 2000; Graber et al.; Theisen & Sandau, 2013). Awareness of the necessary knowledge to effectively provide direct care is pivotal for individual nurses; deficiencies are noted as failure to acquire higher-order thinking skills.

The critical incident exemplar. Although many factors could have influenced the final choice and actions of nurses in the jail, they did not intervene on behalf of the patient. Their behavior could have been influenced by insufficient foundational knowledge of mental health concepts and interventions, addiction treatment, pharmacology, and the urgency of maintaining hemodynamic status. On admission, Mr. Ryan should have received a holistic assessment on which to base a collaborative treatment plan, specifically addressing clinical interventions for his ongoing opioid use. Symptom presentation (increased agitation, physical tremors, nausea, vomiting, and a fall) should have prompted a follow-up assessment to evaluate the appropriateness and effectiveness of the treatment plan. Simply stated, the nursing process was not evident at the most basic level; this prevented an iterative, informed, and relational approach to clinical decision making.

Competence-incompetence is a continuum that is non-binary and temporal in nature. If foundational knowledge was not hindered by external factors, such as lack of staffing and/or physical resources, the question remains: why did it not guide the actions of the witnessing nurses? Perhaps a nurse's response to the situation may have been restricted by overreliance on a biomedical model of care that objectifies clients and views them as their diseases.

Nurses in the critical incident demonstrated an absence of relational competence. Evidence suggests that a lack of identifying and eliminating incompetent nursing actions demonstrates maleficence, injustice, and subjugation, and resulted in the unnecessary death of Mr. Ryan. Each of the nurses failed to intervene in their peer's actions and attempted to cover up their incompetence. They disengaged from their moral commitment to do no harm (ANA, 2015; CNA, 2017; ICN, 2012).

Techne (Action)

Techne, a philosophical term, is grounded in the intentional rationality required to enact knowledge appropriately, efficiently, and effectively (Benner, 2000). The expression of knowledge through actions reflects a continuum from the lowest level of perceiving information by which to enact a response to the ability to create innovative responses to a situation (Hoque, 2016). Nurses' progression from novice to expert clinical practice incorporates coordination and intentionality of movements (Hoque, 2016; Miller, 2010). Action must also be informed by multiple ways of knowing (Roach & Maykut, 2010) and guided by the context of the specific situation (Benner, 2000).

The critical incident exemplar. When reviewing the inaction of the nurses viewed as intentional neglect, RI is noticeably present. The NP prescribed an antiemetic for Mr. Ryan's symptoms, which prevented further episodes of vomiting, yet did not treat the underlying cause of the symptom. Assessing, diagnosing, treating, and evaluating health conditions are within the scope of an NP's mandate. Failure to effectively assess and diagnose prior to prescribing suggests a lack of integrating knowledge into the nursing situation. Although NPs have advanced education, other nurses still have an ethical obligation to question their peer's practice. The other nurses could have intervened by assessing and evaluating the treatment plan and the patient's health status.

Assessment findings (e.g., level of consciousness and vital signs) may have validated the seriousness of Mr. Ryan's condition and prompted activation of a response to transfer him to an outside health care facility. No in-person contacts for over six hours for assessing and monitoring showed a disregard and a failure to adhere to standards of nursing practice and institutional policy. Why the nurses blatantly ignored carrying out minimal expectations for their practice is not known.

Witnessing and failing to intervene may result from numerous factors, including perception of the seriousness of the event, motives of peers, organizational reprisal, patient safety, and culture within the team (Brüggemann et al., 2019; Cerrato, 1998; King, 2001; Price et al., 2014). Witnessing and intervening (educating, supporting, or reporting) are a professional, ethical responsibility of individual nurses. Structural barriers, the cultures of nursing and the health care organization, and the outcomes of intervening (whether punitive or educative in nature) are necessary to understand and respond to situations of RI. A paradigm shift toward relational competence requires movement from a solely individual focus to a collective or community responsibility to ensure that the root causes of RI have been identified and addressed.

Phronesis (Moral Being)

Benner (2000) stressed the importance of moral engagement through relationship and inquiry as vital components for competence. The expression of this domain is in responding to an interpretation of a situation, ranging from feelings to internalizing values and beliefs in the context of the complexity of the environment (Hoque, 2016;

Miller, 2010). To achieve higher performance on the performance continuum (characterizing), an individual's emotional response becomes more intentional and committed to reflecting ethical and moral congruency (Hoque, 2016). Labeling "good versus bad" or "us versus them" restricts nurses' engagement in a caring, supportive relationship with each other as professionals. Lack of moral engagement provides an impetus for not catching near misses, not preventing errors, and/or not supporting each other's continued development as nurses seek to become "the good nurse."

The critical incident exemplar. Bandura (2002) suggested that displacement of responsibility and the diffusion of responsibility are the result of moral justification, minimizing the outcomes of not intervening, and dehumanizing the other. It is difficult to surmise what was in the mind of each nurse in response to the deteriorating condition of Mr. Ryan. Moral engagement was needed to demonstrate a caring response to him in a time of need. Perhaps nurses viewed Mr. Ryan as a culmination of his addictions, crime, and status in the community. Labeling and distancing may have provided the avenue for moral disengagement from providing the relational care necessary for Mr. Ryan's need for sustaining life.

Morality provides a standard that guides nurses' beliefs, values, and actions as humans. As members of the discipline and the profession, nurses are morally obligated to ensure their practice is guided by knowledge, informed by ethics, and enacted through a social justice lens (ANA, 2015; CNA, 2017; ICN, 2012). Moral agency assumes that an individual has the capacity and capability to do and be moral. Moral agency is enacted when nurses make the right choice, while being held accountable for their actions; their capacity is influenced by their code of ethics and supported by sufficient resources (Austin, 2007, 2017). Nurses could act based on their moral foundation, apply sociopolitical insights, and work to understand actions that do not meet practice standards (Benner, 2000; Falk-Rafael, 2005; Iacono, 2019).

PROFESSIONAL WISDOM

Each philosophical expression of competence informs the other to ensure professional practice is safe, competent, compassionate, and ethical, and to shape relational competence. The novice nurse's position of cognitive, affective, and psychomotor domains (remembering, receiving, and perceiving) provides a starting point for exploring and responding to an individual's environment at a superficial level. The other end of the continuum (evaluating, characterizing, and originating) provides an opportunity for social justice, moral agency, and caring actions as nurses become intentionally aware of their responsibility as human beings and nurses. Understanding how *episteme* (knowledge), *techne* (actions), and *phronesis* (moral being) are situated in relation to professional incompetence is critical if nurses intend to mitigate the incompetent clinical practice in nursing.

The critical incident exemplar. What might have been the ending of Mr. Ryan's story if all expressions of competence were embodied by the nurses? Nurses could have utilized foundational knowledge (*episteme*) of well-being, determinants of health, social justice, collaborative teamwork, and code of ethics to inform nursing practice. Any noted deficiencies in knowledge could have been rectified by a collective approach. Actions (*techne*) might have created a space for open dialogue that was respectful and inclusive of the participants (Mr. Ryan and his family, correctional officers, and the team of nurses). Any displacement or diffusion of responsibility would have been addressed by the collective.

Any deviations from practice standards or the code of ethics might have stimulated peer nurses to act. They could have provided education, support, or ultimately report RI. Incompetence is a barrier to fair assessment of nurses' personal capacity and capability. Therefore, the onus of responsibility for RI must lie within the system (both health care and correctional in the case study) and with the team of nurses and correctional officers involved.

Strategies

Table 12 includes resources that address criteria aligned with citations including strategies for change.

Table 12. Strategies to Mitigate Relational Incompetence

Strategies to Effect Change	Evidence-Based Citations
Add affective domain learning experiences to nursing courses	Lachman (2007) Miller (2010) Theisen & Sandau (2013) Valiga (2014)
Increase students' sensitization to negative effects of providers' intentional, harmful actions through course content	Adams & Maykut (2015) Wolf et al. (2019)
Increase nursing staff's knowledge and appreciation of ethical practices in health care settings	Austin (2017) Austin (2007) Brüggemann et al. (2019)
Institute strategies to promote a culture of safety in health care institutions	Hyatt (2017) Pepper et al. (2012) O'Donovan et al. (2019)
Support colleagues demonstrating incompetent clinical behaviors Provide opportunities for development of increased professional competence by attending continuing education programs	Christensen (2019) Croke (2003)
Reinforce leaders' knowledge of moral and ethical behaviors in contexts of cost containment	Maykut (2019)
Examine the moral compass of nurses and the public's trust	Iacono (2019)
Implement educational strategies to increase opportunities to identify oppressive practices and implement actions consistent with social justice	Hutchinson (2015) Landy et al. (2016)

RI must be informed and analyzed through the socio-political influences on nursing practice. Knowledge of the world is acquired and interpreted through nurses' situatedness, including the personal and professional lenses nurses utilize to enact nursing practice. How nurses come to know is influenced by power relations and structural hierarchies and is always social and political.

Nursing Education and Disciplinary Strategies

Nurse education programs must prepare graduates to navigate the dominant bio-medical paradigm and to understand leadership and followership principles, political insight, communication, team building/mentorship, and intersectionality to provide the foundation for care and the development of relational competence grounded in the science of caring. However, knowing is not enough; opportunities for discussing and addressing dark side exemplars provide a context to prepare graduates for the complexities, ambiguities, and human failings in health care delivery systems and nursing practice. Nursing students must have opportunities to apply clinical expertise and to develop professional wisdom (*episteme*, *techne*, and *phronesis*) for their future practice.

The profession of nursing has been associated for some time with the virtues of being a good nurse (Day, 2007; Erichsen et al., 2010; Price et al., 2013). Nightingale's (1859/1946) belief in the necessity of morality to enhance a virtuous woman's capacity is reflected in her treaty:

> She must be a religious and devoted woman; she must have a respect for her own calling, because God's precious gift of life is often literally placed in her hands; she must be a sound, and close, and quick observer; and she must be a woman of delicate and decent feeling [p. 95].

Although Nightingale also spoke of the importance of observing and reporting clinical findings, this limited view of goodness appeared to define nursing for many decades. A proactive response enables nurses to integrate, with intention, the multiple ways of knowing (*episteme*), to guide their actions (*techne*), and to ensure their ethical mandate (*phronesis*) is reached and sustained.

Organizational Leadership Strategies

Leadership is an outward face and representative of the standards and expectations for quality health care delivery. Discursive practices such as Schwartz rounds (Pepper et al., 2012; Thompson, 2013) make moral disengagement visible (by creating opportunities to explore structural barriers such as communication, leadership, allocation of non-human and human resources, and funding models) to eliminate RI.

Not exposing unethical practice allows incompetent nurses to remain in practice, poses a risk for safety violations for patients, and decreases the credibility of the nursing profession. By giving testimony as witnesses, nurses can work collaboratively with leaders to create morally habitable environments in which to enact their moral agency. Balance is needed between the economics of health care delivery and the caring call to ensure authentic, respectful, and dignified connections among all involved. Organizations must create space where clients are encouraged to challenge the status quo when suboptimal care is provided (Austin, 2007, 2017).

Workplace climates must also be developed that support and encourage legitimate concerns with a peer's incompetence. Disinterest or failure to become morally engaged with a peer's practice needs to be addressed as RI with appropriate consequences. Organizations cannot continue to approach the dark side of nursing solely from an individual perspective; to do so perpetuates RI. Outlining responsibilities as an engaged employee, for example through policy development, might provide incentives and boundaries for failing to intervene according to a nurse's professional mandates.

Individual Strategies

Individuals who are incompetent may not have the necessary insight into recognizing their own deficits. Colleague nurses who witness incompetent behavior need to align practice with standards of practice and a code of ethics, a first step in awareness of the complexity of nurses' responsibility to ensure the professional's social mandate. They cannot ignore their responsibility for peer's practice by becoming morally disengaged.

A collective intervention grounded in concerns for patient safety and fear of harm could assist and rectify deficits, reduce the strain on collegial relationships, and uphold the profession's reputation. The managers, leaders, and members of the health care team must own the responsibility of educating, supporting, and reporting peers they deem incompetent.

Situational awareness is best illuminated within a community of practice, which is an example of collective intervention. For relational competence to thrive and be sustained, awareness of diversity and inclusivity must be established by articulating the roles and responsibilities, educational initiatives, protocols, and objectives necessary for sustaining moral engagement with others. Moral engagement creates the space for analyzing nursing actions and behaviors of self and others to ensure fulfillment of the mandates for an ethical, just, and humane society (Austin, 2007, 2017).

Conclusion

Nursing is valued but not always acknowledged as much of the work is invisible. Incompetence, as a construct, cannot be analyzed without addressing power, oppression, avoidance, and linguistic violence. Much literature focuses on power and oppression in nursing practice (administration, education, clinical, and research), with very few citations located on strategies to move the profession forward.

One needed discussion is how labels are attached to individuals, such as "good nurse." Who decides and what entails the labeling of an individual as good? Is it society? Is this part of nursing' social contract? Is the answer: clients (predominantly view us as kind and compassionate), the institution (that is concerned with economics), and peers (the importance of collaboration and patient-centered care)?

Good nurses are committed to do the right thing. Among relational characteristics, described in the findings of Catlett and Lovan's (2011) qualitative, interview study, were caring and caring behaviors and work behaviors with colleagues. In addition to helping others, nurses must be compassionate, helpful, and willing to correct problems, such as intervening when nurse incompetence is demonstrated.

Research on incompetence has focused on *episteme* (knowledge) and *techne* (skill) at the expense of exploring the *phronetic* (moral being) expression. A nurse's professional wisdom, influenced by morals and guided by a code of ethics, dictates actions that will and will not be taken. It is in relationship that nurses honor the other's authenticity and shared humanity congruent with their morals and ethics (Benner, 2000; Maykut, 2018). Instead of identifying incompetent practice as a deficiency or unprofessional (Pitt et al., 2014; Wolf, 2012), it is time to explore witnessing and draw attention to the seriousness of RI as an example of the dark side of nursing.

Nurses need to move past witnessing to intervening; they cannot continue to say,

"It has nothing to do with us, it is happening to someone else." Nurses cannot undo RI; however, they can increase their understanding of it and gain expertise in addressing it through simulated experiences. Rather than stating, "You don't get to not mean it. Just the opposite: you did wrong on purpose because you intentionally ignored what you were morally required to do" (McCann, 2005, p. 746), they could engage in this difficult nursing practice problem. This chapter is a call to critical consciousness to participate, speak, and address RI as one of the dark side exemplars of nursing.

Discussion Questions

1. Is self-regulation, through self-report, enough to support individual competence? What other strategies may assist in developing relational competence both individually and as a team?

2. How can nursing education assist graduates in exercising their moral agency through intervening on a peer's incompetence? How should professional wisdom be actualized in all learning experiences within undergraduate education?

3. What must be in place to ensure witnessing and intervening are educative instead of punitive in nature in all practice settings (administration, clinical, education, policy and research)? What consequences should exist for nurses who witness but fail to intervene? Should there be different levels of consequences based on the severity and number of incidents of incompetence?

4. There is an understood premise to do no harm which is the nurse's social contract with those we care for. This is written negatively—do no harm versus to do good—so our focus on the negative instead of positive has nurses approaching this conversation timidly for fear of being labeled as "that kind of nurse." Why do nurses feel they have to pick sides (we versus they)?

5. There is a paradox of nurses being uncivil to each other but also failing to report incompetency. Why do nurses close ranks (not reporting peers who are incompetent), and how does this inaction perpetuate incompetence, jeopardize patient safety, and challenge the credibility of the nursing profession?

Author Selections

Canadian Nurses Association. (2017). *Ethics for registered nurses* [PDF]. https://cna-aiic.ca/en/nursing-practice/nursing-ethics.

Douglas, M., & Zaentz, S. (Producers), & Forman, M. (Director). (1975). *One flew over the cuckoo's nest* [Film]. Fantasy Films, United Artists.

Einhorn, R. (2009–2015). *Nurse Jackie* [TV series]. HBO Series.

Reiner, R. (Director). (1990). *Misery* [Film]. Columbia Pictures.

Sitzman, K. (2014). *Caring science, mindful practice* [Massive open online course]. https://www.mooc-list.com/course/caring-science-mindful-practice-canvas-net.

Vital Smarts. *Silence kills.* https://www.vitalsmarts.com/resource/silence-kills/.

References

Aäri, R.L., Tarja, S., & Helena, L.K. (2008). Competence in intensive and critical care nursing: A literature review. Intensive Critical Care Nursing, 24(2), 78–89. doi: 10.1016/j.iccn.2007.11.006.

Adams, L., & Maykut, C. (2015). Bullying: The antithesis of caring acknowledging the dark side of the nursing profession. *International Journal of Caring Sciences, 8*(3), 765–773. http://www.internationaljournalofcaringsciences.org/docs/28_Adams_special_8_3.pdf.

American Nurses Association. (2014). *ANA position statement: Professional role competence.* https://www.nursingworld.org/practice-policy/nursing-excellence/official-position-statements/id/professional-role-competence/.

American Nurses Association. (2015) *Code of ethics for nurses with interpretive statements.* https://www.nursingworld.org/practice-policy/nursing-excellence/ethics/code-of-ethics-for-nurses/.

Askola, R., Nikkonen, M., Paavilainen, E., Soininen, P., Putkonen, H., & Louheranta, O. (2018). Forensic psychiatric patients' perspectives on their care: A narrative view. *Perspectives in Psychiatric Care, 54*(1), 64–73. https://doi.org/10.1111/ppc.12201.

Askola, R., Nikkonen, M., Putkonen, H., Kylmä, J., & Louheranta, O. (2017). The therapeutic approach to a patient's criminal offense: In a forensic mental health nurse–patient relationship–The nurses' perspectives. *Perspectives in Psychiatric Care, 53*(3), 164–174. doi: 10.1111/ppc.12148.

Austin, W. (2007). The ethics of everyday practice: Healthcare environments as moral communities. *Advances in Nursing Science, 30*(1), 81–88. https://pdfs.semanticscholar.org/603b/e248e4f6cbdecc735beac4242d3f3cc0bd86.pdf.

Austin, W. (2017). What is the role of ethics consultation in the moral habitability of health care environments? *American Medication Association Journal of Ethics, 19*(6), 595–600. doi: 10.1001/journalofethics.2017.19.6.pfor1–1706.

Báez-Léon, C., Moreno-Jiménez, B., & Aguirre-Camacho, A. (2016). Factors influencing intention to help and helping behaviour in witnesses of bullying in nursing settings. *Nursing Inquiry, 23*(4), 358–367. doi: 10.1111/nin.12149.

Bandura, A. (2002). Selective moral disengagement in the exercise of moral agency. *Journal of Moral Education, 31*(2), 101–118. https://doi.org/10.1080/0305724022014322.

Benner, P. (2000). The roles of embodiment, emotion and lifeworld for rationality and agency in nursing practice. *Nursing Philosophy, 1*(1), 5–19. doi: 10.1046/j.1466–769x.2000.00014.x.

Brüggemann, A.J., Forsberg, C., Colnerud, G., Wijma, B., & Thornberg, R. (2019). Bystander passivity in health care and school settings: Moral disengagement, moral distress, and opportunities for moral education. *Journal of Moral Education, 48*(2), 199–213. doi:10.1080/03057240.2018.1471391.

Canadian Nurses Association. (2004). *Promoting continuing competence for registered nurses* [PDF]. https://www.cna-aiic.ca/~/media/cna/page-content/pdf-fr/ps77_promoting_competence_e.pdf?la=en.

Canadian Nurses Association. (2017). *Ethics for registered nurses* [PDF]. https://cna-aiic.ca/en/nursing-practice/nursing-ethics.

Canadian Nurses Association. (2019). *Regulation of RNs.* https://www.cna-aiic.ca/en/nursing-practice/the-practice-of-nursing/regulation-of-rns.

Canadian Nurses Association and the University of Toronto Faculty of Nursing. (2004). *Nurses and patient safety: A discussion paper* [PDF]. https://www.cna-aiic.ca/~/media/cna/files/en/patient_safety_discussion_paper_e.pdf.

Castledine, G. (2004). Incompetent nurse who failed to acknowledge her limitations. *British Journal of Nursing, 13*(19), 1145. doi: 10.12968/bjon.2004.13.19.16325.

Catlett, S., & Lovan, S. (2011). Being a good nurse and doing the right thing: A replication study. *Nursing Inquiry, 18*(1), 54–63.

Cerrato, P.L. (1998). What to do when you suspect incompetence. *RN, 51*(10), 36–41.

Christensen, S.S. (2019). Escape from the diffusion of responsibility: A review and guide for nurses. *Journal of Nursing Management, 27,* 264–270. doi: 10.1111/jonm.12677.

Coventry, T.H., Maslin-Prothero, S.E., & Smith, G. (2015). Organizational impact of nurse supply and workload on nurses continuing professional development opportunities: An integrative review. *Journal of Advanced Nursing, 71*(12), 2715–2727. https://doi.org/10.1111/jan.12724.

Croke, E.M. (2003). Nurses, negligence, and malpractice. An analysis based on more than 250 cases against nurses. *American Journal of Nursing, 103*(9), 54–63. https://www.doi.org/10.1097/00000446-200309000-00017.

Daibes, M.A., Al-Btoush, M.S., Marji, T., & Rasmussen, J.A. (2017). Factors influencing nurses' attitudes towards patients in Jordanian addiction rehabilitation centres: A qualitative study. *International Journal of Mental Health and Addiction, 15*(3), 588–603. https://link.springer.com/article/10.1007/s11469-016-9682-2.

Day, L. (2007). Courage as a virtue necessary to good nursing practice. American Journal of Critical Care, 16(6), 613–616. https://doi.org/10.4037/ajcc2007.16.6.613.

Donkin, K., & Smith, C. (2019, July 10). Death of sick inmate at Saint John jail 'a pretty significant failure,' ombud says. *CBC News.* https://www.cbc.ca/news/canada/new-brunswick/jeffrey-ryan-investigation-report-1.5203710.

Dunning, D., Johnson, K., Ehrlinger, J., & Kruger, J. (2003). Why people fail to recognize their own incompetence. *Current Directions in Psychological Science, 12*(3), 83–87. https://doi.org/10.1111/1467-8721.01235.

Erichsen, E., Danielsson, E.H., & Friedrichsen, M. (2010). A phenomenological study of nurses' understanding of honesty in palliative care. *Nursing Ethics, 7*(1) 39–50. doi: 10.1177/0969733009350952.

Expósito, J.S., Costa, C.L., Agea, J.L.D., Izquierdo, M.D.C., Rodriguez, D.J. (2018). Ensuring relational competency in critical care: Importance of nursing students' communication skills. Intensive and Critical Care Nursing, 44, 85–91.

Falk-Rafael, A. (2005). Speaking truth to power: Nursing's legacy and moral imperative. *Advances in Nursing Science, 28*(3), 212–223. https://insights.ovid.com/pubmed?pmid=16106151.

Gardner, A., Hase, S., Gardner, G., Dunn, S.V., & Carryer, J. (2008). From competence to capability: A study of nurse practitioners in clinical practice. *Journal of Clinical Nursing, 17*(2), 250–258. http://dx.doi.org/10.1111/j.1365-2702.2006.01880.x.

Garside, J.R., & Nhemachena, J.Z.Z. (2013). A concept analysis of competence and its transition in nursing. *Nursing Education Today, 33*(5), 541–545. doi: 10.1016/j.nedt.2011.12.007.

Gluyas, H. (2015). Effective communication and teamwork promote patient safety. *Nursing Standard, 29*(49), 50–57. doi: 10.7748/ns.29.49.50.e10042.

Government of Canada. (2019). *Determinants of health.* https://www.canada.ca/en/services/health/determinants-health.html.

Graber, M.L., Rencic, J., Rusz, D., Papa, F., Croskerry, P., Zierler, B., Harkless, G., Giuliano, M., Schoenbaum, S., Colford, C., Cahill, M., & Olson, A.P.J. (2018). Improving diagnosis by improving education: A policy brief on education in healthcare professions. *Diagnosis, 5*(3), 107–111. https://doi.org/10.1515/dx-2018-0033.

Hinrichs, K.T., Wang, L., Hinrichs, A.T., & Romero, E.J. (2012). Moral disengagement through displacement of responsibility: The role of leadership beliefs. *Journal of Applied Social Psychology, 42*(1), 62–80. doi: 10.1111/j.1559-1816.2011.00869.x.

Hoque, M.E. (2016). Three domains of learning: Cognitive, affective and psychomotor. *The Journal of EFL Education and Research (JEFLER), 2*(2), 45–52. www.edrc-jefler.org.

Hutchinson, J.S. (2015). Anti-oppressive practice and reflexive lifeworld-led approaches to care: A framework for teaching nurses about social justice. *Nursing Research and Practice, 2015,* Article ID: 18750. http://dx.doi.org/10.1155/2015/187508.

Hutchinson, M., Higson, M., Cleary, M., & Jackson, D. (2016). Nursing expertise: A course of ambiguity and evolution in a concept. *Nursing Inquiry, 23*(4), 290–304. doi: 10.1111/nin.12142.

Hyatt, J. (2017). Recognizing moral disengagement and its impact on patient safety. *Journal of Nursing Regulation, 7*(4), 15–21. https://doi.org/10.1016/S2155-8256(17)30015-7.

Iacono, M.V. (2019). Nursing integrity: A moral imperative. *Journal of PeriAnesthesia Nursing, 34*(1), 220–222. doi: 10.1016/j.jopan.2018.12.002.

International Council of Nurses. (2012). *ICN Code of Ethics for Nurses* [PDF]. https://www.icn.ch/sites/default/files/inline-files/2012_ICN_Codeofethicsfornurses_%20eng.pdf.

Jones, E.S., & Wright, K.M. (2017). "They're Really PD Today": An exploration of mental health nursing students' perceptions of developing a therapeutic relationship with patients with a diagnosis of antisocial personality disorder. *International Journal of Offender Therapy and Comparative Criminology, 61*(5), 526–543. doi: 10.1177/0306624X15594838.

King G., III (2001). Perceptions of intentional wrongdoing and peer reporting behavior among registered nurses. *Journal of Business Ethics, 34,* 1–13. https://doi.org/10.1023/A:1011915215302.

Kruger, J., & Dunning, D. (1999). Unskilled and unaware of it: How difficulties in recognizing one's own incompetence led to inflated self-assessments. *Journal of Personality and Social Psychology, 77*(6), 1121–1134. doi: 10.1037//0022-3514.77.6.1121.

L'Abate, L.L., Cusinato, M., Maino, E., Colesso, W., & Scilletta, C. (2010). *Relational competence theory: Research and mental health applications.* Springer Science & Business Media.

Lachman, V.D. (2007). Moral courage: A virtue in need of development? *MEDSURG Nursing, 16*(2), 131–133. http://test.nursingworld.org/~4af2ed/globalassets/docs/ana/ethics/moral-couragevirtue.pdf.

Laing, P. (2013, September 27). Incompetent nurses can no longer be struck off, says health watchdog. *Deadline News,* 13. http://www.deadlinenews.co.uk/2013/09/27/incompetent-nurses-can-no-longer-be-struck-off-says-health-watchdog/.

Landy, R., Cameron, C., Au, A., Cameron, D., O'Brien, K., Robrigado, K., Baxter, L., Cockburn, L., O'Hearn, S., Olivier, B., & Nixon, S. (2016). Educational strategies to enhance reflexivity among clinicians and health professional students: A scoping study. *Forum Qualitative Sozialforschung / Forum: Qualitative Social Research, 17*(3), Article 14. http://eprints.lse.ac.uk/68328/7/Au_Educational%20strategies%20to%20enhance.pdf.

Latané, B., & Darley, J.M. (1969). Bystander "apathy." *American Scientist, 57*(2), 244–268. https://faculty.babson.edu/krollag/org_site/soc_psych/latane_bystand.htm.

Létourneau, D., Cara, C., & Goudreau, J. (2017). Humanizing nursing care: An analysis of caring theories through the lens of humanism. *International Journal of Human Caring, 21*(1), 32–40. doi: 10.20467/10 91–5710.21.1.32.

Maykut, C. (2018). DASEIN: A celebration of caring science scholars in communion. *International Journal for Human Caring, 22*(1), 20–25. doi: 10.20467/1091–5710.22.1.pg56.

Maykut, C. (2019). Skillful moral leadership: Collective action to foster moral habitability. Nurse Leader, *18*(5), 491–496. https://doi.org/10.1016/j.mnl.2019.09.020.

McCann, H.J. (2005). Intentional action and intending: Recent empirical studies. *Journal of Philosophical Psychology, 18*(6), 737–748. https://doi.org/10.1080/09515080500355236.

McIntosh, E. (2019). The implications of diffusion of responsibility on patient safety during anaesthesia, "So that others may learn and even more may live"–Martin Bromiley. *Journal of Perioperative Practice, 29*(1), 341–345. doi: 10.1177/1750458918816572.

Meyer, E.C., Sellers, D.E., Browning, D.M., McGuffie, K., Solomon, M.Z. & Truog, R.D. (2009). Difficult conversations: Improving communication skills and relational abilities in health care. *Pediatric Critical Care Medicine, 10*(3), 352–359.

Miller, C. (2010). Improving and enhancing performance in the affective domain of nursing students: Insights from the literature for clinical educators. *Contemporary Nurse, 35*(1), 2–17. doi: 10.5172/conu.2010.35.1.002.

Niederberger, U., Masche, J.G., & Holmberg, U. (2013). Relational competency theory: Can respect, authenticity, and responsibility for the relationship predict relationship quality? *Examensarbete,* 1–15. https://familylab.de/files/Grundlagen/23_Bachelors_Thesis_Ueli_Niederberger.pdf.

Nightingale, F. (1859/1949). *Notes on nursing. What it is, and what it is not.* J.B. Lippincott.

O'Donovan, R., Ward, M., De Brún, A., & McAuliffe, A. (2019). Safety culture in health care teams: A narrative review of the literature. *Journal of Nursing Management, 25*(5), 871–883. doi: 10.1111/jonm.12740.

Pepper, J.R., Jagger, S.I., Mason, M.J., Finney, S.J., & Dusmet, M. (2012). Schwartz rounds: Compassion in modern healthcare. *Journal of the Royal Society of Medicine, 105*(3), 94. doi: 10.1258/jrsm.2011.110231.

Pitt, V., Powis, D., Levett-Jones, T., & Hunter, S. (2014). Nursing students' personal qualities: A descriptive study. *Nurse Education Today, 34*(9), 1196–1200. https://doi.org/10.1016/j.nedt.2014.05.004.

Price, L., Duffy, K., McCallum, J., & Ness, V. (2014). Are theoretical perspectives useful to explain nurses' tolerance of suboptimal care? *Journal of Nursing Management, 23*(7), 940–944. doi: 10.1111/jonm.12239.

Price, S.L., Hall, L.M., Angus, J.E., & Peter, E. (2013). Choosing nursing as a career: A narrative analysis of millennial nurses' career choice of virtue. *Nursing Inquiry, 20*(4), 305–316. https://doi.org/10.1111/nin.12027.

Roach, M.S. (2002). *Caring, the human mode of being: A blueprint for the health professions* (2nd Rev. ed.). CHA Press.

Roach, M.S. (2013). Caring, the human mode of being: A blueprint for the health professions. In M.C. Smith, M.C. Turkel, & Z.R. Wolf, *Caring in nursing: An essential resource* (pp. 165–170). Springer Publishing.

Roach, M.S., & Maykut, C.A. (2010). Comportment: A caring attribute in the formation of an intentional practice. *International Journal for Human Caring, 14*(4), 22–26. doi: 10.20467/1091–5710.14.4.22.

Sutton, G., Liao, J., Jimmieson, N.L., & Restubog, S.L.D. (2011). Measuring multidisciplinary team effectiveness in a ward-based healthcare setting: Development of the Team Functioning Assessment Tool. *Journal for Healthcare Quality, 33*(3), 10–24. https://doi.org/10.1111/j.1945-1474.2011.00138.x.

Tenkanen, H., Tiihonen, J., Repo-Tiihonen, E., & Kinnunen, J. (2011). Interrelationship between core interventions and core competencies of forensic psychiatric nursing in Finland. *Journal of Forensic Nursing,7*(1), 32–39. doi: 10.1111/j.1939–3938.2010.01093.x.

Theisen, J.L., & Sandau, K.E. (2013). Competency of new graduate nurses: A review of their weaknesses and strategies for success. *Journal of Continuing Education in Nursing, 44*(9), 406–414. https://doi.org/10.3928/00220124-20130617-38.

Thomas, K.A., De Freitas, J., DeScioli, P., & Pinker, S. (2016). Recursive mentalizing and common knowledge in the bystander effect. *Journal of Experimental Psychology: General, 145*(5), 621–629. http://dx.doi.org/10.1037/xge0000153.

Thompson, A. (2013). How Schwartz rounds can be used to combat compassion fatigue. *Nursing Management, 20*(4), 16–20. doi: 10.7748/nm2013.07.20.4.16.e1102.

Valiga, T.M. (2014). Attending to affective domain learning: Essential to prepare the kind of graduates the public needs. *Journal of Nursing Education, 53*(5), 247. doi: 10.3928/01484834–20140422–10n.

Whittaker, S., Smolenski, M., & Carson, W. (2000, June 30). Assuring continued competence—Policy questions and approaches: How should the profession respond? *Online Journal of Issues in Nursing, 5*(3). www.nursingworld.org/MainMenuCategories/ANAMarketplace/ANAPeriodicals/OJIN/TableofContents/Volume52000/No3Sept00/ArticlePreviousTopic/ContinuedCompetence.aspx.

Wolf, Z.R. (2012). Nursing practice breakdowns: Good and bad nursing. *MEDSURG Nursing, 21*(1), 16–36. https://search.proquest.com/docview/922981856?pq-origsite=gscholar.

Wolf, Z.R. (2019). The dark side of nursing [Editorial]. *International Journal for Human Caring, 23*(1), 1–3. http://dx.doi.org/10.20467/1091–5710.2.3.1.1.

Wolf, Z.R., Donohue-Smith, M., & Wolf, K.C. (2019). Nurses who murder or who are accused of murder. *International Journal for Human Caring, 23*(1), 51–70.

Zhang, Z., Luk, W., Arthur, D., & Wong, T. (2001). Nursing competencies: Personal characteristics contributing to effective nursing performance. *Journal of Advanced Nursing, 33*(4), 467–474. https://doi.org/10.1046/j.1365-2648.2001.01688.x

Zhao, H., & Xia, Q. (2019). Nurses' negative affective states, moral disengagement, and knowledge hiding: The moderating role of ethical leadership. *Journal of Nursing Management, 27*(2), 257–370. https://doi-org.dbproxy.lasalle.edu/10.1111/jonm.12675.

Multiple-Choice Questions

1. Which of the following theorists on caring in nursing addresses nurse competency?
- A. Watson
- B. Neuman
- C. Roach
- D. Duffy

2. Which of the following descriptions characterizes an attribute of incompetent nursing care?
- A. Inadvertently not performing nursing care functions
- B. Inability to provide timely, relevant, and ethical nursing care
- C. Intentionally failing to perform nursing care that is required
- D. Deliberately avoiding nursing care due to bias against a patient

3. What is an outcome of crowd behavior associated with witnessed, incompetent performance?
- A. Failing to intervene
- B. Fearing reprisal
- C. Lacking knowledge
- D. Expressing sympathy

4. Which of the following descriptions highlight the double threat of incompetent nurses?
- A. Inability to carry out nursing's social contract with society
- B. Lack awareness of inappropriate and dangerous nursing actions
- C. Refusal to admit knowledge and skill shortcomings
- D. Superficial knowledge of how to act in patient care situations

CHAPTER 10

Reckless Nursing Care

Zane Robinson Wolf, PhD, RN,
CNE, FCPP, ANEF, FAAN

Objectives

1. Describe behaviors that illustrate reckless nursing care.
2. Compare accidents to at-risk and reckless behavior.
3. Examine how blurring of clinical responsibilities for nurse and physician providers creates a context for reckless behaviors.
4. Explore the ethical principles violated by reckless nursing care.

Critical Incident

A charge nurse was pressured by the post-anesthesia care unit (PACU) to admit a patient following cardiac surgery to an intensive care unit (ICU). Beds were full, yet one patient was cleared to be transferred to another unit. However, the patient's blood pressure was low and fluctuated. The patient's primary nurse did not think that it would be safe to transfer the patient. The charge nurse overrode the primary nurse's assessment, administered a 250 mL bag intravenous (IV) infusion, and transferred the patient based on the increased blood pressure that resulted from the IV. There was no order for the infusion. The short-term change in the patient's blood pressure may or may not have been sustained following transfer out of the ICU. The charge nurse violated nursing's scope of practice, perhaps because of a sense of being an autonomous nurse, having established competence in critical care nursing, and a willingness to risk a negative outcome for the patient. The major reason for the behavior was the pressure to make room for a new postoperative patient following cardiac surgery.

Reckless nursing care has been described as professional misconduct; case studies appear in nursing journals as nursing alerts. For example, one case involved an ICU nurse who changed a patient's tracheostomy tube for the first time and did not carry out the procedure or written policy (Anonymous, 1999). Her breach of the code of professional conduct was reviewed by a professional conduct organization in the United Kingdom. The nurse's name was removed from the register. Still another case described a nurse's failure to restock a crash cart following use of a laryngoscope for a patient earlier in a shift, so that a medium blade laryngoscope was not located on the cart later when a patient needed to be reintubated (Austin, 2001). The patient died. Both situations could be classified as reckless behavior, because procedures were not followed. The first example showed intent; the second was a lapse, perhaps due to the pressures of a busy unit. Another example of reckless misconduct was provided (Fiesta, 1996): a nursing assistant slapped the face of a long-term care resident during bathing; a background check would have revealed a prior criminal conviction. The last example is an assault, and contrasts with reckless behavior.

Background

At-risk and reckless behavior demonstrated by health care providers is hazardous (Marx, 2007) and threatens patient safety. At-risk behavior is defined as a behavioral choice that increases risk where risk is not recognized or is mistakenly believed to be justified (Marx, 2007). Reckless behavior is defined as a behavioral choice to consciously disregard a substantial and unjustifiable risk (Marx, 2007). Reckless behavior is a direct violation of clinical practice ethics and is deliberate or intentional (Taxis & Barber, 2003).

In contrast, reckless behavior differs from disruptive behavior. Clinicians display disruptive behavior by intimidating employees at work, thus undermining organizational culture and the culture of safety (Petrovic & Scholl, 2018). Disruptive behavior categories include a pattern of passive-aggressive behavior, physical or verbal threats, verbal abuse, physical violence, harassment, intimidation, bullying, and discrimination (Petrovic & Scholl, 2018).

Health care errors result from reckless behavior and endanger the lives of patients. Nursing practice breakdowns typically include errors that are accidental and may or may not cause harm in patients. Reckless behavior is not accidental, chiefly because of intent. One interpretation is that the person knew or should have known that an action was likely to result in harm (Thompson Reuters, 2019, para. 2). The distinction is debatable. Reckless nursing care plays out in a context much larger than that of patient care units and homes. The complexity of health care delivery activities and the multiple interactions of patients, family members, friends, and numerous health care providers and other employees provide numerous situations in which reckless behavior can be enacted.

The public's trust in nurses may erode because of identified nursing practices labeled as reckless. Loss of trust in the caring relationship between nurses and patients means that the "virtues of caring, honesty, and responsibility, which speak to the character of a community or society" (Lagana, 2000, p. 6) may be vacated by reckless nurses. Moreover, nurses are accountable for clinical nursing practice.

It is important that professional nurses acknowledge the phenomenon of reckless nursing practice in health care agencies and wherever nursing care is delivered. Reckless behaviors must also be analyzed by administrators of health care organizations aimed at the status and accomplishments of a high reliability organization. Disciplinary procedures need to be carried out for those committing blameworthy acts to assure patient trust (Chassin & Loeb, 2013).

Reckless behavior might be managed by remedial or punitive action (Marx, 2007) meted out by managers, administrators, and human resource personnel of health care agencies, state boards of nursing, or courts. Professional regulations structure responses to reckless behavior, consistent with aims to ensure the delivery of safe, ethical, competent care. Reasons to report nurses to state boards of nursing are motivated by concerns that nurses are "not safe to practice after internal attempts to address the practice issue have failed" (Pugh, 2011, p. 28).

Nursing care, as nurses' professional responsibility, is high-consequence health care. Nursing interventions definitively affect patient safety and other patient and institutional outcomes. The consequences of nursing care actions, direct or delegated, are serious for patients in danger of poor health outcomes, for the staff and for the liability of health care institutions.

Ethical Considerations

As humans, nurses are never perfect. They are implicated in health care mistakes classified as errors of omission or commission. Many nurses work in institutions in which various factors, including human and systems problems, have been linked with nursing practice errors that are accidental. However, reckless behavior by nurses is unacceptable. It violates two of the three duties of a just culture: the duty to avoid causing unjustified risk or harm; the duty to produce an outcome; and the duty to follow a procedural rule (Marx, 2007). A just culture is characterized as a work environment that is open, fair, and just and represents a learning culture in which safe systems are designed and behavioral choices are managed (Marx, 2007).

Reckless nursing care violates several ethical principles that coincide with personal, professional, and organizational ethical values. One major principle is beneficence (obligation to help others and promote their welfare) (Pugh, 2011); patients might be harmed by reckless nursing care. Individual autonomy and justice for patients are violated by reckless behavior; patients are often powerless and very dependent on the care of nurses and other health care providers. The Advisory Committee on Human Radiation Experiments (1994–1996) proposed the following six principles, aimed chiefly at research but applicable to health care overall:

> One ought not to … treat people as mere means to the ends of others; to deceive others; to inflict harm or the risk of harm…. One ought to promote welfare and prevent harm (beneficence); treat people fairly and with equal respect (justice); respect the self-determination of others (autonomy) [Devettere, 2016, p. 477].

The Joint Commission (TJC, 2016) has published principles that constitute that organization's code of conduct. Principle 7 targets workplace conduct and employment practices. In addition to the ethical standard for a workplace safety culture, the standard expects TJC's employees to comport themselves professionally and mentions disciplinary or contractual action for inappropriate behavior. Leaders at TJC are responsible for promoting ethical conduct. Many of these notions are easily applied to health care practices. Reckless behavior fails to demonstrate a regard for standards of care and "can be seen as morally reprehensible" (Lagana, 2000, p. 5).

Codes of conduct influencing services of health care systems are many. They consist of federal, state, and local laws, professional organization codes for ethical and research conduct, standards of care in organizations, protocols, algorithms, policies, procedures, and so on. Guidelines also shape health care providers' behaviors and attitudes.

Literature

Different databases were searched to locate studies on reckless nursing behavior. CINAHL, PubMed, Medline, PsychInfo, Google, and Summon databases netted few studies on reckless behavior. Several studies were located that included minimal information on reckless nursing behavior. The following selections address aspects of reckless behavior.

State Board Disciplinary Action

State boards of nursing in the U.S. publish monthly reports naming nurses whose conduct has been reviewed because of allegations that they have violated state law. Names, types of infractions, and judgments are published. Institutions in countries across the world publish similar reports. In addition to these reports and professional journal accounts, research has been conducted on disciplinary data. Conduct that illustrates reckless nursing care can be inferred from studies describing nurses' characteristics when disciplined by state boards of nursing.

For example, an observational study (Carruth & Booth, 1999) was conducted to compare disciplined nurse characteristics and non-disciplined nurses in Louisiana with permission of the Louisiana State Board of Nursing. A random selection of nurse violators ($N = 249$) from 1991 to 1995 was obtained. The mean age of the sample was 42.4 years, and 59.8 percent were nurses longer than 10 years at the time of the event. Females comprised 81.9 percent of the sample; 58.2 percent were disciplined by suspension, and 30.9 percent were on probation. Of the disciplined nurses, 41.3 percent held associate degrees. Males were disproportionately disciplined compared to females; associate degree-prepared nurses were disproportionately represented compared to those with baccalaureate degrees. The age range of 40–49 was proportionately more likely be disciplined than those 50–59 years. Chemical dependency and violated recovering nurse programs were the most reported types of infractions of the state nurse practice act. Nurses may have been charged with more than one violation. The researchers suggested that high acuity units and easier access to narcotics might provide opportunities to divert narcotics. The results showed that the assumption of young, inexperienced nurses being frequently disciplined was not upheld in the sample. Diversion of narcotics is criminal behavior. When nurses use opioids and are working, their behavior is reckless.

State boards of nursing also discipline nurses for unprofessional conduct outside of the workplace. For example, alcohol and drug abuse, failing to pay child support, harassment, and stalking are examples of unprofessional behavior (Lilly, 2015). A misdemeanor or any other criminal conviction might result in a state board charge for a nurse because unprofessional behavior resulted in an accident that placed the public in harm's way. The morals of professional nursing were violated. Other examples result in state board of nursing sanctions. State board of nursing and regulatory agencies require that nurses perform board requirements, whether a result of health care agency or personal charges; not to comply leads to additional sanctions.

Professional Boundaries and Reckless Nursing

The boundaries between nursing and medicine are frequently examined in professional literature and research. Medical sociologists have explored the work of nurses and physicians at the intersections of care. For instance, part of a hospital ethnographic study (Liberati, 2016) examined the social, contextual, and organizational factors directly affecting the negotiation of the medical-nursing boundary and nurses and physicians that functioned in different care settings. Three wards were the sites chosen: neurology, neurosurgical, and intensive care units. Surgeons, neurologists, intensivists, and nurses participated. Different degrees of physician attendance, levels of acuity, and patient turn-over were noted in comparisons across ward contexts and different negotiations operated among unit clinicians.

Nurse and physician work differed in the neurology ward (Liberati, 2016). Nurses adhered to their formal role. The surgical ward was described as having few surgeons present; nurses performed surgeons' tasks, including prescribing drugs, contacting consultants, and handling surgical wounds. Nurses replaced surgeons and expanded their practice when carrying out medical functions in the surgical ward. Surgeons relied heavily on nurses for patient information. Nurses replaced surgeons on the ward, blurring the boundary between surgeon and nurse. In the ICU, boundaries were further blurred and physicians and nurses double-checked others' actions; their functions intersected. ICU clinical boundaries were the most blurred.

The level of acuity, including turnover, emergencies, and severity of patients' conditions affected the medical-nursing boundary (Liberati, 2016). Patient interaction also affected boundary; ICU patients were unconscious or did not often respond. Holistic versus specialized clinical approaches differed among narrowed clinical approaches, for example neurology showed more restricted practices than the more holistic ICU care. Intensivists considered themselves different from other physicians. In ICUs, collaborative uses of power were linked with boundary blurring. Perhaps boundary blurring functions to "encourage or make it virtually impossible for nurses to act strictly within their formal jurisdictions" (Liberati, 2016, p. 142). The findings of this study suggest that blurring might foster a unit culture in which reckless behavior might flourish among nurses or illustrate a pervasive team culture. Finally, although legislation regulates each role, practice changes are often enacted prior to modifications of laws by state legislatures.

Dekker (2009) observed that adaptations in clinical settings, such as procedural violations, are used in actual clinical situations. Dekker proposed that accounts of the same act vary depending on questions asked of clinicians and could be explained either as evil or weakness of behavior. Stories or versions describing clinical failures (errors or procedural violations) can structure subsequent actions.

Accounts of clinicians' failures are socially constructed. The social constructivist analysis of Dekker (2009) on failures at work confirmed that at-risk or procedural violations are difficult to judge. The outcomes of these events depend on the storyteller or individual, such as who writes an incident report in a health care organization. He suggested that peers need to be included in writing reports on these narratives. Dekker also proposed that individuals work in discretionary space. For example, they decide to act during a crisis in a patient care situation. They are responsible and can be held accountable for a course of action even though they did not have the authority to act. Dekker noted that accountability, although often backward-looking, is best forward-looking. Forward-looking approaches are not retributive; they are organizational, operational, technical, educational, or political. Judicial and professional sanctions vary. The line gets drawn by different bodies, legal, professional groups, or peer staff. Dekker implicitly supported systems solutions to failures, since it is difficult to draw the line between at-risk behavior and procedural violations:

> The socially constructed judgment of the line means that its location will forever be more unpredictable than relatively stable arrangements among stakeholders about who gets to draw the line, with or without help from others [p. 184].

In contrast, a grounded theory study (Pugh, 2011) sampled 21 Australian registered nurses to obtain accounts of their experiences when reported to nurse regulatory authorities for unprofessional conduct allegations. Interviews were analyzed using grounded theory methods. Review panels did not uphold all the allegations. Some nurses were disciplined by license suspension and requirements for additional education. According to Pugh, nurses experienced transformed personal identities following allegations and requirements mandated by regulatory processes. They were vulnerable and changed the way they saw nursing work. The transformational process included being confronted, assuming a stance, going through it, living the consequences, and revisioning.

Findings (Pugh, 2011) were categorized as overall personal and professional vulnerabilities, framed by individual and contextual causal attributes of unprofessional conduct. The individual and contextual domains were interrelated between and within nine properties. The individual causal attribute of professional vulnerability, working around standards, was emphasized in this chapter. This property, working around standards, consisted of unknowingly or knowingly bending the rules, reckless nursing behavior. Participants knew that their practice differed from established standards. They justified the working around property by meeting patients' immediate needs; they felt obligated to violate a nursing practice standard.

Responsible Subversion and Rule Bending

Nurses who provide direct care to patients often make clinical decisions in the moment. Their intent is to provide the best care for patients. Nurses bend the rules or work around policies and procedures to achieve what they consider to be the best interests of patients. Nurses' advocacy for patients, therefore, differs from organizational policies and procedures (Hutchinson, 1990). Clinical judgment overrides institutional structures in rule-bending instances.

It is difficult to quantify how often nurses make decisions that bend the rules. Of greater concern is attempting to estimate the outcomes of risky behaviors for patients and nurses. Rule bending carries the potential for negative outcomes.

Hutchinson provided a theory to explain nurses' rule-bending process. Based on data from a larger study, the experiences of nurses when bending the rules to benefit patients were described (Hutchinson, 1990). Interviews and participant observation data (300 hours) were analyzed using grounded theory design. Additional focused interviews were conducted with 21 nurses. Hutchinson represented the basic social-psychological problem and process as responsible subversion. Nurses were responsible when using their best clinical judgment within the context of rules imposed in the clinical setting.

The resulting substantive theory included the following conditions for nurses: knowledge (assessment-based decision making), ideology (commitment and patient advocacy), and experience (unit-based knowledge and knowledge of health care providers)

(Hutchinson, 1990). The simultaneously occurring phases consisted of evaluating, predicting, rule bending, and covering. The evaluating phase incorporated patient (physical and psychological assessment), context (unit history and patient history on unit), rules (reasons for the rules), and nurses' motives (patient versus nurse needs). Predicting was used as nurses rapidly gauged the consequences of risk of rule bending for patients, nurses, and hospital rule-makers. Rules may be implicit or explicit. Timing of the rule bending and controlling information are linked to nurses being persuaded by patients' desires. Nurses may have exaggerated or lied about clinical symptoms or interpreted medication orders flexibly. Covering, as the last phase of responsible subversion, included nurses redefining their behavior based on a rationale. They also may collude with physicians and family members. Secrets are kept, documentation protects rule-bending actions, and the invisible practice of rule bending continued.

Responsible subversion was explained by nurses upholding patients' right to autonomy and self-determination and nurses' commitment to beneficence or doing good for patients. Yet the consequences of responsible subversion were both positive and negative (Hutchinson, 1990). Actions may not be discovered, a questionable positive result. However, institutional rules may be changed by persistent rule bending. For example, in another positive result, visiting hours, originally subverted, were formally changed. Institutional rule-makers, becoming angry and alarmed, might complete incident reports or report nurses by submitting complaints to state boards of nursing, examples of negative results.

When reviewing this study, Munhall (1990) questioned whether nurses considered ethical principles when bending the rules. She also asked if alternate actions were possible during these decisions and whether institutional rules might be based on law and should not be broken. Munhall asked if institutional ideologies differed and compared military institutions versus hospice settings. She directed nurses to gain increased understanding of this complex clinical phenomenon.

Next, Collins (2012) examined rule bending and identified related constructs: workplace deviance and violations of workplace organizational norms. She labeled rule bending a deliberate violation of professional conduct. Institutional contexts of operating procedures, codes of practice, rules, and regulations provided a social environment for violations, according to the researcher. Rule bending may be tolerated and become socialized behavior for staff, and ultimately the drift becomes the norm. She also shared that workarounds block the accomplishment of a work goal. In contrast, Hutchinson's (1990) findings on the theory of responsible subversion process were noted to frame nurses' behavior as having good intent and thus justified.

Collins (2012) presented a model explaining nurses' recognition and management of error in the clinical setting. She discussed nurses' tolerance of rule bending and described it as socialized deviant behavior. Collins represented it as a nurse practice act violation. Labels included bad apples, impaireds, incompetents, criminals, rule benders, and good nurses having a bad day. She also reported on a pilot study that developed an instrument with three subscales based on her model, literature, and findings from a previous study.

The survey results showed that rule bending was practiced frequently by respondents. Reasons were categorized as personal drivers (time, workload, personal needs, and disagreement with rules) and environmental drivers (staffing, medication and supply, physician and staff response, conflict, and communication issues) (Collins 2012).

The highest percentage on the "Often" response to items was: Allow visitors contrary to the facility's policy; Administer medication at a different rate than ordered; and Borrow supplies from one patient to use for another patient. The three highest percentages on examples for "Sometimes" included: Delayed ordered treatment for a patient; Allow children to visit contrary to the facility's policy; and Initiate treatment for a patient without an order, and when ancillary services and staff are slow to respond. Highest-percentage reasons for bending the rules were to ease the workload, to save time, when there were insufficient supplies, and when there was not enough non-nursing support staff. Items were further classified through the lenses of responsible subversion theory and Collins' tolerance for rule bending model.

Reckless nursing can be described by a number of phrases. These are bending the rules, workaround nursing, and responsible subversion. The motivation of all nurses who bend the rules, according to literature, is beneficence, that is, decisions made for the good of patients. Nonetheless, the legal implications of bending the rules can be severe for nurses, and have a potential for negative, personal outcomes for patients.

Patient Safety: Implications for Reckless Nursing

Patient safety initiatives continue to be implemented in U.S. health care agencies and worldwide. Organizations implement strategies, such as safety net software, to encourage employees to report potential safety threats and errors. The culture of blame, whereby punishment and disapproval were targeted at improving performance, was replaced with the no blame culture. Experienced nurse administrators reacted; the no blame culture did not fit practice environments, since staff behavior required management strategies and performance improvement. Thereafter, the Just Culture approach was introduced. The Just Culture is based on Reason's (1990) theory and Marx's (2007) methods of addressing safety in health care organizations. Increased safety has been attributed to the Just Culture approach (Marx, 2007).

Health care practitioners have used Reason's (1990) human error theory (HET) as a framework for understanding health care errors and organizational failures. According to Reason (2000), two approaches explain errors and procedural violations: person and system. The person approach relies on a reporting culture; individuals targeted for being responsible for errors may not report them, thus limiting analysis and opportunities to address safety threats. The person approach restricts safety efforts. Blame of an individual does not necessarily result in improved patient safety. Systems problems require a multifaceted approach. A systems analysis of safety threats separates blameless from blameworthy actions.

Active failures and latent conditions allow holes in Reason's (1990) Swiss cheese model so that holes align and errors result. Active failures are defined as "the unsafe acts committed by people who are in direct contact with the patient or system" (Reason, 2000, p. 769); they include slips, lapses, fumbles, mistakes, and procedural violations (Reason, 1990). Latent conditions are associated with the system. Decisions on workplace design, spatial building structure, and procedures are examples of safety threats and may be dormant until an accident occurs.

Workplace conditions need to include administrator commitment to safety, clear safety responsibilities, team training, and education to reduce deficiencies in system defenses. Reason's (1990) classification of error types includes three categories:

skill-based slips (errors in execution); rule-based mistakes (errors in planning); and knowledge-based mistakes (errors in planning). Violations are deliberate and can become routine activities for health care providers. The last category is no error. HET helps to explain health care errors and provider performance. Working conditions need to be changed to increase patient safety. Of note is that Reason's (1990) theory introduced the concept of procedural violations. This concept provides a basis for distinguishing errors from reckless practices.

In contrast, the American Organization of Nurse Executives (AONE, 2019) created a series of guiding principles to support nurse leaders facing health care challenges. Citing literature in which egregious behavior by nurses who killed patients was described, AONE produced a guiding principle aimed at protecting patients from reckless behavior by registered nurses. Major recommendations include effective recruitment, screening, and hiring practices; and ensuring effective clinical onboarding (competency assessment, monitoring behavior, culpability assessment). However, murder is the most extreme example of reckless behavior.

The intents of AONE's (2019) guiding principles were applications to identify and mitigate the behavior of registered nurses/advance practice registered nurses whose actions are harmful to patients. Monitoring performance was essential, accomplished by analysis of the performance of permanent and temporary staff. Data sources include incident reports, sentinel events, complaints, grievances, near miss data, claims data, quality audits, and chart or electronic health record audits. Analysis of data recorded in these documents requires staff to track emerging risk patterns. Risk management, quality improvement, patient safety, mortality and morbidity, and other committees are examples of institutional structures and personnel that monitor safety patterns and identify risk.

The question of whether or not to discipline nurses, other health care providers, and health care staff that violate procedures has challenged administrators of health care institutions. Nurse leaders may think that discipline is justified. In the context of the just culture, reckless behavior is considered a professional violation. "Accountability for behavioral choices dictates accountability" (Pastorius 2007, p. 24, citing Smetzer) according to an expert, and:

> Only if the nurse purposely disregarded a substantial and justifiable risk might disciplinary actions be warranted. Even if the nurse held a mistaken belief that the risk was justified. In a just culture, the nurse would be coached about safer behavioral choices, but not subjected to disciplinary actions [Pastorius, 2007, p. 24 citing Smetzer].

The Institute for Safe Medication Practices (ISMP, 2012), citing selected findings from the Agency for Healthcare Research and Quality Hospital Survey on Patient Safety Culture, pointed out that humans practice at-risk behaviors when they justify them. At-risk behaviors may persist and become normative behavior in groups. In addition to shortcuts, policies are violated. Reckless behavior, such as violations of policies, needs to be called out by staff at all levels to alert colleagues, managers, and administrators to safety threats. According to ISMP, peer coaching was preferable to counseling from managers for helping to eliminate risky behavior.

Amori and Curtin (Relias Media, 2006) reported survey results on risk managers' survey responses. The 30 randomly selected hospitals sampled had established non-punitive policies to encourage staff to report safety issues, including near misses and error events. They presented findings at the annual meeting of the American Society for Healthcare Risk Management. Amori noted that the nonpunitive approach to health care errors resulted in staff "disregard for rules and policies because they think they won't be disciplined for their actions" (Relias Media, 2006, para. 4). Neither the blame nor the no blame approaches to staff-involved errors were advocated. The Just Culture (Marx, 2007) approach promotes the reporting of safety threats. It also takes violators of procedures to task by remediation or disciplinary processes.

An alternative approach to remediation was described by Matthews, Benton, Moreland, and Wagner (2019) for nurses sanctioned for practice violations. The Knowledge, Skills, Training, Assessment & Research (KSTAR) Nursing Pilot Program was implemented by the Texas Board of Nursing. The program included a course on nursing jurisprudence and ethics and a reflective exercise. A comprehensive assessment and analysis of the practice breakdown used cognitive testing and a simulated clinical patient scenario based on nurses' practice settings. Nurse competencies were tested to identify potential gaps. Nurses in the pilot study did not differ in recidivism at 24 months after they completed the program when compared to the standard program.

Summary

Health care providers and other health care agency staff that violate procedures threaten patient safety. As framed by Just Culture approaches (Marx, 2007), the line between at-risk and reckless behavior is fluid. It is then difficult for administrators and clinical colleagues to evaluate the intent of nurses who violate procedures and to provide an opportunity for them to modify their behavior. Violators make an intentional, personal decision; these judgments cannot be measured directly during clinical nursing situations.

Administrative decisions for nurses' performance judged as reckless must be made in health care institutions to assure patient safety. Administrators may prefer to respond to reckless behavior in-house rather than lodge complaints to state boards of professional nursing practice for review. Employees are required to participate in remediation or disciplinary actions for continued employment in health care institutions.

Counseling and disciplinary requirements become part of nurses' permanent record in a health care institution. However, administrative decisions that result in internal solutions to reckless behavior, by not reporting violations of professional practice standards to state boards of nursing or the criminal justice system, may not be under the control of the health care institution. Health care provider violations and poor patient outcomes might become public regardless of administrator decisions. The difference between error as a mistake or a crime could be decided in the criminal justice system. A case illustrates this issue. Kelman (2019) reported on a registered nurse charged with reckless homicide and impaired adult abuse as a result of a medication error in which a patient received a dose of a paralyzing drug, vecuronium, instead of versed, obtained from a prescribing cabinet. The nurse's intent to harm was absent.

The blurred boundaries of nurses and physicians in clinical settings most likely provide an opportunity for nurses to step outside their scope of practice. Despite on-the-job training for nurses that provides local certifications for high-acuity patient care, such as caring for ICU patients needing ECMO (extracorporeal membrane oxygenation), boundary violations might be tolerated by unit nursing staff and other health care providers.

Nurses are autonomous persons who practice in different settings. Their work environment constitutes discretionary space for clinical decisions (Dekker, 2009). Nurses' autonomy provides a space for reckless behavior to occur, as does their commitment to beneficent practice. Nurses who break the rules threaten patient safety. Furthermore, nurse managers who discipline nursing staff for reckless behavior are obligated to monitor them over time.

Some unit cultures demonstrate procedural violations as normative. The responsibility of health care providers, such as nurses, is to report at-risk behaviors or procedural violations of coworkers. This charge remains despite a conspiracy of silence (Boothman, 2016).

Strategies

Strategies to support nurses involved in reckless nursing care situations are presented in Table 13. Activities are supported by research and evidence-based citations with a caring focus.

Table 13. Strategies to Change Reckless Behavior and Support Involved Nurses

Strategies to Effect Change	Evidence-Based Citations
Theory-based education of nursing staff following administration and analysis of Collins' (2012) survey on bending the rules, conducted in their workplace, followed by intermittent workshops at least twice a year	Ray et al. (2011)
Nursing grand rounds on caring in the human health experience, moral action, and the ethics of caring: applied to reckless nursing practice; crucial conversation on bending the rules start with sharing stories and analysis of ethical principles	Chinn (2011)
Leadership conference on causal explanations for responsible subversion based on analyzing nurse caring and environmental drivers of bending the rules (Collins, 2012); annual conferences	Ray (2013)
Monitor statistical patterns to identify risk patterns framed by the professionalism caring attribute, preventing harm, and outcomes following development of healing relationships	Roach (2002) Halldorsdottir (1991) Watson (2005)
Counsel nurses using lovingkindness so that demonstration of their high risk, reckless behavior is mitigated	Watson (2007)
Discipline nurses using lovingkindness so that high risk, reckless behavior is mitigated	Watson (2006) Watson (2007)
Do not publicly shame nurses but guide them as an application of respect for their dignity and well-being and an investment in compassion	Swanson (1991) Watson (2002; 2007)
Provide educational sessions to develop competence and in recognition of their frame of reference	Roach (2002) Watson (2007)

Strategies to Effect Change	Evidence-Based Citations
Conduct thorough investigations of failures; listen to both sides and consider both perspectives	Watson (2005) Watson (2007)
Share relevant information about reckless, performance-related situations with entire team and maintain provider anonymity	Watson (2007)
Report unprofessional conduct to state board of nursing, other regulatory agency, or professional organization	Halldorsdottir (1991)

Conclusion

Nurses who bend the rules take risks that put patients and themselves into situations that initially center on a decision intended to benefit patients. However, the outcomes of this risky behavior cannot be predicted. A crucial conversation needs to be held on bending the rules or responsible subversion.

Intentionally breaking rules is deviant behavior and creates error-prone situations. Other approaches are available to initiate policy and procedure change in health care institutions when rules need to be replaced. Education of nursing staff on responsible subversion provides opportunities for discussion and suggestions for different decisions and actions.

Discussion Questions

1. What is the main distinguishing characteristic that differentiates bending the rules from accidental errors?

2. What are the cultural characteristics of units in which the norm for nursing practice is bending the rules?

3. Describe how procedural violations fit into the literature on bending the rules and the Just Culture theory (Marx, 2007).

4. Explain the basic social-psychological process of responsible subversion related to health care agency rules as explained by Hutchinson (1990).

5. What are the positive and negative outcomes for patients and nurses of bending the rules?

AUTHOR SELECTION

Hutchinson, S. (1990); Responsible subversion: A study of rule-bending among nurses. *Scholarly Inquiry for Nursing Practice, 4*(1), 3–17.

REFERENCES

American Organization of Nurse Executives. (2019). *AONE Guiding Principles: To Protect Patients from Reckless Behavior by Registered Nurses.* http://www.aone.org/resources/reckless-behavior.pdf.

Anonymous. (1999). Case 6: Tracheostomy Care: Intensive care sister who did not follow unit guidelines. *British Journal of Nursing, 8*(11). 707.

Austin, S. (2001). Policies and procedures: Friend or foe? Part 3. *Nursing Management, 32*(3). 22–23.

Boothman, R.C. (2016). Breaking through dangerous silence to tap an organization's richest source of information: its own staff. *Joint Commission Journal on Quality and Patient Safety, 42*(4), 147–148.

Carruth, A.K., & Booth, D. (1999). Disciplinary actions against nurses: Who is at risk? *Journal of Nursing Law, 6*(3), 55–62.

Chassin, M.R., & Loeb, J.M. (2013). High-reliability care: Getting there from here. *Milbank Memorial Quarterly, 91*(3), 459–490.

Chinn, P.L. (2019). The evolution of nursing's ethics of caring. In W. Rosa, S. Horton-Deutsch, & J. Watson (Eds.), *A handbook for caring science: Expanding the paradigm* (pp. 37–52). Springer Publishing.

Collins, S.E. (2012). Rule bending by nurses: Environmental and personal drivers. *Journal of Nursing Law, 25*(1), 14–26.

Dekker, S.W. (2009). Just culture: Who gets to draw the line? *Cognition, Technology & Work, 11*, 177–185.

Devettere, R.J. (2016). Medical and behavioral research. In R.J. Devettere, *Practical decision making in health care ethics* (pp. 463–528). Georgetown University Press.

Fiesta, J. (1996). Legal issues in long-term care–Part II. *Nursing Management, 27*(2), 18–19.

Hader, R. (2006). Put employee termination etiquette to practice. *Nursing Management, 37*(12), 6.

Halldorsdottir, S. (1991). Five basic modes of being with another. In D.A. Gaut, & M. Leininger (Eds.), *Caring: The compassionate healer* (pp. 37–49). National League for Nursing.

Hutchinson, S. (1990); Responsible subversion: A study of rule-bending among nurses. *Scholarly Inquiry for Nursing Practice, 4*(1), 3–17.

Institute for Safe Medication Practices. (2012, May 17). *Just culture and its critical link to patient safety (part I).* https://www.ismp.org/resources/just-culture-and-its-critical-link-patient-safety-part-i.

Joint Commission. (2016, May). *Code of Conduct.* https://www.jointcommission.org/assets/1/18/Code_of_Conduct_2016.pdf.

Kelman, B. (2019, February 4). Vanderbilt ex-nurse indicted on reckless homicide charge after deadly medication swap. https://www.tennessean.com/story/news/health/2019/02/04/vanderbilt-nurse-reckless-homicide-charge-vecuronium-versed-drug-error/2772648002/.

Kunyk, D., Milner, M., & Overend, A. (2016). Disciplining virtue: Investigating the discourses of opioid addiction in nursing. *Nursing Inquiry, 23*, 315–326.

Lagana, K. (2000). The "right" to a caring relationship: The law and ethic of care. *Journal of Perinatal & Neonatal Nursing, 14*(2), 12–24.

Liberati, E.G. (2016). Separating, replacing, intersecting: The influence of context on the construction of the medical-nursing boundary. *Social Science & Medicine, 172*, 135–143. http://dx.doi.org/10.1016/j.socscimed.2016.11.008.

Lilly, L.L. (2015). Risky business: Your personal conduct outside of work can lead to discipline from the nursing boards. *West Virginia Nurse, March/April*, 7. https://d3ms3kxrsap50t.cloudfront.net/uploads/publication/pdf/1137/West_Virginia_Nurse_2_15.pdf.

MacLean, L., Coombs, C., & Breda, K. (2016). Unprofessional workplace conduct: Defining and defusing it. *Nursing Management, 47*(9), 30–34.

Marx, D. (2007). *Patient safety and the "Just culture"* [PowerPoint slides]. Outcome Engineering. https://www.unmc.edu/patient-safety/_documents/patient-safety-and-the-just-culture.pdf.

Matthews, D.W., Benton, D., Moreland, S.C., & Wagner, T. (2019). Addressing nursing practice breakdown: An alternative approach to remediation. *Journal of Nursing Regulation, 10*(1), 28–34.

Michael, J.E. (2004). Investigate thoroughly to avoid wrongful termination suits. *Nursing Management, 35*(5), 20, 22, 53.

Munhall, P.L. (1990). Response to "Responsible Subversion: A Study of Rule-Bending Among Nurses." *Scholarly Inquiry for Nursing Practice, 4*(1), 19–22.

Pastorius, D. (2007). Crime in the workplace, part 1. *Nursing Management, 38*(10), 18, 20, 22, 24, 26–27.

Petrovic, M.A., & Scholl, A.T. (2018). Why we need a single definition of disruptive behavior. *Cureus*. doi: 10.7759/cureus.2339.

Pugh, D. (2011). A fine line: The role of personal and professional vulnerability in allegations of unprofessional conduct. *Journal of Nursing Law, 14*(1), 21–31.

Ray, M.A. (2013). The Theory of Bureaucratic Caring for Nursing Practice in the organizational culture. In M.C. Smith, M.C. Turkel, & Z.R. Wolf (Eds.), *Caring in nursing classics: An essential resource* (pp. 309–320). Springer Publishing.

Ray, M.A., Turkel, M.C., & Cohn, J. (2011). In A.W. Davidson, M.A. Ray, & M.C. Turkel, *Relational caring complexity: The study of caring and complexity in health care hospital organizations* (pp. 93–124). Springer Publishing.

Reason, J. (1990). *Human error.* Cambridge University Press.

Reason, J. (2000). Human error: Models and management. *BMJ, 320*, 768–770.

Relias Media. (2006, January 1). *Defining reckless behavior hard with just culture.* https://www.reliasmedia.com/articles/120628-defining-reckless-behavior-hard-with-just-culture.
Relias Media. (2006, January 1). *"Just culture" model called better, allows discipline for reckless behavior.* http://www.reliasmedia.com/articles/120636-just-culture-model-called-better-allows-discipline-for-reckless-behavior.
Roach, S.M. (1990, December 5–8). Creating communities of caring [Paper]. *Curriculum revolution: Community building and activism* (pp. 123–138). Scottsdale, AZ. National League for Nursing Conference.
Roach, S.M. (2002). Caring: The human mode of being (2nd ed.). Canadian Healthcare Association.
Swanson, K.M. (1991). Empirical development of a middle range theory of caring. *Nursing Research, 40*, 161–166.
Taxis, K., & Barber, N. (2002). Causes of intravenous medication errors: An ethnographic study. *Quality and Safety in Health Care, 12*(5), 343–347. doi: 10.1136/qhc.12.5.343.
Thompson Reuters. (2019). *Recklessness.* FindLaw. https://injury.findlaw.com/accident-injury-law/recklessness.html.
Watson, J. (2002). Intentionality and caring-healing consciousness: A practice of transpersonal nursing. *Holistic Nursing Practice, 16*(4), 12–19.
Watson, J. (2005). *Caring science as sacred science.* F.A. Davis.
Watson, J. (2006). Caring theory as an ethical guide to administrative and clinical practices. *Nursing Administration Quarterly, 30*(1), 48–55.
Watson, J. (2010). *Core Concepts of Jean Watson's Theory of Human Caring/Caring Science.* https://www.watsoncaringscience.org/files/PDF/watsons-theory-of-human-caring-core-concepts-and-evolution-to-caritas-processes-handout.pdf.
Wolf, Z.R., Donohue-Smith, M., & Wolf, K.C. (2019). Nurses who murder or who are accused of murder. *International Journal for Human Caring, 23*(1), 51–70.

Multiple-Choice Questions

1. **What is the difference between at-risk and reckless behavior shown by health care providers?**
   A. Mistakenly justified
   B. Deliberately disregards risk
   C. Intentionally disruptive
   D. Verbally aggressive

2. **What does reckless behavior of health care staff require administrators to do with reckless staff?**
   A. Counsel
   B. Fire
   C. Discipline
   D. Discuss

3. **When do state boards of nursing need to be involved in responding to nurses deemed to be reckless?**
   A. As soon as reckless behavior is identified
   B. When the reckless behavior begins to be abandoned
   C. When internal institutional strategies fail to change behavior
   D. During the process of documenting reckless behavior

4. **What is one result for nurses of being disciplined by state boards of nursing following allegations of misconduct?**
   A. Used rule bending
   B. Kept their former personal identities
   C. Convinced them to change work sites
   D. Changed the way they saw nursing work

CHAPTER 11

Missed Nursing Care

A Covert Error of Omission

Joanne R. Duffy, PHD, RN, FAAN

Objectives

    1. Analyze the extent and occurrence types of missed nursing care.

    2. Examine the relationship of missed nursing care to important health care outcomes.

    3. Contrast evidence-based explanations for missed nursing care.

    4. Compare the theoretical, ethical, and regulatory consequences of missed nursing care.

    5. Defend strategies for reducing missed nursing care.

Critical Incidents

Several years ago, a story broke about a hospital that agreed to a $2.7-million out-of-court settlement, but denied wrongdoing, related to nurses not noticing a 61-year-old woman's deteriorating condition (Curtin, 2011). In this case, the woman was admitted with pneumonia and gradually became short of breath, resulting in a resuscitation attempt that left her with severe brain damage, unable to care for herself. Although assessment and routine monitoring of hospitalized patients are nursing standards (American Nurses Association [ANA], 2015), the nurses accused in the case attributed their lack of appropriate assessment and monitoring to short staffing. The plaintiff's attorneys used that explanation to argue that inadequate nurse staffing levels led directly to the permanent brain damage the woman suffered. This settlement was extremely large, to put it mildly, because at the time the range for hospital out-of-court settlements was $125,000 to $235,000. Moreover, the family refused to agree to any conditions that the settlement remain confidential, and the case was broadcast on national news channels, including CBS's *60 Minutes*, and was published in *Reader's Digest* and several large newspapers. Thus, not only did the health system incur outrageous costs, but it also suffered serious damage to its image and credibility as a health system that provides excellent patient care.

Although the above incident was serious, costly, and widely publicized, similar, but less obvious, incidents occur daily in hospitals. For example, busy hospital registered nurses (RNs) working on medical-surgical units regularly delegate vital signs to assistive personnel (e.g., nursing assistants). Without adequate follow-up of nursing assistants, a rising temperature, for example, might be missed or inaccurately documented, providing the set up for an untreated infection. Another almost obscure example relates to accurate and timely communication between hospital nurses and physicians. Often RNs find participation in clinical rounds to be challenging because they cannot leave their patients unattended. Without adequate communication, however, physicians are sometimes left uninformed about a patient's changes in status, leading to undiagnosed or untreated conditions. Other scenarios, similar but not as shocking as the former lawsuit example, include gradually deteriorating changes in patients' conditions (e.g., slowly decreasing levels of consciousness, drops in blood pressure or unobserved post-operative retroperitoneal bruising) that go unnoticed in the busyness of simultaneously providing care to several acutely ill persons. Unfortunately, clinical worsening could be present for many hours and the clinical response might be delayed or not provided at all. This represents a dangerous scenario in light of the evidence that shows that 80 percent of patients who suffer in-hospital cardiac arrest exhibited signs of deterioration in the hours preceding the event (Stevenson et al., 2016).

Background

The literature has been replete in recent years with persistent incidences of inadequate performance of routine standards of nursing care by hospital-based RNs (Duffy et al., 2018; Hessels, 2019; McMullen, 2017). For example, patient falls (some with injury), catheter-associated urinary tract infections (CAUTIs), pressure injuries, problems related to transitions in care, struggles with facilitating patients' early mobility, inadequate medication teaching, poor hand hygiene, reports of discontinuity of nursing care, and poor oral hygiene practices in hospitalized elders continue to plague hospitals, nursing homes, schools, and outpatient facilities (Coker et al., 2017; Manojilovich et al., 2017; Yakusheva et al., 2017). Websites have sprouted up for patients to relay their hospital horror stories, and noted clinicians have authored books (Rosenthal, 2018) and websites to help patients protect themselves when hospitalized.

In just the last 18 months, this author alone has witnessed numerous instances of inadequate nursing care. For example, several clinical nurses at a mid-sized community Magnet® hospital allowed a confused patient to go unmonitored for over 18 hours despite physician orders for telemetry monitoring. The patient arrested and died at the hospital, and both the nurses and the hospital are facing a large lawsuit. In a peer review analysis of this case, unit nurses explained that it was acceptable nursing practice to leave monitoring leads off a confused patient who continued to disconnect them. When asked if the decision to discontinue monitoring the patient should have been discussed with the physician team, the nurses stated that they did not ask the physicians for permission to discontinue monitoring.

In another incident, an emergency department (ED) nurse failed to properly assess a woman with neurological symptoms who was labeled a drinker by an EMT. The patient subsequently suffered a stroke and was left unable to work. The nurse and the health system settled the case out of court for several million dollars. In this case, the ED nurse mistook the woman's neurological symptoms to be those related to alcohol intake as she had been told. However, she failed to use her own nursing assessment skills, accepting the label of drinker which had been relayed to her by the EMT, and in the process, undermined important treatment decisions that risked the patient's prognosis.

In another occurrence, a frustrated physician reported hospital nurses' failure to ambulate one of his post-operative patients to The Joint Commission (TJC). According to his complaint, he had tried several times to communicate the importance of ambulation to the nurses, the nurse manager, and even wrote the order, ambulate 3 × daily, in the patient's record to no avail. The hospital was required to communicate a remediation plan to TJC, and the patient was transferred to a nursing home for extended rehabilitation for deconditioning. The patient's family filed a lawsuit against the hospital that is now pending. Nurses and nursing assistants on the unit as well as the nurse manager have been disciplined, and the story was published in the local newspaper. Finally, issues of improper delegation to unlicensed personnel and even falsification of records related to basic nursing care have been observed.

Most nurses would agree that these situations are not optimal care, but are not medical errors per se. In fact, many people and several shifts may overlook such occurrences as they are taking place. Thus, it conveys the impression that no one person is responsible. In the instances cited above, no one interfered with or called attention to the provision of nursing care during the process; rather, it was only after a lawsuit was filed that a retrospective examination of the incidences occurred.

Most often what emerges during after-the-fact discussions of such incidences are claims of system problems. In most instances, these system problems are tolerated. Often nurses explain these forms of omissions with statements such as "You can't expect this level of care when we are understaffed" or "Suzie is a new nurse and is trying to learn how to prioritize." Some nursing leaders also rationalize missed nursing care with statements such as "Many nurses are in orientation" or "After we finish upgrading the electronic health system, we will concentrate on this." Although they are not considered errors of commission (doing something that does not follow the standard of care), they do represent errors of omission (failing to act according to the standard of care) (Kalish, 2016).

A common theme in these examples is lacking, limited, or missed basic or fundamental nursing care. Missed nursing care is defined as any aspect of required patient care that is omitted (either in part or in whole) or delayed (Kalisch et al., 2009). Using this definition, missed nursing care can be thought of as a subset of the medical error category known as error of omission. Errors of omission are incidences of failing to do the right thing, such as not ambulating a patient, failing to reposition a patient to prevent skin breakdown, failing to carry out ordered interventions, or failing to administer medications on time that lead to adverse outcomes or have significant potential for such outcomes. An error of omission occurs when a health care professional fails to act as a reasonably prudent professional would in the same case (Scruth & Pugh, 2018). These errors occur from an action not taken or when an appropriate action is left out from a process. For example, using the ANA's *Nursing Scope and Standards of Practice* (2015) as a guide, errors of omission may include:

- failing to holistically assess a patient or prioritize patient assessment based on patients' immediate conditions or anticipated needs AND failing to convey assessment data to facilitate safe transitions and continuity in care delivery.

- neglecting to collaborate with patients to define expected outcomes, integrating the health care consumer's culture, values, and ethical considerations OR generating a time frame for the attainment of these outcomes.
- failing to use caring behaviors with patients and families to develop therapeutic relationships.
- overlooking the person, task, direction, communication, supervision, or evaluation of nursing care when it is delegated to others [ANA, 2015].

Errors of omission diminish the ability of the nurse to provide a safe environment, and some errors may even lead to disciplinary action. For example, the Texas Board of Nursing Rule 217.11(1) (B) states that each nurse must implement measures to promote a safe environment for all patients and others (Texas Board of Nursing, 2019). Nursing errors of omission can have significant consequences for patients, their family members, health systems, and nurses themselves. The impact of these errors on nurses may include moral distress, decreased job satisfaction and turnover (Larrabee et al., 2003), compassion fatigue and burnout (Kalisch, 2016). "Errors of omission can influence whether a nurse is meeting the minimum standard of care and competency requirements to provide safe and effective care to patients" (Laws & Hughes, 2018, p. 5).

Malpractice claims (Reising & Allen, 2007) often involve examples of missed nursing care. They are often filed to recover compensation for health care errors, including those of omission. Such claims are intended to recover past, current, and future medical expenses, lost wages, costs associated with disability and disfigurement, rehabilitation expenses, and estimated costs of pain and suffering as a result of the omitted care.

Although most lawsuits involving health care errors are against hospitals and health systems, increasingly, legal cases against individual nurses are occurring (Nursing Service Organization, 2015). Moreover, incidences of missed nursing care and their consequences impact one's own sense of professionalism, value to the health system, and enthusiasm for continued engagement in the work.

Literature

Occasionally labeled rationing of nursing care, RNs who perceive limited resources such as time or inadequate work environments or who have underdeveloped skills, are forced to ration their attention across patients in their care by using their clinical judgment to prioritize assessments and interventions, which may increase the risk of negative patient outcomes (Schubert et al., 2008). Differences in individual RN abilities, such as time management skills or lack of understanding of the importance of certain responsibilities, may also influence missed nursing care.

In the hospital environment, RNs plan, deliver, and evaluate patients' symptoms and responses to care, alleviate suffering, and advocate for and promote health and healing (ANA, 2015). RNs also coordinate, provide, and evaluate many interventions linked to the work of other health professionals, supervise unlicensed personnel, and participate in unit governance, often creating competing demands (Duffy, 2018). Because RNs coordinate, provide, and evaluate interventions prescribed by others as well as plan, deliver, and evaluate their own nurse-initiated interventions, it is not hard to imagine that occurrences of missed nursing care have developed in hospitals, representing an enormous problem with serious consequences for patients, nurses, and health systems.

In the last two decades, a number of areas of missed nursing care were recognized, such as inadequate patient mobilization, poor thorough assessments, insufficient hygiene and feeding processes, scanty communication, patient teaching and discharge planning, and ineffective surveillance and care documentation (Recio-Saucedo et al., 2018). Offering psychological and emotional support to patients, parental support, and teaching have also been reported missing (Rochefort & Clarke, 2010; Schubert et al., 2008). In fact, assessment was reported to be missed by 44 percent of respondents while interventions, basic care, and planning were reported to be missed by over 70 percent of the survey respondents. A review of 17 quantitative studies by Papastavrou et al. (2014) concluded that negative consequences for both patients and nurses were associated with rationed or missed care. Reasons reported for missed nursing care across 10 hospitals were reported as inadequate labor resources (93.1 percent), followed by material resources (89.6 percent) and communication (81.7 percent). Thus, the prioritization strategies of some RNs leave patients vulnerable to unmet educational, emotional, physical, and psychological needs.

Individual nurse characteristics, such as work experience or communication ability, and organizational features of the work environment that may contribute to missed nursing care are important to consider since their presence (or absence) may generate or even predict the conditions for missed nursing care.

Individual Factors

Kalisch et al. (2006) identified individual nurse characteristics, such as demographics, work experience, decision-making abilities, work habits, understanding of responsibilities, and values/beliefs as antecedents of missed nursing care. Differences in these characteristics may influence the process of care, in particular its timeliness, completeness, and consistency. Sadly, as nurses deliver substandard care over time, evidence has linked it to job dissatisfaction, plans to leave, and absenteeism. In fact, in one study, 58 percent of the variance in intent to leave was accounted for by missed nursing care (Tschamen et al., 2010).

Although limited by the design and the Australian/Tasmanian sample, Blackman et al. (2015) used structural equation modeling to demonstrate significant direct relationships between individual RNs' characteristics and missed nursing care. In this study, health professional communication, nurses' level of work (dis)satisfaction, and intent to leave, directly contributed to the overall variance of missed nursing care. These results are somewhat consistent with Kalisch et al.'s work, although they explain only 30 percent of the variance in reported missed nursing care (Kalisch et al., 2011).

Organizational Factors

Nurses' work environment is defined as an organizational characteristic that facilitates or constrains professional nursing practice (Lake, 2002). The complexity and demands of the current hospital work environment on professional nurse responsiveness to changing patient needs, relationships with leaders and other health professionals, access to adequate resources, and nurses' perception of their practice autonomy may intensify occurrences of missed nursing care. Thus, along with individual nurse factors, organizational factors may contribute to missed nursing care. Organizationally, inadequate human resources, insufficient teamwork, unavailability of supplies, ineffective delegation, and long working hours have been linked to missed nursing care (Kalisch, 2016). In Kalisch et al.'s 10-hospital study, labor resources, material resources, and communication were common reasons cited for missed nursing care, but shift work, absenteeism, perceived staffing adequacy, and patient workloads were also significantly associated with missed nursing care (Kalisch et al., 2011). A more recent study of three hospitals in North Carolina found similar results; however, the sample and low response rate (27.3 percent) limited results (Maloney et al., 2015). Blackman et al. (2015) and Jones et al. (2015) demonstrated adequacy of resources as the strongest predictor of missed nursing care. Finally, nurse staffing continues to be associated with missed nursing care, and omission rates were high as reported in the systematic review of Griffiths et al. (2018). Elements of planning and communication were more often missed than clinical care. The researchers suggested that objective measures of care should also be studied.

In summary, although evidence exists that describes the phenomenon of missed nursing care, its associated reasons, and some influencing factors, measurement and sampling concerns have limited results. Better evidence is needed to understand the antecedents and consequences of missed nursing care to design targeted strategies and/or innovations that improve patient and system outcomes.

Professional Standards and Nursing Theory

The American Nurses Association's publication, *Nursing Scope and Standards of Practice* (2015), defines professional nursing and guides nurses in practice. Furthermore, it specifies duties and competencies that all registered nurses, regardless of role, population, or specialty, are expected to perform. The main purpose of these standards is to direct and maintain safe and clinically competent nursing practice. Violating a professional standard can expose nurses and their workplaces to liability and potential loss of licensure.

Meanwhile, the *Code of Ethics for Nurses with Interpretive Statements* (ANA, 2015) is a document that includes the ethical obligations and duties of all professional nurses that coincide with the standards of practice. It is the profession's nonnegotiable norms of behavior that guide nurses in understanding their commitment to society. It discusses the primacy of the nurse's commitment to the patient and the protection of patients' health, safety and rights. It also describes nurses' responsibility and accountability for individual nursing practice as well as the appropriate delegation of tasks consistent with the obligation to provide optimum patient care. The ANA Code of Ethics states that "[individual] registered nurses (RNs) bear primary responsibility for the nursing care their patients receive and are individually accountable for their own practice" (ANA, 2015, p. 2).

The *Code of Ethics for Nurses with Interpretive Statements* (ANA, 2015) is based on sound ethical principles of autonomy (the right of patients to retain control over their body); beneficence (intention to do the most good); nonmaleficence (do no harm); and justice (fairness). As important members of the health care team, RNs who fail to exercise their responsibility and accountability related to important health care decisions may be in violation of the code of ethics and could be liable for damages.

To that end, Kalisch and colleagues developed the Missed Nursing Care Model (2009) after extensive examination of the topic. The model is a middle-range theory that depicts components involved in missed nursing care. Those components are the care environment that facilitates or inhibits the practice of nursing (such as labor resources); the nursing process; internal perceptions and decision processes of the nurse (such as habits, values, and beliefs); care that is provided as planned; and care that is delayed or omitted and consequential patient outcomes. Omissions or delays in care may occur at any stage of the nursing process and may be influenced by factors within the care environment that facilitate or inhibit the practice of nursing, such as demands for patient care, resource allocation, and professional relationships. The model can be used as a guide for understanding the factors that contribute to missed nursing care and resultant patient outcomes, and to stimulate future research.

The Quality Caring Model© (Duffy, 2018), on the other hand, is a middle-range theory that has been adopted in over 56 hospitals nationwide as the basis for professional nursing practice. The model calls attention to the persistent crisis of health care quality in America. Although many nursing theories have spoken to nursing's inherent relationship to quality of care, Duffy's model explicitly ties nurse caring to patient quality. In this middle-range theory, nursing is viewed as a valuable, but often hidden, contributor to patient and health system value. The theory espouses that, although many health professionals are caring, registered nurses maintain 24/7 presence, have the most direct contact with patients and families, are a stabilizing force in the disjointed health care system and are influential in the prevention of adverse outcomes. They do this in the context of caring relationships where routine everyday behaviors (such as assessments, re-positioning, mobility, hygiene care, and health counseling), together with the perceived more challenging nursing behaviors (such as managing patients' endotracheal tubes, titrating multiple vasoactive intravenous medications, delivering end-of-life discussions, and treating dysrhythmias), form the process of nursing care. Both are tied to quality patient outcomes, especially in the hospital environment where patients are most vulnerable.

Duffy maintained that when nurses practice from a caring theoretical base, patient, nurse, and system outcomes advance. Unfortunately, in the last few years, the highly technological, cure-oriented, and financially driven hospital environment has contributed to the notion that routine basic nursing care is not significant (Duffy, 2018). Thus, it is delegated to others and, although RNs remain responsible for its provision, it is not always tracked or followed through for adequate and timely delivery.

Accrediting Agencies, Quality Organizations, and Databases

Several accrediting agencies and reimbursement organizations (e.g., Centers for Medicare and Medicaid Services [CMS]) have issued standards for safe and quality care. For example, TJC requires an RN to supervise all nursing care 24/7; assess and reassess patients as conditions change; and address important patient safety goals (TJC, 2019).

The National Quality Forum (NQF), a not-for-profit, nonpartisan, membership-based organization, works to catalyze improvements in health care. The Department of Health and Human Services relies on the guidance of NQF's quality measures in federal programs that provide health coverage for Americans. Today, about 300 NQF-endorsed measures are voluntarily used nationwide to publicly report and/or reimburse health systems. Fifteen of these are nursing sensitive (NQF, 2004). Since 2004, these measures have been voluntarily applied in health systems, and in 2014, improvement was shown in the areas of patient falls with injury, nurse turnover, and increase in nurse time spent at the bedside (NQF, 2014). However, recent NQF reports on nursing quality in the last five years could not be found.

The National Database of Nursing Quality Indicators measures nursing quality through evidence-based, nursing-sensitive quality indicators. Participation in this database provides hospitals with unit-level performance comparisons (Press-Ganey, 2019). Although this database does not provide data on missed nursing care, it does report data that are known consequences of missed nursing care, such as pressure ulcer and patient fall rates.

It is interesting that missed nursing care is not routinely reported as a nursing-sensitive quality measure per se because the evidence points to its growing existence. However, because it represents a negative aspect of nursing that reflects on nurses, nurse leaders, and health systems, it is not surprising.

Regulation of Nursing Practice

Each jurisdiction (state) legislates nurse practice acts, which are enforced by each state's board of nursing. These laws regulate nurses' qualifications for licensure and the titles they are certified to use and stipulates their scope of practice. Boards of nursing hold nurses accountable for conduct based on legal, ethical, and professional standards. Nursing regulation uses evidence-based standards of practice, advances in technology, and demographic and social research in its mission to protect the public. Nurses are required to comply with the law and related rules to maintain their licenses.

Pertinent to this chapter, the National Council of State Boards of Nursing (NCSBN) convened two panels of experts representing education, research, and practice to discuss delegation in 2015. As a result, the National Guidelines for Nursing Delegation provides clarification on the responsibilities associated with delegation (NCSBN, 2016). Additionally, these guidelines are meant to address delegation with respect to the various levels of nursing licensure (i.e., APRN, RN, and LPN/VN, where the state NPA allows).

In essence, the document reaffirms that nurses delegate the responsibility for a given task but maintain overall accountability for the patient. In other words, the nurse is responsible for ensuring an assignment given to a delegatee is carried out completely, accurately, and efficiently. Furthermore, the nursing functions of clinical reasoning, nursing judgment, or critical decision making cannot be delegated.

In this document, it is important to distinguish between the terms delegated responsibility and accountability. A delegated responsibility refers to a nursing activity, skill or procedure that is transferred from a licensed nurse to a delegate. Accountability, on the other hand, refers to owning one's behaviors or obligations to oneself and others for one's own choices, decisions and actions as measured against a standard (American Nurses Association, 2015, p. 41). Although the terms accountability and responsibility are often used interchangeably, they are not synonyms. Responsibility relates to what a person is required to do or the performance of specific duties, tasks, or roles. Accountability means being answerable for the decisions made in one's professional practice. One way to understand the difference is to recognize that an individual is responsible *for* something (e.g., administering prescribed medications) and accountable *to* something (e.g., to oneself, society, professional standards). Nursing departments and individual RNs can be held accountable for those activities over which they have autonomy.

In the bulleted sections that follow, the NCSBN provided national guidelines for nursing delegation (NCSBN, 2016). The NCSBN listed five responsibilities of nurses related to delegation:

- The nurse determines when and what to delegate based on the practice setting, the patients' needs and condition, the state/jurisdiction's provisions for delegation, and the employer policies and procedures regarding delegating a specific responsibility.
- The nurse must communicate with the delegatee who will be assisting in providing patient care.
- The nurse must be available to the delegatee for guidance and questions, including assisting with the delegated responsibility, if necessary, or performing it him/herself if the patient's condition or other circumstances warrant doing so.
- The nurse must follow up with the delegatee and the patient after the delegated responsibility has been completed.
- The nurse must provide feedback information about the delegation process and any issues regarding delegatee competence level to the nurse leader.

The delegatee also has responsibilities:

- The delegatee must accept only the delegated responsibilities that he or she is appropriately trained and educated to perform and feels comfortable doing given the specific circumstances in the health care setting and patient's condition.
- The delegatee must maintain competency for the delegated responsibility.
- The delegatee must communicate with the licensed nurse in charge of the patient.
- Once the delegatee verifies acceptance of the delegated responsibility, the delegatee is accountable for carrying out the delegated responsibility correctly and completing timely and accurate documentation per facility policy.

Finally, the NCSBN provides guidelines for employers/nursing leaders:

- The employer must identify a nurse leader responsible for oversight of delegated responsibilities for the facility.
- The designated nurse leader responsible for delegation, ideally with a committee (consisting of other nurse leaders) formed for the purposes of addressing delegation, must determine which nursing responsibilities may be delegated, to whom, and under what circumstances.
- Policies and procedures for delegation must be developed.
- The employer/nurse leader must communicate information about delegation to the licensed nurses and UAP and educate them about what responsibilities can be delegated.
- All delegatees must demonstrate knowledge and competency on how to perform a delegated responsibility.
- The nurse leader responsible for delegation, along with other nurse leaders and

administrators within the facility, must periodically evaluate the delegation process.

• The employer/nurse leader must promote a positive culture and work environment for delegation [NCSBN, 2016].

In 2019, the NCSBN and the ANA released a Joint Position Paper on Delegation (NCSBN, 2019) that further verifies the nursing delegation process. In this position paper, the fact that a nurse is still responsible for determining patient needs and when to delegate, evaluating delegated outcomes, and ensuring overall accountability for delegated nursing responsibilities is reiterated. The delegatee bears the responsibility for accepting activities based on their competency level, for maintaining competence for delegated responsibilities, and for being accountable for carrying out delegated activities completely and correctly. Finally, the nursing leadership responsibilities are highlighted and repeated.

Thus, delegation of all aspects of nursing care remains an important nursing responsibility for which registered nurses are held accountable (NCSBN, 2016). Reports of unprofessional conduct in terms of delegation can be reported to state boards of nursing. State boards of nursing administer and enforce the state nurse practice act and its rules in their ongoing effort to protect the public from unsafe and/or incompetent practitioners. They respond to complaints, provide guidance and, when necessary, enforce disciplinary action.

The model presented by Collins and Mikos (2008) helps to organize situations of unprofessional conduct performed by nursing staff. Two domains in the model are relevant to missed nursing care. In the professional credentialing domain, professional misconduct is a violation of social policy, codes of ethics, or professional standards and is established by competencies and certifications by professional credentialing bodies. In the civil law domain, professional negligence is demonstrated by the breach of professional duty through violation of the standards of care causing harm, prompting a civil lawsuit and the award of money damages to compensate the patient for injury.

The consequential results of nurse practice violations in the case of missed nursing care may include employment actions (such as educational remediation, progressive discipline, and even termination). In severe cases, licensure disciplinary actions may occur when standards of care are breached even in the absence of harm to a patient.

Summary

Missed nursing care is a serious and growing adverse outcome of hospitalization and long-term care organizations. Its occurrence has been rising internationally, and influencing factors have been documented. For example, individual nurses' decision-making and communication habits, attitudes and beliefs about nursing responsibilities as well as organizational factors, such as available resources, team norms and unit culture have been tied to missed nursing care (Recio-Saucedo et al., 2018). A theory of missed nursing care has been developed and professional standards exist to guide nursing practice. Many hospitals use professional practice models and quality data to guide and improve nursing practice. Finally, state regulations exist that hold nurses accountable for their professional conduct.

Despite these available resources, many of today's practicing RNs face difficulties balancing the needs of individual patients, the demands of their employers, their professional values, and the obligations of their profession. This situation is not purely organizational- or systems-related; however, since judgments are made daily by nurses in terms of how nursing care is to be distributed. There is clearly a need for a more thorough understanding of how nurses and nurse leaders experience missed nursing care, how it is evaluated and improved, and how it relates to the obligations inherent in professional nursing practice.

Consistent reports of missed nursing care have questioned whether it is becoming normalized, gradually accepting missed nursing care as the social norm (Duffy, 2018). Such a practice reflects poorly on a profession that is trusted by patients and families, but has also been linked to poor patient outcomes, has become the basis of lawsuits, and generates feelings of dissatisfaction among its own, who face important decisions daily.

Strategies

Various strategies have been proposed to reduce missed nursing care, although none have undergone robust evaluation. For example, increasing teamwork, improving patient engagement, and requiring greater attention of nursing leaders (Duffy, 2018) have been recommended. Categories of suggestions born out of research studies that have been recommended for reducing missed nursing care are presented next.

- Because the day-to-day work environment of hospitals and nursing homes is complex and rushed, omitting basic nursing care may seem insignificant. However, lasting effects on patients and families show otherwise. Thus, rearranging the nursing workload to accommodate these aspects of care, including attending to an adequate and competent appropriate skill mix, reducing interruptions, or attending to the availability of supplies, seems to be necessary to effectively prioritize nursing care.
- Re-educating frontline nursing staff and nursing leaders on the need to effectively delegate nursing care (NCSBN, 2019) is recommended. Re-emphasize that professional accountability is universal and reciprocal. Follow up with case studies and other work-related continuing education.
- Include missed nursing care as a department indicator and routinely review at hospital quality improvement meetings. The MISSCARE Survey (Kalisch & Williams, 2009) is available for use in this regard and has implications for constructing databases for organizations and the profession that could be used as a critical measure for improving quality. Periodically, examining missed care data as well as having the ability to follow long-term trends for the improvement of such patterns provides important patient quality and safety information.
- Enhance organizational culture to maintain patient safety and quality. Although errors of commission are routinely documented and discussed, errors of omission are often not talked about nor reported during shift change or patient hand offs. Leaving this important information out of regular communication among nurses and other health professionals' information stream may have disastrous consequences to patient quality and safety. Use more transparent methods to communicate important aspects of patient care,

including that which is left undone (e.g., culture of safety) (Hessels et al, 2019). Such communication allows for early remediation.

- Because the nursing practice environment has been significantly and inversely linked to missed care, nurse leaders have a tremendous opportunity to facilitate reductions in missed care. For example, in Hessel's (2015) work, findings indicated that the amount of missed nursing care in hospitals can be decreased by 7.3 percent to 13.5 percent simply through improvements in the nursing practice environment. Although the study had some limitations, including the cross-sectional design and self-reported survey data, its findings offer nurse leaders much to act on. Specific interventions aimed at improving any one of the dimensions of the nursing work environment can be used to reduce the amount of missed nursing care.

- Historically, patients have been passive recipients of care, but recent attention to patient-centeredness has increased appreciation of this important aspect of nursing. Kalisch (2015) suggested that nurses advocate for patient involvement by promoting liberal visitation, conducting interprofessional rounds at the patient's bedside, including family members in rounds, and providing patients with access to and the ability to write on their own health care record. Other methods to consider are providing patients with electronic methods for educating and monitoring their own participation in care, creating patient councils, involving patients and families in health care organizational committees, and giving patients responsibilities for their own care.

- Another option for addressing missed nursing care is technology. There is little research that demonstrates how the use of technology can reduce the incidence of missed nursing care; however, some studies have suggested the use of electronic reminders as a method for reducing missed nursing care (Piscoty & Kalisch, 2014; Piscoty et al., 2015). Recently, the use of artificial intelligence (AI) in the form of "service robots" has facilitated delivery of basic nursing care in Japan (Topol, 2019). To meet the needs of an increasingly aging population, the Japanese government subsidized the development costs of robot nurse assistants. These robots can collect patient data and vital signs, deliver meals, and even combat loneliness, allowing nurses more time to spend with patients and families.

- Closer attunement to the structural components of nursing practice is needed by nursing leadership. For example, establishing clear professional role expectations, providing specific direction on how nursing work should be accomplished, performing frequent monitoring using established metrics for judging role performance, fostering teamwork and recognition, and building sustainable positive ownership cultures that apply high expectations for self and others, while continuously observing and perfecting the work, require relentless leadership attention (Duffy, 2018).

- In schools of nursing, enhancing nursing students' awareness of and openness to discussions about missed nursing care is needed (Bagnasco et al., 2017). Also recommended is an increase in critical reflections about collaboration between instructors and clinical sites.

- Although it has been suggested that errors of omission outnumber errors of commission, errors of omission are not yet studied as extensively as errors of commission. However, studies are beginning to emerge. In 2017, Poghosyan et al. published a study looking at errors of omission in primary care, with findings similar to Kalisch's work. In this study, the authors found that omitting patient teaching, patient follow-up, emotional support, and mental health needs were the predominant topics of missed care in the primary care setting. Thus, serious agreement on the problem of missed care upholds the need for continued research, specifically to develop and test nursing interventions to reduce missed care and ultimately correcting the negative patient outcomes known to result from missed nursing care. Just as testing interventions are appropriate to the prevention of errors of commission, they are also appropriate to protect against and prevent errors of omission.

See Table 14 for a list of recommendations for reducing missed nursing care.

Table 14. Overall Strategies for Reducing Missed Nursing Care

Strategies to Effect Change	Evidence-Based Citations
Rearrange nursing workload to accommodate all patient needs	Tubbs-Cooley et al. (2015)
Re-educate frontline and nursing leaders on appropriate delegation techniques	Sager & AbuAlRub (2018) Du et al. (2020)
Use missed nursing care as a quality indicator; routinely measure, monitor, and report findings for improvement	Jones et al. (2019)
Instill cultures of safety where transparency of communication is valued	Hessels et al. (2019)
Increase patient engagement in their care	Tobiano et al. (2015)
Leverage technology to assist with patient care needs	Piscoty & Kalisch (2014)
Increase nursing leadership attention to role expectations, teamwork, and empowerment	Bagnasco et al. (2020)
Introduce the concept of missed nursing care in schools of nursing	Bagnasco et al. (2017)
Investigate specific nursing interventions to reduce missed care and its consequences	Schubert et al. (2020)

Conclusion

Although evidence highlights the incidence and consequences of missed nursing care, staff nurses and nursing leaders may not act on it. Data on missed nursing care are often not obvious; thus, quality improvement departments may not be aware of its frequency and intensity. Individual nurses may not recognize the possibility that unlicensed persons working with them do not complete or even start basic nursing care or even worse, falsify records of this care. Lacking awareness of this possibility may hinder nurses' ability to properly delegate nursing duties and/or to perform accountably. In certain situations, it is not until a lawsuit occurs that administrators and nursing leaders take the necessary steps to examine and reduce missed nursing care in their institutions.

Sometimes, even in such situations, missed nursing care continues to plague nurses, health systems, and patients.

The implications of the errors of omission for nurses are numerous. Research has shown that nurses want to provide quality nursing care, but organizational restraints may sometimes hinder these efforts. Addressing errors of omission improves patient safety while upholding minimum standards of nursing care. As patient advocates, nurses must adhere to professional standards and coordinate with appropriate members of the health care team to meet the care needs of all patients. When those needs are not being met, nurses must take action to resolve issues that prohibit safe and quality care. Nursing leaders must sustain cultures of safety where cohesive teams of clinicians who communicate regularly leverage their collective knowledge and skills to meet all patient needs. Patients trust and expect nurses to do the right thing, including preventing errors of omission.

Discussion Questions

1. Contrast errors of omission with errors of commission. Why is missed nursing care considered an error of omission?

2. What individual and organization factors influence missed nursing care?

3. What delegating responsibilities do nurses have related to transferring nursing work to assistive personnel?

4. How might nurses and nursing leaders regularly monitor missed nursing care for hospital units?

5. What delegating responsibilities do employers and nursing leaders have related to transferring nursing work to assistive personnel?

AUTHOR SELECTION

Longfellow, H.W. (2000). Something left undone [Poem]. In *Longfellow: Poems and other writings* (p. 352). Penguin Putnam Inc.

REFERENCES

American Nurses Association. (2015). *Code of ethics for nurses with interpretive statements.* https://www.nursingworld.org/practice-policy/nursing-excellence/ethics/code-of-ethics-for-nurses/.

American Nurses Association. (2015). Nursing: scope and standards of practice (3rd ed.). https://www.nursingworld.org/practice-policy/scope-of-practice/.

Bagnasco, A., Catania, G., Zanini, M., & Sasso, N. (2020). Are data on missed nursing care useful for nursing leaders? The RN4CAST@IT cross-sectional study. *Journal of Nursing Management, 18*(8), 2136–2145. https://doi-org.dbproxy.lasale.edu/10.1111/jonm.13139.

Bagnasco, A., Timmins F., de Vries, J.M.A., Aleo, G., Zanini, M., Catania, G., & Sasso, L. (2017). Understanding and addressing missed care in clinical placements–Implications for nursing students and nurse educators. *Nurse Education Today, 56,* 1–5. https://doi.org/10.1016/j.nedt.2017.05.015.

Blackman I., Henderson, J., Willis, E., Hamilton, P., Toffoli, L., Verrall, C., Abery, E., & Harvey, C. (2015). Factors influencing why nursing care is missed. *Journal of Clinical Nursing, 24*(1–2), 47–56. https://doi.org/10.1111/jocn.12688.

Coker, E., Ploeg, J., Kaasalainen, S., & Carter, N. (2017). Observations of oral hygiene care interventions provided by nurses to hospitalized older people. *Geriatric Nursing, 38*(1), 17–21.

Collins, S.E., & Mikos, C.A. (2008). Evolving taxonomy of nurse practice violators. *Journal of Nursing Law, 12*(2), 85–91.

Curtin, L. (2011). Ethics case study: Poor staffing results in brain-damaged patient. *American Nurse Today, 6*(12).

Du, H., Yang, Y., Wang, X., Zang, Y. (2020). A cross-sectional observational study of missed nursing care in hospitals in China. *Journal of Nursing Management, 29*(7), 1578–1588. https://doi-org.dbproxy.lasalle.edu/10.1111/jonm.13112.

Duffy, J. (2018). *Quality caring in nursing and health systems: Implications for clinical practice, education, and leadership* (3rd ed.). Springer Publishing.

Duffy, J., Culp, S. & Padrutt, T. (2018). Description of and factors associated with missed nursing care in a community hospital. *Journal of Nursing Administration, 48*, 361–367.

Griffiths, P. Recio-Saucedo, A., Dall'Ora, C., Briggs, J., Maruotti, A., Meredity, P., Smith, G.B., Ball, J., & Missed Care Study Group. (2018). The association between nurse staffing and omissions in nursing care: A systematic review. Journal of Advanced Nursing, 74, 1474–1487. doi: 10.1111/jan.13564.

Hessels, A., Paliwal, M., Weaver, S., Siddiqui, D., & Wurmser, T. (2019). Impact of patient safety culture on missed nursing care and adverse patient events. *Journal of Nursing Care Quality, 34*(4), 287–294.

Hessels, A.J., Flynn, L., Cimiotti, J.P., Cadmus, E., & Gershon, R.R.M. (2015). The impact of the nursing practice environment on missed nursing care. *Clinical Nursing Studies, 3*(4), 60–65.

Joint Commission. (2019). *For nurses.* https://www.jointcommission.org/nurses.aspx.

Jones, C., Chesak, S., Forsyth, D., & Meiers, S. (2019). Missed nursing care as a quality indicator during transition to a dedicated education unit model. *Nursing Education Perspectives, 40*(2), 105–106. https://doi.org/10.1097/01.NEP.0000000000000364.

Jones, T.L., Hamilton, P., & Murry, N. (2015). Unfinished nursing care, missed care, and implicitly rationed care: State of the science review. *International Journal of Nursing Studies, 52*, 1121–1137.

Kalisch, B. (2006). Missed nursing care: A qualitative study. *Journal of Nursing Care Quality, 21*(4), 306-313.

Kalisch, B., Landstrom, G., & Hinshaw, A. (2009). Missed nursing care: A concept analysis. *Journal of Advanced Nursing, 65*(7), 1509–1517.

Kalisch B., & Lee K.H. (2010). The impact of teamwork on missed nursing care. *Nursing Outlook, 58*(5), 233–241.

Kalisch B., Tschannen D., & Lee, H. (2011). Does missed nursing care predict job satisfaction? *Journal of Healthcare Management, 56*(2), 117–134.

Kalisch, B., & Williams, R. (2009). Development and psychometric testing of a tool to measure missed nursing care. *Journal of Nursing Administration, 39*(5), 211–219.

Kalisch B.J. (2016). *Errors of omission: How missed nursing care imperils patients.* American Nurses Association.

Kalisch, B.J., Tschannen D., Lee H., & Friese C.R. (2011). Hospital variation in missed nursing care. *American Journal of Medical Quality, 26*(4), 291–299.

Lake, E.T. (2002). Development of the practice environment scale of the Nursing Work Index. *Research in Nursing and Health, 25*(3), 176–188.

Larrabee, J.H., Janney, M.A., Ostrow, C.L., Withrow, M.L., Hobbs, G.R., & Burant, C. (2003). Predicting registered nurse job satisfaction and intent to leave. *Journal of Nursing Administration, 33*(5), 271–283.

Laws, L., & Hughes. C. (2018). Errors of omission in nursing care and its impact on patient care. *Texas Board of Nursing Bulletin.* https://link.gale.com/apps/doc/A537205093/HRCA?u=iulib_iupui&sid=HRCA&xid=959332fd.

Maloney S., Fencl, J.L., & Hardin, S.R. (2015). Is nursing care missed? A comparative study of three North Carolina hospitals. *MEDSURG Nursing, 24*(4), 229–235.

Manojlovich, M., Ratz, D., Miller, M.A., & Krein, S.L. (2017). Use of daily interruption of sedation and early mobility in US hospitals. *Journal of Nursing Care Quality, 32*(1),71–76.

Marx, D. (2007). *Patient safety and the "Just culture"* [PowerPoint slides]. Outcome Engineering. https://www.unmc.edu/patient-safety/_documents/patient-safety-and-the-just-culture.pdf.

McMullen, S.L., Kozik, C.A., Myers, G., Keenan, K., Wheelock, M., & Kalman, M. (2017). Improving nursing care: Examining errors of omission. *MEDSURG Nursing, 26*(1), 9–14, 19.

National Council of State Boards of Nursing. (2016). *National Guidelines for Nursing Delegation.* https://www.ncsbn.org/NCSBN_Delegation_Guidelines.pdf.

National Council of State Boards of Nursing. (2019). *National Guidelines for Nursing Delegation.* https://www.ncsbn.org/NGND-PosPaper_06.pdf.

National Quality Forum. (2004). *National Voluntary Consensus Standards for Nursing-Sensitive Care: An Initial Performance Measure Set.* https://www.qualityforum.org/Publications/2004/10/National_Voluntary_Consensus_Standards_for_Nursing-Sensitive_Care__An_Initial_Performance_Measure_Set.aspx.

National Quality Forum. (2014). *Improving Care Through Nursing.* https://www.qualityforum.org/improving_care_through_nursing.aspx.

Nursing Service Organization. (2015). *Nurse Professional Liability Exposures: 2015 Claim Report Update.* https://aonaffinity-blob-cdn.azureedge.net/affinitytemplate-dev/media/nso/images/documents/cna-nurse-claim-report-101615.pdf?refID=iiWLTNPi.

Papastavrou E., Andreou, P., Tsangari, H., & Schubert, M. (2014). Rationing of nursing care within professional environmental constraints: a correlational study. *Clinical Nursing Research, 23*(3), 314–335.

Piscoty, R., & Kalisch, B. (2014). The relationship between electronic nursing care reminders and missed nursing care. *Computers, Informatics, Nursing, 32*(10), 475–481.

Piscoty, R., Kalisch, B., & Gracey-Thomas, A. (2015). Impact of healthcare information technology on nursing practice. *Journal of Nursing Scholarship, 47*(4), 287–293.

Poghosyan L., Norful A.A., Fleck, E., Bruzzese J.M., Talsma, A., & Nannini, A. (2017). Primary care providers' perspectives on errors of omission. *Journal of the American Board of Family Medicine, 30,* 733–742.

Pugh, D. (2011). A fine line: The role of personal and professional vulnerability in allegations of unprofessional conduct. *Journal of Nursing Law, 14*(1), 23–31.

Recio-Saucedo, A., Dall'Ora, C., Maruotti, A., Ball, J., Briggs, J., Meredith, P., Redfern, O.C., Kovacs, C., Prytherch, D., Smith, G.B., & Griffiths, P. (2018). What impact does nursing care left undone have on patient outcomes? Review of the literature. *Journal of Clinical Nursing, 27,* 2248–2259. doi: 10.1111/jocn.14058.

Reising, D.L., & Allen, P.N. (2007, February 11). Protecting yourself from malpractice claims. American Nurse. https://www.myamericannurse.com/protecting-yourself-from-malpractice-claims/.

Rochefort, C.M., & Clarke, S.P. (2010). Nurses' work environments, care rationing, job outcomes, and quality of care on neonatal units. *Journal of Advanced Nursing, 66*(10), 2213–2224.

Rosenthal, E. (2018). *An American sickness: How healthcare became big business and how you can take it back.* Penguin Press.

Sager, T.J., & AbuAlRub, R.F. (2018). Missed nursing care and its relationship with confidence in delegation among hospital nurses. *Journal of Clinical Nursing, 27*(13–14), 2887–2895. https://doi-org.dbproxy.lasalle.edu/10.1111/jocn.14380.

Schubert, M., Ausserhofer, D., Bragadóttir, H., Rochefort, C.M., Bruyneel, L., Stemmer, R., Andreou, P., & Leppée, M. (2020). Interventions to prevent or reduce rationing or missed nursing care: A scoping review. *Journal of Advanced Nursing.* Advance online publication. https://doi-org.dbproxy.lasalle.edu/10.1111/jan.14596.

Schubert M., Glass T.R., Clarke S.P., Aiken, L.H., Schaffert-Witvliet, B., Sloane, D.M., & De Geest, S. (2008). Rationing of nursing care and its relationship to patient outcomes: The Swiss extension of the International Hospital Outcomes Study. *International Journal of Quality Health Care, 20*(4), 227–237.

Scruth, E.A., & Pugh, D. (2018). Omission of nursing care: An international perspective. *Clinical Nurse Specialist, 32*(4), 172–174.

Stevenson, J.E., Israelsson, J., Nilsson, G.C., Peterson, G.I., & Bath, P.A. (2016). Recording signs of deterioration in acute patients: The documentation of vital signs within electronic health records in patients who suffered in-hospital cardiac arrest. *Health Informatics Journal, 22*(1), 21–33.

Texas Board of Nursing Administrative Code. (2019). *Rule 217.11- Standards of Nursing Practice.* http://www.bon.texas.gov/rr_current/217-11.asp.

Tobiano, G., Bucknall, T., Marshall, A., Guinane, J., & Chaboyer, W. (2015). Nurses' views of patient participation in nursing care. *Journal of Advanced Nursing, 71*(12), 2741–2752. https://doi-org.dbproxy.lasalle.edu/10.1111/jan.12740.

Topol, E. (2019). *Deep medicine: How artificial intelligence can make healthcare human again.* Basic Books.

Tschannen, D., Kalisch, B., & Lee, K. (2010). Missed nursing care and nurse turnover and intent to leave. *Canadian Journal of Nursing Research, 42*(4), 22–39.

Tubbs-Cooley, H.L., Pickler, R.H., Mark, B.A., & Carle, A.C. (2015). A research protocol for testing relationships between nurse workload, missed nursing care and neonatal outcomes: the neonatal nursing care quality study. *Journal of Advanced Nursing, 71*(3), 632–641. https://doi-org.dbproxy.lasalle.edu/10.1111/jan.12507.

Yakusheva, O., Costa, D.F., & Weiss, M. (2017). Patients negatively impacted by discontinuity of nursing care during acute hospitalization. *Medical Care, 55*(4), 421–427.

Multiple-Choice Questions

1. Missed nursing care represents which of the following categories of health care error?

    A. Commission

    B. Omission

    C. Adverse event

    D. Lapse

2. **Which of the following factors is often cited as a cause of missed nursing care?**
    A. Violation of professional challenges
    B. Health care quality challenges
    C. Technologic distractions
    D. Perceived inadequate staffing

3. **What does Duffy emphasize about basic, routine nursing care's connection to missed nursing care? Select all that apply.**
    A. Importance
    B. Necessity of tracking
    C. Effect on quality outcomes
    D. Immeasurable

4. **Which of the following databases measures nursing quality through evidence-based, nursing-sensitive quality indicators?**
    A. National Quality Forum
    B. Institute for Healthcare Improvement
    C. Agency for Healthcare Research and Quality
    D. Patient Safety Network

CHAPTER 12

Shielding from Bad News

Mary L. Wilby, PhD, MSN,
MPH, RN, CRNP, ANP-BC

Objectives

1. Discuss the barriers that interfere with delivery of bad news in health care settings.

2. Identify possible ethical dilemmas encountered during communication of bad news.

3. Discuss the responsibilities inherent in the role of health care providers when communicating bad news to patients and families.

4. Identify models developed to assist health care providers with effective delivery of bad news.

Critical Incident

The patient is someone I'll never forget. She was an older woman with three young grandchildren. She had been diagnosed with cancer three years before and had been undergoing chemotherapy for a second recurrence. With each cycle of treatment, she was becoming weaker and recovering from the side effects was becoming more and more difficult for her. Her oncologist had not told her the prognosis clearly and continued to offer treatment even though the cancer had metastasized to her liver and lungs and there was no hope of a cure. Both the disease and the treatment were taking their toll on her. I had known her since the first day she came to the hospital for her diagnosis and she trusted me. As we sat together in the infusion center, at the completion of her treatment she said, "I think I'm dying. Do you think I'm dying? Please tell me I'm not dying, I'm not ready." She looked at me with an expression that seemed to ask me to tell her the truth. I did not know what to say. I struggled with giving her my honest answer, that yes, I thought the treatment was doing more harm than good and taking away the last good days she might have. I had seen many patients in situations like this and the outcomes were always the same. But then, I thought, "Well, she says she's not ready, so maybe she doesn't really want to know." I awkwardly told her, "No, I don't think you're dying and this is something you need to talk with the doctor about." I dodged the bullet that day avoiding that difficult conversation, but I could never look at her again in the same way when she came to the clinic. I hadn't told her the truth and it made my heart feel heavy. I wondered who I was protecting, her or me? I felt like I had let her down and when she died a few months later, I cried for the whole day.

The incident described above illustrates some problems inherent in giving and not giving bad news. The nurse missed an opportunity to explore what the patient understood about her illness and prognosis and to explore her fears about what lay ahead. It is unclear what she had been told by her health care team and what her understanding of that information was. Unclear expectations about her future may have caused more worry and denied her the opportunity to prepare herself and her family for her inevitable disease progression and death. Moreover, the nurse missed a chance to address her own thoughts and feelings about the death of a patient and perhaps her own fears about serious illness and death.

Collaboration with others on the health care team may have created an opportunity for all members to address their concerns as well as those of the patient. A unified approach to addressing the patient's concerns may have allayed some of her fears and offered team members the support they needed to care for the patient more effectively. An example of team collaboration was provided by Bowman et al. (2018) who described a collaborative practice model created to improve the delivery of bad news on an in-patient medical oncology unit. They administered an interdisciplinary survey of daily practice patterns and perceived barriers to communicating bad news. An interdisciplinary group reviewed the baseline survey's findings, examined best and evidence-based practices, and identified workflow routines to develop the collaborative practice model intervention. Barriers included "failure of nurse participation; failure of provider to include the nurse; inadequate planning for bad news delivery time; inadequate coverage for participation of the nurse; and failure to provide staff follow-up when unplanned bad news decisions occur" (Bowman et al., 2018, p. 25). Of concern was the barrier of nurses feeling unprepared to support patients with the crises evoked by receiving bad news. Types of bad news events for the unit included patients' nonresponse to treatment or hospice being initiated.

Stakeholder involvement fostered model development; advanced practice nurses were key in literature synthesis, survey development, work group planning, auditing progress, and role-modeling the collaborative practice model use (Bowman et al., 2018). The work group derived a collaborative practice model flow chart and implemented the model. Staff were trained on best practices for communication of bad news. Champions advocated for change as did work group members. Six months post implementation results showed that 85 percent of the time the intervention model was used, and statistically significant improvements resulted. Clinically significant findings in this before-and-after study were noted in the medical team's improvement of communication skills, including the nurse in delivering bad news, and notifying the nurse about imminent bad news events. Application of a collaborative practice model across oncology and other patient units might help with standardizing care and building communication skills. As an evidence-based practice model, it could foster therapeutic relationships and staff accountability for providing patient-centered care during and in the aftermath of receiving bad news. Team collaboration holds promise for continued improvement of strategies to communicate bad news to patients.

Background

Offering bad news is a responsibility that challenges many health care providers. All health care providers, including nurses, are involved in delivering bad news in different forms in many practice settings. It is not surprising that nurses and other health care providers fear both planned and unanticipated, unplanned situations when they have difficult conversations with patients, family members, and friends (Martin et al., 2015). Such situations may be influenced by caregiver perceptions and fears of finding the right words. Additionally, patient, family member, and provider judgments about how well the bad news was delivered might be shaped by care providers' and care recipients' misperceptions and cultural influences. The success of difficult communication episodes affects patients' and families' evaluation of the quality of care delivered (Martin et al., 2015).

The emotions experienced by health care providers may influence them to shield patients from bad news (Martin et al., 2015). However, not providing truthful information about patients' difficult circumstances can affect care delivery. Patients' understanding of their impending death, for example, could be hindered by health care professionals' personal conflicts about apprehensions about death and dying (McLeod-Sordjan, 2014).

Health care professionals have struggled for decades with identifying the most effective manner for dealing with this challenge. In the current health care environment, the roles of the nurse and advanced practice nurse often include giving bad news in long-term care facilities, hospice programs, intensive care units, private oncology practices, and in small hospitals where 24-hour medical staff coverage is absent (Corey & Gwyn, 2016; Curtis et al., 2011; Lorenz, 1997). Bad news, at times termed difficult communications or difficult health care conversations, is often described as information that can alter someone's view of the future in a negative manner (Berkey et al., 2018; Buckman, 1984; Martin et al., 2015; Shildmann et al., 2012). Types of bad news include a diagnosis of serious illness, life-threatening illness, or reports of a death (Ayers et al., 2017); difficult communications may also consist of information that a chronic condition has worsened or that options for treatment are limited (Bumb et al., 2017).

When patients are gravely ill and unable to participate in conversations about their conditions, bad news is conveyed to family members or other loved ones. Once bad news has been conveyed, additional challenges of understanding the concerns of patients and their families emerge. Patients and families frequently have inadequate understanding of medical information. It has been noted that this is because providers seldom offer information coupled with the time necessary to absorb information with its complex concepts, answer questions, and offer clarification of misunderstandings (Gutierrez, 2010). An adequate amount of time spent by physicians during a visit in which bad news is delivered is important for patients (Sobczak et al., 2018). Providing additional information and repeating the bad news is a role frequently undertaken by nurses. The delivery of distressing news is seldom a one-time event. Repeated discussions to allow processing of information and reinforcement are often required (Bumb et al., 2017).

Literature

Most available literature about delivering bad news comes from oncology and emergency medicine where it is not uncommon to offer a diagnosis of serious or advanced illness or that someone has died. Research about the roles played by nurses in the delivery of bad news is limited (Dewar, 2000). The following databases were searched to locate literature on the delivery of bad news: Cochrane Library, PubMed, CINAHL, ProQuest Dissertation and Theses, and SUMMON.

Barriers to Delivering Bad News

Barriers to providers offering bad news successfully include both inadequate education on effective communication and personal responses about the meaning of bad news for patients and providers. Providers may fear being the target of blame when delivering bad news. Although this is not always the case, physicians and others often fear the repercussions of being blamed. It is important that providers are supported in facing their fears and that placing blame is a common response that should not be taken personally. Dealing with unfamiliar situations and those perceived to be uncomfortable naturally may cause feelings of inadequacy and anxiety (Buckman, 1984). Providers also identify varying opinions about their responsibilities in giving bad news and in helping patients and families cope with their emotional responses. Each member of the health care team can have a role in the process; a coordinated team-based approach may be useful in sharing responsibility and assisting patients and families as well as each other (Myers, 2010).

Preliminary goals when delivering bad news include achieving a mutual understanding of the problem, attending to information needs, providing the opportunity for an emotional response, responding to immediate discomfort, addressing immediate medical needs including risk for suicide, providing a plan for follow-up, and reducing feelings of isolation and abandonment (Rabow & McPhee, 1999).

The approach to delivery of bad news can have a significant impact on the receiver's ability to cope or can result in increased anguish and distress. When giving bad news, it is critical that providers consider the impact of the news for patients and their loved ones. It is essential that providers consider how their authentic presence can enhance the recipient's ability to cope in an effective manner when delivering potentially devastating news (Lorenz, 1997).

Situations in which bad news is delivered are often complex. In addition to providing the necessary information in a way that is understood by all parties involved, the emotions of the patient and loved ones must also be considered. Although it is ideal to have an established relationship with the patient, this is not always possible, particularly in the acute care settings where palliative care teams and hospitalist services are often involved in patient care (Baile et al., 2000; Rosenzweig, 2012). It can be difficult to anticipate how news will be perceived and interpreted by the patient and his or her family (Bumb et al., 2017). Communication can be derailed by emotional distress experienced by patients and their families as well as members of the health care team, leading to misperceptions about prognosis, goals of treatment, and expectations for the future. The task of breaking bad news can be especially challenging for inexperienced clinicians (Baile et al., 2000).

Ethical Concerns

Ethical questions may arise when there are conflicting cultural values between providers and patients and families. While the principle of autonomy affirms the value of truth-telling (veracity), other essential principles, including beneficence, nonmaleficence, and justice, must also be considered in these sensitive situations (Taher, 2019).

Telling the truth about bad news is addressed in various ways in different countries and there is no universal agreement on this issue. Although trends worldwide lean toward offering more information, providers are often conflicted about how much and whom to tell. Withholding information may conflict with ethical values and may also compromise relationships between providers and patients when trust is broken (Sarafis et al., 2014).

To explore ethical challenges associated with communicating bad news, researchers (Rejnö et al., 2016) intended to deepen the understanding of truth-telling in end-of-life care members of a stroke team. The researchers acknowledged patients' reduced consciousness at acute stroke onset and their resulting inability to communicate their needs. In these situations, health care providers typically approached relatives as surrogates. Providers assumed that relatives shared patients' interests. The researchers emphasized that trust and intent not to harm were important ethical imperatives and that lying could impact provider and family relationships; however, providers at times shared half-truths.

This qualitative design study focused on caregivers' ways to manage ethical problems (Rejnö et al., 2016). Participants included physicians, registered nurses, and enrolled nurses working in stroke unit teams. Fifteen female members of an interdisciplinary team participated. Interview guides consisted of 24 expressions of ways to handle ethical problems. Reasons for truth-telling and reasons against truth-telling were analyzed from a caring and ethical perspective. Findings from interviews revealed that caregivers shared similar views about truth-telling. The *Truth above all* category included subcategories of *a value in itself* and *to establish trust*. Honesty was essential in relationships with relatives and truth-telling was factual. *Truth above all* represented an intrinsic value and framed caregivers' actions.

The *Hide truth to protect* category included subcategories of *not add extra burden in the sorrow*, *awaiting the timely moment*, and *not being a messenger of bad news*. Caregivers were motivated to avoid giving bad news and protect themselves by hiding the truth. They realized that truth could be harmful. Truth was sometimes hidden, or parts of the truth were shared strategically. Health care providers might lie about patients' diagnostic study results, whether inconclusive or negative. Caregivers reasoned that they were not lying or being dishonest. *Awaiting the timely moment* could result from experience; experienced clinicians are effective at assessing timely moments to share difficult information. Truth-telling in health care requires that cultural norms must be considered. The researchers recommended more research and the sharing of knowledge among the professions.

Individual Preferences and Cultural Considerations

Among cancer patients, studies have suggested, despite what providers and family members might think, that the majority of patients want to be told their diagnosis. However, there is a sizable minority of patients for whom this is not the case. There is sometimes a belief that giving news of a serious diagnosis, such as cancer, will cause overwhelming distress and can have an impact on quality of life and survival in some individuals. There is resistance to disclosure of a serious diagnosis and prognosis in some cultures with some patients not willing or able to hear such news. Alternatively, they may prefer that family members receive the initial diagnosis. This makes the decision to tell or not to tell difficult in some cases yet disclosing bad news can be important in helping patients to engage in complex medical decisions, including whether resuscitation and mechanical ventilation in the event of a cardiac or pulmonary arrest is desired (Abbszadeh et al., 2014; Arabi et al., 2010; Taher, 2019). Some evidence suggests that not knowing the diagnosis and prognosis may contribute to uncertainty and increased anxiety (Sarafis et al., 2014).

In the United States and many other Western cultures, most providers tell patients their diagnosis. However, in some Asian, Latin American, and Islamic cultures, providers take a more paternalistic approach and are less likely to openly discuss diagnosis of serious illness or poor prognosis with patients (Rising, 2014, 2017; Sarafis et al., 2014). Latin Americans often seek to protect family members from bad news and may believe that this shields their loved one from psychological harm.

In contrast, Chinese patients and families may approach offering bad news from a point of view based in Confucianism, deferring to family to decide if and when bad news should be conveyed to the patient (Rising, 2017). The Chinese perspective on breaking bad news was described by Tse and Chong (2017). They pointed out that autonomy varies among cultures and shared that Chinese families do not wish patients to be told a bad diagnosis or prognosis and that the family's preferences might take precedence in the disclosure. As part of family units, Chinese patients make decisions in harmony and in cooperation with other persons. Veracity, another ethical concept, suggests in the Chinese culture if patients ask for the truth (bad news), providers are obligated to tell it. Additionally, paternalism results in subgroups of the family protecting other family members from information that could be interpreted as harmful. Nonetheless, false information is not at all condoned. The authors advised that the words *death*, *fatal illness*, or *cancer* should be avoided with patients and that more tacitly or euphemistically couched communication is preferred.

In a contrasting example from another culture, Ayers et al. (2017) examined managing emotions when communicating about life-threatening illness in palliative care settings, using a focused ethnography. The care context was an early, national effort for palliative care, combined with the collective responsibility of Ethiopians with family at the center of decision making when caring for sick and dying people. The study's purpose was to examine how dying patients, palliative care staff, and family caregivers communicated about life-threatening illness in palliative care settings, including homes and in-patient settings. The researchers used non-participant observation with immersive field observations and interviews with palliative care staff, patients, family caregivers, and spiritual leaders. Findings included palliative care staff protecting patients from receiving distressing, painful details of illness and providing communication episodes that included small amounts of information. It was important to family caregivers that their emotions were suppressed. Professional caregivers deferred to the family and asked for clarification from patients and family members about which details they would like to know. Termed a *to-follow* strategy, a slow approach was espoused in that a tactful, culturally acceptable way shaped disclosure of distressing information. Patients and family members could control how much information then was shared. Open-ended questions were posed to patients so that they were encouraged to express preferences for treatments such as radiation and chemotherapy. *Not wanting to upset* was the predominant cultural dynamic.

Providers must understand and be prepared to address cross-cultural differences.

Tailoring information to individuals based on cultural preference is a process that requires preparation and knowledge of effective communication techniques as well as cultural humility. These beliefs can vary, and nurses and others must not assume to understand the values of patients and families without personalized assessment (Bumb et al., 2017; Rising, 2017; Taher, 2019).

Provider Style and Education

Difficulty engaging in conversations about death and dying and acknowledging ambiguity challenge providers as well as patients and their loved ones. Communication style often varies among providers with some more adept at communicating sensitive information than others. When considering patients' perspectives on receiving bad news, Swingmann et al. (2017) conducted a prospective, experimental, factorial design study to determine anxiety, negative affect, and trust in the physician communicating a cancer diagnosis to adults. Participants were obtained by convenience; adult ($N = 189$) cancer patients ($N = 97$) and unaffected persons ($N = 92$) of both sexes were sampled. Block randomization with stratification (age) was performed. Groups were similar demographically. Participants were randomized to an empathic or nonempathic intervention group to compare the anxiety and negative affect participants would experience when viewing a video showing disclosure of a cancer diagnosis. One standardized video showed a physician displaying an empathic, enhanced patient-centered communication style; another standardized video showed a nonempathic, low patient-centered communication style. Trust (trust in physician subscale), anxiety (State-Trait Anxiety Inventory-State scale), negative affect (Befindlichkeits-Skala adjective checklist), and premeasure (T1) and post-measure (T2) time were also compared, as was previous experience receiving a cancer diagnosis versus no experience and according to sex and age. State anxiety (T1 & T2) and negative affect (T1 & T2) increased in all participants regardless of video style. The physician's style moderated the response. Those viewing the empathic style video were less anxious than the nonempathic style video. Trust was also more positive regarding the empathic style video. The magnitude of the anxiety response to empathic or nonempathic style did not differ by participants' experience with cancer, as did sex and age. Physician style was important for patients facing a life-limiting diagnosis. The researchers suggested that experiential teaching be implemented, whereby clinicians use their own patient vignettes and develop awareness of their own emotional involvement, so that empathy might be experienced. Nurse style may also contribute to patients' responses to receiving difficult information about their health status. Caring and empathic behaviors could foster less anxiety and negative affect and increase trust.

Inadequate provider education regarding communication of bad news has left many providers ill-prepared for engaging in these challenging conversations and in coping with their own and patient and family members' responses to the possibility of death and dying (Gutierrez, 2010). Health professions' education has begun to address providers' delivery of bad news, but more work and research on best practices is needed. Many clinicians report feeling ill-prepared to communicate bad news. Only recently have schools of nursing and medicine incorporated training in breaking bad news into their curricula, and clinician groups have targeted the need to improve notification of bad news (Servotte et al., 2019). Even when content about communicating distressing news is provided, it may be difficult to put knowledge into practice without adequate guidance (Bays et al., 2014; Farber et al., 2003; Reitschuler-Cross et al., 2017).

Shildmann et al. (2012) conducted an intervention study in Germany to examine changes in communication competencies of third-year medical students ($N = 37$) on breaking bad news in a before-and-after study. The teaching module was delivered following baseline measures. No communication skill training with standardized patients (SP) was used prior to the study. Course theory (introduction, basics of doctor-patient communication, ethical and legal aspects of informed consent, ethical case study) and practice (role-play with feedback demonstrated before and after the intervention: videotapes = 47) were presented in the course. Role play with a trained SP and the SPIKES-protocol structured discussions on breaking bad news. An SP interaction was required; students disclosed a diagnosis of cancer, with 1 of 4 post–SP scenarios randomly allocated; cancer vignettes differed from the first student-SP interaction. Independent raters used a modified breaking bad news assessment scale (BAS) and a global rating scale version of the BAS. BAS domains include introduction, disclosing bad news, eliciting concerns, providing information, and general aspects, scaled at *very good* = 1 and *very poor* = 5. Interrater reliability was 0.86. Overall breaking bad news competencies improved significantly after course content ($p<0.001$). Four of the five domains improved. The eliciting concerns domain did not change. Global competencies differed significantly ($p<0.001$) in all five domains. The researchers advocated that faculty reflect on methods to teach and evaluate breaking bad news competencies. It is not surprising that perceptions of empathic or caring style affects perception of how bad news is delivered.

The need to develop advanced communication skills in adult acute care nurse practitioner students stimulated Rosenzweig et al. (2008) to develop a communication simulation laboratory with collaborating nursing and medicine faculty. The intervention aimed at affecting perceived confidence and skill in difficult communication. The faculty team created four cases addressing breaking bad news, empathetic communication, motivational interviewing, and the angry patient. Students had completed two clinical practicums prior to the intervention. A short presentation published articles on exact skills, and PowerPoint slides were provided. SPs were oriented to the two-hour simulations carried out in exam rooms, and cases were developed with matching checklists for SPs to provide verbal and written feedback to students and faculty. Students ($N = 38$) completed 12-minute communications following a general introductory session. They followed the rotation schedule; reflection and debriefing sessions were held on three cases. A Likert-scaled questionnaire elicited perceptions of confidence and skill. Immediate and four-month post confidence and overall ability to communicate improved at a statistically significant level ($p = .001$) on before and after simulation scores. Students were enthusiastic about the experience yet indicated that the motivational interviewing scenario required more time than the others. SP personnel costs were a continuing issue. A train-the-trainer program was implemented for nursing faculty and future workshops were planned.

Baer and Weinstein (2013) recognized that oncology nurses might benefit from an educational project created to improve therapeutic communication skills during discussions with patients with cancer and families on treatment options and how they connect to goals of care and on giving bad news. Avoidance of emotional cues and superficial levels of communication were identified as nurse challenges. The researchers noted the American Association of Colleges of Nursing's leadership in developing nurse competencies in communicating effectively and compassionately at end of life. A communication series of three, one-hour sessions was developed by a collaborative team: nurse educator, outpatient staff nurse, and palliative care physician. Social workers and nurses attended at different sites using the institution's learning management system. Presentations included "general communication skills content, giving bad news, goals of care with specific 'pearls and pitfalls'" (Baer & Weinstein, 2013, p. E47). Class 1 ($N = 16$) was structured by the SPIKES (setting, patient perception, invitation, knowledge, emotions, summary, and strategy) protocol and the NURSE (name, understand, respect, support, explore) method of responding with empathy to patient emotion. Class 2 ($N = 14$) provided goals of care and giving bad news. Class 3 ($N = 8$) on difficult conversations included techniques of Tell-Me-More, Ask/Tell-Ask, SPIKES, and NURSE methods. Post-program evaluations were positive. Small group practice sessions with feedback, regular team conferences, meetings with families, and psychosocial rounds were suggested to continue progress with communication skills.

Addressing barriers to effective communication is not an insurmountable task. Nurses and other health professionals can receive education, such as in the selected example cited, and guided experience in communicating bad news. Formalizing education is essential to encouraging providers to recognize that this is a vital aspect of their professional responsibilities. Mentoring by more experienced providers can assist novice clinicians in coping with their fears about blame, dealing with discomfort with their own thoughts and feelings about death and dying, and learning to help others cope with their feelings.

Processes for Delivering Bad News

Several protocols for delivering bad news have been suggested as models to ease the burdens of providers and patients. The SPIKES model offers a mnemonic that outlines a structured process for delivering bad news to patients and their families (Baile et al., 2000; Kaplan, 2010). The SPIKES model was developed in the field of oncology for initiating discussions about the diagnosis of cancer. **Setting** involves selecting an appropriate location where the patient and family can have privacy.

Understanding the patient's and family's knowledge and **perceptions** of the situation combine as a necessary step before presenting any additional information and proposing a plan of care (Baile et al., 2000; Kaplan, 2010). **Invitation** or **information** directs the provider to identify how much and what kind of information would be helpful for the patient and family according to their needs and reactions. This step offers a framework for providing additional information. **Knowledge** is the step in which the bad news is communicated. Information about the patient's condition, including the stage of the disease and plan of care is offered clearly and truthfully in small portions, avoiding the use of medical terminology. Throughout the conversation the provider should make certain that the patient and family members understand what is being said and offer additional clarification. **Empathy** requires recognizing the patient's and family's emotional reactions throughout the discussion and responding to them in a way that conveys empathy. **Summarizing** or **strategizing** requires that the provider presents information in understandable terms and language (Baile et al., 2000). Once the news is summarized, the provider can begin to discuss the plan of care and treatment options with the patient and family.

The PEWTER model provides another example of structured process to convey bad news. Created as a tool to be used by mental health workers and school counselors, the PEWTER model has also been used in clinical settings to present difficult information to patients (Keefe-Cooperman & Brady-Amoon, 2013; Nardi & Keefe-Cooperman, 2006). The first step in the process is to **prepare**, which includes establishing which information will be presented and understanding how to offer it in clear language that can be easily understood. Preparation also includes creating a private and uninterrupted setting for meeting with the person or persons receiving the news. **Evaluate** refers to the evaluation of what the patient and family members already understand or believe and should include the patient's physical, cognitive, and psychological condition. Additionally, the provider delivering the news should be aware of their own emotions, posture, and facial expressions. **Warning** refers to giving the patient and/or family an indication that serious news will be discussed. The warning should allow for a brief pause for all involved to prepare before the provider proceeds with delivering the news. **Telling** involves delivery of the information in a direct and honest manner. It is recommended that the information be given in small pieces, with no more than three pieces of information given at a time. The provider should validate understanding of the information at each step of the process. Limiting information allows the patient and family to process each portion of the information and reduce the feeling of being inundated. **Emotional** response requires that the provider assess the patient's or family's response to the bad news. If they are overwhelmed, it may be necessary to have more than one meeting to continue the discussion. The final step in the process, **regrouping** involves collaboration between the provider and patient and family to respond to the bad news. This phase can be critical in offering hope. While hope for cure is not possible, hope for treatment, hope for maintaining the patient's quality of life, and hope that the patient's wishes can be upheld may be discussed without being unrealistic (Nardi & Keefe-Cooperman, 2006). Being hopeful involves remaining engaged in identifying and working toward new, often revised, goals. Offering hope is not appropriate in all situations (Bruininks & Malle, 2005).

The ABCDE mnemonic can guide providers to offer support during the delivery of bad news to patients (Rabow & McPhee, 1999). **Advance planning** includes clarifying what is known about the situation and how the patient copes with challenges. Additionally, arranging to have family or other support persons present, and selecting a time that will be uninterrupted are critical. Planning should include selecting the words to be used during the conversation, even writing them down if needed, and rehearsing the delivery of the news for those who are less experienced. **Building a therapeutic environment and/or relationship** requires providing a private place for meeting with enough seats for all involved, sitting close enough to offer supportive touch, if needed. Offering reassurance about pain, suffering, and abandonment can be important. **Communicating well** includes being direct, avoiding use of euphemisms, medical jargon, and abbreviations. Using terms including *death* and *cancer* avoid confusion. Allowing silence to process information is often necessary. Communication is a two-way process; it is important to have members of the group repeat their understanding of the information provided. Repetition may be necessary so follow-up meetings and writing information down can be beneficial. **Dealing with patient and family reactions** is a challenging but necessary part of the process. Assessing the range of responses, both physical and psychological, is important. Listening to responses, exploring feelings, and demonstrating concern can make a significant difference for all involved. **Encouraging and validating emotions** is the final part of the process. Correcting any misunderstandings and evaluating responses to the news can be followed by appropriate referrals for additional support for immediate and future needs. Assessment for suicidality may be needed. It is also important that providers process their own feelings and reactions to each situation.

Although there are differences among these three models, there are also similarities. Advance preparation to provide an appropriate environment for the conversation is a common feature. Setting the stage for such an important conversation is critical. Assessing the patient's/family's knowledge about the situation to be discussed is necessary so all the details of care can be covered and that any misunderstandings can be addressed. Providing information in a direct, honest, yet empathetic manner is an important aspect of developing and maintaining the trust of everyone involved as is responding to the patient's/family's reaction to the news. Also, educational resources offering training in the *how to* of having difficult conversations are available for clinicians and institutions through organizations. Examples include VitalTalk (n.d.) and the Center to Advance Palliative Care (n.d.).

There is currently no consensus about which one model is superior to another. Providers may choose to incorporate elements of the models when communicating bad news or supporting patients and families. Using frameworks such as these can promote the comfort and confidence needed to engage in difficult conversations (Dias et al., 2003). It should be noted that these guidelines are primarily based on expert opinion and not empirical evidence. Studies evaluating protocols for delivering bad news are limited. In one study assessing patient satisfaction with the delivery of bad news using the SPIKES protocol, less than half of patients were completely satisfied with the way the news of a cancer diagnosis had been given to them. Moreover, it was also noted that the delivery of the news was often contrary to patient preferences, and the SPIKES protocol did not match with patient priorities (Seifart et al., 2014).

For providers, the goal is to become comfortable in the delivery and discussion of bad news. As the provider becomes more comfortable with breaking bad news, it is believed that the experiences become more satisfying and perhaps even positive (Dias et al., 2003). Being focused, thorough, therapeutic, and effective while breaking bad news requires preparation, a review of current evidence, and a communication model for practice.

Girgis and Sanson-Fisher (1995) presented consensus guidelines for medical practitioners when breaking bad news to patients. The consensus process involved 28 panel members: medical oncologists, general practitioners, surgeons, nurse consultants, social workers, clergy, and human rights representatives. A draft of guidelines, based on evidence-based literature, was presented to the panel and 100 cancer patients. The guidelines were amended. The researchers emphasized that situations varied among patients and were steps to consider. The principles included the following:

1. One person only should be responsible for breaking bad news.
2. The patient has a legal and moral right to information.
3. Primary responsibility is the individual patient.
4. Give accurate and reliable information.
5. Ask people how much they want to know.
6. Prepare the patient for the possibility of bad news as early as possible.
7. Avoid giving the results of each test individually if several tests are being performed.

8. Tell the patient his/her diagnosis as soon as it is certain.

9. Ensure privacy and make the patient feel comfortable.

10. Ideally, family and significant others should be present.

11. If possible, arrange for another health professional to be present.

12. Inform the patient's general practitioner and other medical advisers of level of development of patient's understanding.

13. Use eye contact and body language to convey warmth, sympathy, encouragement, or reassurance to the patient.

14. Employ a trained health interpreter if language differences exist.

15. Be sensitive to the person's culture, race, religious beliefs, and social background.

16. Acknowledge your own shortcomings and emotional difficulties in breaking bad news (Girgis & Sanson-Fisher, 1995, p. 2453).

These guidelines provide a series of recommendations that could be reviewed periodically by clinicians, despite being disseminated over 20 years ago.

Summary

Breaking bad news to patients and their loved ones is fraught with challenges and nurses have varying roles and responsibilities in doing so. Unfortunately, few nurses have been adequately prepared during their formal education to address this issue. Nurses and other providers charged with delivering difficult news must face their own feelings about death and dying and be prepared to present the facts of the situation. Although it is important to be knowledgeable about the medical aspects of patient care, nurses must be compassionate and pay attention and respond to the emotional reactions of their patients and families. This can be especially challenging for inexperienced providers. While truth-telling is valued in our society, there may be times when differing cultural beliefs and values may pose additional challenges.

Strategies

The following strategies are proposed to support nurses and other health care providers to become more effective and comfortable with providing bad news to patients and families. Table 15 includes models that might be implemented to improve the sharing of bad news.

Table 15. Models to Frame Sharing Bad News

Strategies to Effect Change	Evidence-Based Citations
SPIKES model	Baile et al. (2000)
PEWTER model	Keefe-Cooperman & Brady-Amoon (2013) Nardi & Keefe-Cooperman (2006)
ABCDE model	Rabow & McPhee (1999)

These models offer guidance to nurses and other health care professionals that may structure delivering bad news in a thoughtful, respectful, and sensitive manner. The models are based primarily on expert opinion, making further study of best practices necessary. The frameworks are useful in helping nurses and other providers become more comfortable in delivering bad news.

Conclusion

Nurses perform many roles. They may be the first person to offer news of a death of a patient to the family and other loved ones in the hospice and long-term care setting. APRNs may present the diagnosis of cancer or other serious illness or disease progression in the inpatient and outpatient setting. Nurses often provide reinforcement of news given by physicians or other providers when information needs to be repeated or explained in different terms to facilitate understanding.

Discussion Questions

1. Describe similarities among the models for breaking bad news.
2. What types of barriers can prevent providers from communicating bad news in an effective manner?
3. Describe how differing cultural values may create an ethical dilemma when delivering bad news.
4. What are barriers that interfere with patients and families obtaining adequate information about medical conditions?
5. What roles can nurses play in breaking bad news to patients and their families?

AUTHOR SELECTIONS

Books

Abbey, A. (2019). *Seven signs of life: Unforgettable stories from an intensive care doctor.* Vintage UK.
Case, M. (2019). *How to treat people: A nurse's notes.* W.W. Norton & Company.
Gawande, A. (2014). *Being mortal: Medicine and what matters in the end.* Picador.
Kleinman, A. (2019). *The soul of care: The moral education of a husband and a doctor.* Viking.
Puri, S. (2019). *That good night: Life and medicine in the eleventh hour.* Viking.

Documentary Films

Cunningham, S.S. (Producer/Director). (2017). *The nurse with the purple hair* [Film]. Crystal Lake Entertainment.
Mucciolo, L. (Producer), & Jennings, T. (Producer/Director). (2015). *Being mortal* [Film]. Frontline.
O'Connor, P. (Producer/Director). (2016). *The invisible patients: Life at the edges of the health care system* [Film]. Whetstone Road Productions.

REFERENCES

Abbaszadeh, A., Ehsani, S.R., Begjani, J., Kaji, M.A., Dopolani, F.N., Nejati, A., & Mohammadnejad, E. (2014). Nurses' perspectives on breaking bad news to patients and their families: a qualitative content analysis. *Journal of Medical Ethics and History of Medicine, 7*(18), 1–7.

Arabi, M., Roozdar, A., Taher, M., Arjmand, M., Mohammadi, M.R., Nejatisafa, A., & Rozzdar, A. (2010). How to break bad news: Physicians' and nurses' attitudes. *Iranian Journal of Psychiatry, 5*(4), 128–133.

Ayers, N.E., Vydelingum, V., & Arber, A. (2017). An ethnography of managing emotions when talking about life-threatening illness. *International Nursing Review, 64*, 486–493.

Baer, L., & Weinstein, E. (2013). Improving oncology nurses' communication skills for difficult conversations. *Clinical Journal of Oncology Nursing, 17*(3), E45-E51. doi: 10.1188/13.CJON.E45-E51.

Baile, W.F., Buckman, R., Lenzi, R., Glober, G., Beale, E.A., & Kudelka, A.F. (2000). SPIKES–A six-step protocol for delivering bad news: Application to patients with cancer. *Oncologist, 5*, 302–311.

Bays, A.M., Engelberg, R.A., Back, A.I., Ford, D.W., Downey, L., Shannon, S.E., & Curtis, J.R. (2014). Interprofessional communication skills training for serious illness: Evaluation of a small-group, simulated patient intervention. *Journal of Palliative Medicine, 17*(2), 159–166.

Berkey, F.J., Wiedemer, J.P., & Vithalani, N.D. (2018). Delivering bad or life-altering news. *American Family Physician, 98*(2), 99–104. https://www.aafp.org/afp/2018/0715/afp20180715p99.pdf.

Berlacher, K., Arnold, R.M., Reitschuler, E., Teuteberg, J., & Teuteberg, W. (2017). The impact of communication skills training on cardiology fellows' and attending physicians' perceived comfort with difficult conversations. *Journal of Palliative Medicine, 20*(7), 767–769.

Bowman, P.N., Slusser, K., & Allen. D. (2018). Collaborative Practice Model: Improving the delivery of bad news. Clinical Journal of Oncology Nursing, 22(1), 23–27. doi: 10.1188/18.CJON.23–27.

Bruininks, P., & Malle, B. (2005). Distinguishing hope from optimism and related affective states. *Motivation and Emotion, 29*(4), 327–355.

Buckman, R. (1984). Breaking bad news: Why is it still so difficult? *British Medical Journal, 288*, 1597–1599.

Bumb, M., Keefe, J., Miller, L., & Overcash, J. (2017). Breaking bad news: An evidence-based review of communication models for oncology nurses. *Clinical Journal of Oncology Nursing, 21*(5), 573–580.

Center to Advance Palliative Care. (n.d.). *Welcome to the Center to Advance Palliative Care.* https://www.capc.org/.

Corey, V.R., & Gwyn, P.G. (2016). Experiences of nurse practitioners in communicating bad news to cancer patients. *Journal of Advanced Practitioner in Oncology, 7*, 485–494. doi: 10.6004/jadpro.2016.75.2.

Curtis, J.R., Nielsen, E.L., Treece, P.D., Downey, L., Dotolo, D., Shannon, S.E., Back, A.L., Rubenfeld, G.D., & Engelberg, R.A. (2011). Effect of a quality-improvement intervention on end-of-life care in the intensive care unit: A randomized trial. *American Journal of Respiratory and Critical Care Medicine, 183*, 348–355.

Dewar, A. (2000). Nurses' experiences in giving bad news to patients with spinal cord injuries. *Journal of Neurosciences Nursing, 32*(6), 324–330.

Farber, N.J., Friedland, A., Aboff, B.M., Ehrenthal, D.B., & Bianchetta, T. (2003). Using patients with cancer to educate residents about giving bad news. *Journal of Palliative Care, 19*(1), 54–57.

Girgis, A., & Sanson-Fisher, R.W. (1995). Breaking bad news: Consensus guidelines for medical practitioners. *Clinical Journal of Oncology Nursing, 13*(9), 2449–2456.

Gutierrez, K.M. (2010). Communication of prognostic information in an ICU at end of life: Practices among and between nurses, physicians and family members. (UMI No. 3411843). [Dissertation, University of Minnesota]. ProQuest Dissertations and Theses Global Database.

Kaplan, M. (2010). SPIKES: A framework for breaking bad news to patients with cancer. *Clinical Journal of Oncology Nursing, 14*(4), 514–516. doi: 10.1188/10.CJON.514–516.

Keefe-Cooperman, K., & Brady-Amoon, P. (2013). Breaking bad news in counseling: Applying the PEWTER model in the school setting. *Journal of Creativity in Mental Health, 8*(3), 265–277. doi: 10.1080/15401383.2013.821926.

Lorenz, E.V. (1997). Giving bad news: Nurses' perspective. (UMI No. 1390256). [Master's thesis]. ProQuest Dissertations and Theses Global Database.

Martin. E.B., Mazzola, N.M., Brandano, J., Luff, D., Zurakowski, D., & Meyer, E.C. (2015). Clinicians' recognition and management of emotions during difficult healthcare conversations. *Patient Education and Counseling, 98*, 1248–1254.

McLeod-Sordjan, R. (2014). Death preparedness: A concept analysis. *Journal of Advanced Nursing, 70*(5), 1008–1019. doi: 10.1111/jan.12252.

Myers, K.R. (2010). Emergency department staff adherence to bad news delivery recommendations. (ProQuest No. 3721186). [Dissertation]. ProQuest Dissertations and Theses Global Database.

Nardi, T., & Keefe-Cooperman, K. (2006). Communicating bad news: A model for emergency mental health helpers. *International Journal for Emergency Mental Health, 8*(3), 203–2017.

Rabow, M.W., & McPhee, S.J. (1999). Beyond breaking bad news: How to help patients who suffer. *Western Journal of Medicine, 17*(1), 260–263.

Rising, M.L. (2017). Truth telling as an element of culturally competent care at end of life. *Journal of Transcultural Nursing, 28*(1), 48–44.

Rosenzweig, M., Hravnak, M., Magdic, K., Beach, M., Clifton, M., & Arnold, R. (2008). Patient communication simulation laboratory for students in an acute care nurse practitioner program. *American Journal of Critical Care, 17*(4), 364–372.

Rosenzweig, M.Q. (2012). Breaking bad news: A guide for effective and empathetic communication. *Nurse Practitioner, 37*(2), 1–4. doi: 10.1097/01.NPR.0000408626.24599.9e.

Sarafis, P., Tsounis, A., Malliarou, M., & Lahana, E. (2014). Disclosing the truth: A dilemma between instilling hope and respecting autonomy in everyday clinical practice. *Global Journal of Health Sciences, 6*(2), 128–137.

Seifart, C., Hofmann, M., Bar, T., Riera Knorrenschild, J., Seifart, U., & Rief, W. (2014). Breaking bad news–what patients want and what they get: Evaluating the SPIKES protocol in Germany. *Annals of Oncology, 25*, 707–711.

Servotte, J-C., Bragard, I., Szyld, D., Van Ngoc, P., Scholtes, B., Van Cauwenberge, I., Donneau, A-F., Dardenne, N., Manon, G., Pilote, B, Guillaume, M., & Ghuysen, A. (2019). Efficacy of a short role-play training on breaking bad news in the emergency department. *Western Journal of Emergency Medicine, 20*(6), 893–902. doi: 10.5811/westjem.2019.8.43441.

Shildmann, J., Kupfer, S., Burchardi, N., & Vollmann, J. (2012). Teaching and evaluating breaking bad news: A pre-post evaluations study of a teaching intervention for medical students and a comparative analysis of different instruments and raters. *Patient Education and Counseling, 86*, 210–219.

Sobczak, K., Leoniuk, K., & Janaszyk, A. (2018). Delivering bad news: Patient's perspectives and opinions. *Patient Preference and Adherence, 12*, 2397–2404. doi: 10.2147/PPA.S183106.

Taher, A.F. (2019). A patient-centered approach to the ethical dilemma of breaking bad news to cancer patients: Recommendations for better communication strategy. *Advances in Cancer Research & Clinical Imaging, 1*(2). doi: 10–33552/ACRCI2019.01.00510.

VITALtalk (n.d.). *VitalTalk makes communication skills for serious illness learnable.* https://www.vitaltalk.org/.

Zwingmann, J., Baile, W.F., Schmier, J.W., Gernhard, J., & Keller, M. (2017). Effects of patient-centered communication on anxiety, negative affect, and trust in the physician in delivering a cancer diagnosis: A randomized, experimental study. Cancer, 123, 3167–3175. doi: 10.1002/cncr.30694.

Multiple-Choice Questions

1. Barriers to delivery of bad news include which of the following?
A. Over conscientiousness of health care providers
B. Immediacy of patients' current health care needs
C. Repercussions from health care administrators
D. Feelings of inadequacy of health care providers

2. What do nurses often experience when communicating with patients following a health provider's delivery of bad news to patients and family members?
A. Deciding not to disclose the information again
B. Repeating the nature of the bad news again
C. Referring patients' questions to the first provider
D. Being personally concerned to get the message right

3. What is a common strategy identified in the models for communicating bad news to patients?
A. Providing a private setting
B. Validating emotions
C. Warning the patient about bad news
D. Avoiding medical terminology

4. Which of the following goals does Dias et al. (2003) suggest for providers delivering bad news?
A. Using opportunities to consider options
B. Becoming comfortable in the delivery and discussion
C. Considering the first discussion a time-limited event
D. Correcting all inadequacies with practice

CHAPTER 13

Failure to Report Abuse
and Whistleblowing

Denise Nagle Bailey, EdD, RN,
MEd, MSN, CSN, FCPP

Objectives

1. Identify and analyze examples of patient abuse in varied clinical settings.
2. Describe factors that contribute to nurse failure in reporting patient abuse.
3. Examine behavioral characteristics that contribute to increased incidents of patient abuse.
4. Compare strategies and interventions used to identify and reduce abuse in clinical settings.

Critical Incident

T.F. was a 92-year-old male with a significant medical history including hyperlipidemia, coronary artery disease (CAD), myocardial infarction (MI) requiring quintuple coronary artery bypass grafting (CABG), and subsequent multiple stent placements post–CABG. T.F. also had a concomitant diagnosis of mild dementia. T.F. and his wife of 63 years resided at his childhood home until his wife could no longer be cared for in the home environment. Subsequently, the family placed her in a local long-term care facility where he visited her daily. After his wife was transferred to the facility, it became apparent to the family that T.F.'s declining cognitive status intensified to the point that he was no longer able to function independently. This was despite efforts of family members to provide a safety net of in-home care through agency placement of nurses and aides.

Consequently, T.F. was placed in the same long-term care facility as his wife, sharing a room. Initially, this placement worked well, and nurses and health care staff were responsive to his care requirements and requests. T.F. was pleasant and cooperative. Over the course of several months, his cognitive function deteriorated quickly, and as a result of this marked decline in mental status, he became increasingly more dependent upon nurses and staff to assist him with activities of daily living (ADLs). T.F. also demonstrated verbal signs of agitation when he did not understand prescribed treatments and procedures related to his care. Increasing fear and paranoia developed while he was adjusting to his new and unfamiliar environment.

As the months passed, nurses and health care staff were observed by family members to be less involved in his overall care. Interaction between care providers and T.F. appeared to be minimal. Meal trays were placed on the bedside table, but little or no assistance in cutting food, opening milk containers, or unwrapping food on meal tray was provided by health care staff. Lack of assistance in feeding during meals eventually led to significant weight loss, increased isolation, and withdrawal. The family noticed his oral care was extremely poor; toileting and basic assistance with hygiene was deplorable with visible signs of dried feces frequently observed under fingernails and on hands or clothing. Family members also noted soiled undergarments with visible dried urine or feces and accompanying excoriation of surrounding skin. Disposable pull-up diapers were provided by the family, with infrequent changing by nurses and staff. Family members noted that he did ask for assistance, as several nurses were observed walking past his room after he called out for help. Family members overheard staff discussing how they handled him when assigned, admitting among themselves that they assist "only when they have to." Nurses and staff complained to the nursing home administrator of the facility, stating they feared providing care to him.

T.F. was subsequently referred to an in-patient behavioral health facility for adjustment of his psychiatric medications and evaluation, eventually returning to the long-term care facility. T.F. continued his daily life in increasing isolation except for the presence of his wife, who provided him with a sense of security, comfort, and familiarity. Nurses and staff continued to avoid interacting with him, which led to a poor patient outcome and continued downward spiral in the quality of his care.

T.F.'s wife became increasingly concerned, mentioning to family members that her husband was the recipient of harsh verbal reprimands from several nurses and staff members who entered the room in pairs when changing or providing basic care to him. She also stated that the nurses did not take the time to greet him or explain the purpose of the intended encounter. Caregivers quickly performed each task (for example, change his diaper) while holding his arms firmly in place until the particular task was completed. T.F.'s wife informed family members, who were assured by the charge nurse that she was not aware of any incidents or concerns of abuse or neglect by nurses or staff members but would "look into it." Lacerations and bruising of arms were noted on several occasions by family members, but they were never able to determine the origin of these injuries.

Ultimately, the administrator approached the family after meeting with the charge nurse and staff, informed the family that she did not feel he was a candidate for placement in their on-site Alzheimer's unit, and recommended that he be placed in a county-funded facility that had a dedicated Alzheimer's unit that "could better meet his growing needs." The family complied. Shortly after the administrator met with the family, T.F. was transferred to the county-funded facility, where he died within weeks after admission. During this period at the facility, he received adequate care from nurses and other caregivers. Although the charge nurse contacted the family to obtain permission to use restraint mittens during waking hours, T.F.'s attending physician discontinued the mittens after he observed T.F. wearing this restraining device while sitting in the hallway, commenting that implementing this measure stripped the patient of any remaining dignity.

The scenario presented above gives rise to serious concerns related to the obligation of professional nurses and other health care professionals to report acts of verbal or physical abuse toward patients entrusted in their care. This case study captures a subtle, yet alarming example of nurses who violate ethical principles and disregard regulatory mandates for practice under individual state boards of nursing and the American Nurses Association's (ANA's) Code of Ethics (2015). More serious examples involving failure to report abuse appear in the literature.

Background

This chapter examines patient abuse and whistleblowing in health care situations, both of which address issues related to the failure of reporting abuse in institutional settings. The first topic speaks to concerns and consequences encountered when nurses fail to report abuse. The second topic brings forth problems and considerations related to whistleblowing in the health care arena and the obstacles that nurses encounter as they resort to this uncomfortable activity of reporting abuse.

Patient Abuse: Case Examples

In *Kim v. Lakeside Adult Family Home*, No. 91536–9, S. Ct. Wash., May 12, 2016, the Washington Supreme Court rendered an opinion that extended the potential liability in a nursing home abuse lawsuit involving nurses who were mandated to report "discovered" instances of abuse in a nursing home but failed to disclose discovered information. After review of the case, the court determined that under the Revised Code of Washington's Abuse of Vulnerable Adults Act (AVAA), RCW 74.34, a state-enacted law to protect the elderly, there is a separate cause of action against individuals who are mandated to report nursing home abuse but fail to disclose such abuse.

The plaintiffs in this legal action are the surviving "loved ones" of an elderly female who was given a lethal dose of morphine. The drug was not ordered by a physician; however, it was administered by a nurse who was not named a party in this case.

The defendants were two nurses who were not employed by the nursing home where the deceased older person had been a resident and were not responsible in any way for her care. The defendants were providing care for another patient at the facility at the time and observed what they perceived as lapses in care of the deceased prior to her death. On one occasion, one of the defendants witnessed the elderly woman lying on the floor. That defendant confronted the patient's nurse caregiver, who conveyed to the defendant that the patient had a history of frequent falls and "falls a lot."

The following day, the second defendant was caring for an unrelated patient at the same facility, when she learned that the nurse, who was providing care to the woman prior to her death, administered a dose of morphine. The second defendant attempted to contact the Department of Human Services by phone but was unable to get through to speak directly to an intake person; however, she did leave a message regarding her concerns. Eventually, the patient died as a result of a deliberate and lethal overdose of morphine. The family of the deceased filed a lawsuit naming both nurses who witnessed the lapses in patient care, asserting a failure to take immediate action through reporting the incident.

The seminal issue at trial was whether the two nurse defendants, who were not responsible for the care of the deceased patient, were liable under the AVAA, RCW 74.34, for failing to report and follow up upon the observed abuse of the deceased. It was not disputed that the defendants were mandatory reporters under the Act, as they were required to report discoverable abuse during the course of their employment at the facility. What had not been previously decided was whether the defendants could be held personally accountable for their failure to do so.

The court determined that any failure to report abuse by an individual or party who is a mandated reporter can result in liability. The court further articulated that the intent of the AVAA, RCW 74.34, was to fashion a cause of action for failure to report abuse, although it was not expressly stated in the statute's language. As a result of this ruling, the plaintiffs were permitted to bring a cause of action against the nurse defendants.

Another lawsuit involving health care workers and the failure to report abuse is addressed in *Burr Road Operating Company II, LLC v. New England Health Care Employees Union, District 1199* (Appellate Court of Connecticut, No. 33954, January 26, 2016). Among other issues the court addressed in this matter was a nurse's obligation to report abuse pursuant to Connecticut law. The Burr Road Operating Company (Plaintiff) operated a skilled nursing facility. The employee nurse (Nurse) was employed by Plaintiff as a certified nursing assistant for eight years until her termination. The events that resulted in the Nurse's termination occurred while the Nurse was working a night shift. The Nurse overheard a conversation between two coworkers, which caused the Nurse to conclude a resident had been the subject of abuse. She also believed that the incident might have involved abuse. The Nurse failed to report her suspicions immediately, because, as found by the initial arbitrator fact finder, "[she] didn't know for sure that there had been abuse" (Burr, supra.). The Nurse was terminated for failure to report abuse.

Upon completion of the initial arbitration hearing, the arbitrator concluded that the Nurse did fail to make a timely report of what she had learned during the referenced night shift, and she was aware of the rule that required her to report abuse immediately. However, the arbitrator concluded that the Plaintiff had just cause to suspend the grievant without pay for one month and to issue her a final warning but not terminate the Nurse's employment.

The Plaintiff (employer) challenged, through a series of court appeals, the arbitrator's rulings, arguing that the Nurse's termination was justified and therefore the arbitrator abused its discretion in disallowing the termination for failure to report suspected abuse of a resident. The various courts that reviewed this matter universally agreed that the Nurse's failure to report suspected abuse was egregious and violated her employment rules and abuse reporting regulations. Ultimately the appellate court confirmed the arbitrator's decision, finding that when arbitration clauses are included in the contracts of parties, they supersede the more formalistic rules that are observed in a courtroom setting and defer to the judgment of the arbitrator in considering what is fair. Although the employee (Nurse) was reinstated with a suspension due to vague language in the collective bargaining agreement, a health care worker's obligation to report suspected or perceived abuse is considered a seminal duty.

Literature

Abuse of patients by health care professionals and the subsequent failure of those who witness abusive acts are unfortunate and troublesome realities that occur within institutional settings including hospitals, long-term care facilities, and other outpatient facilities where patient care is delivered. The negative outcomes experienced by patients, as they endure abuse at the hands of health care providers, give pause for nurses to seriously examine factors that contribute to abuse and formulate appropriate measures that could be implemented to reduce or eliminate negative behaviors in the clinical setting.

The body of literature located on the topic of failure of nurses to report abuse was meager, even after searching ProQuest, PubMed, National Library of Medicine (NLM), Google Scholar, and Medline; nonetheless, an emerging pattern was identified revealing that intentional acts of abuse by nurses resulted in negative patient outcomes. Incidents varied in severity from feelings of humiliation when being cared for to seminal events involving murder or wrongful death. This observation is supported in the research of others in this general topic area (National Council of State Boards of Nursing [NCSBN], 2011; Wolf, 2012). Issues relating to reporting abuse in the institutional setting are more readily available in the topic area of whistleblowers in health care when compared to the reporting of abuse in clinical settings.

The area of elder abuse is one topic area that has expanded and garnered increasing attention of researchers; however, most extant research focuses on the abuse of elderly individuals residing in community-based settings. Modest research has been conducted on the identification of characteristics and risk factors inherent to this subset of the population in nursing homes. Payne and Fletcher (2005) noted that research on this topic area has increased, with the caveat that as the topic evolved, little attention has been dedicated to the abuse of patients within this unique institutional setting.

Institutional Culture: Care Challenges

The need for administrators and nurses to place patient abuse at the forefront of their agendas is obvious as patient harm violates moral, ethical, and professional obligations that serve as sacred, foundational elements guiding a profession that incorporates elements of caring into daily practice. Ensuring the safety and welfare of vulnerable patients, incorporating appropriate measures to reduce patient harm, and encouraging an institutional culture that supports nurses who witness and report abuse could reduce nurse hesitancy in reporting abusive acts and ultimately improve outcomes related to patient care and safe practice (Malmedal et al., 2014).

Changing institutional culture is a critical component in the reduction of patient abuse. When negative patient outcomes are identified within the clinical setting, it is easy for administrators to blame the RN, technician, physician, or other member of the health care delivery team who is directly involved in the care of the patient who experienced abuse (Albina, 2016). However, the condoning of disrespectful or disturbing employee conduct clearly demonstrates a need for immediate change in the culture of the health care institution. Albina (2016) stated that finger-pointing does not solve the more pressing issue.

Hospital employees must function as change agents within the workplace milieu in order to foster a culture that halts abusive behaviors when they are witnessed. Albina (2016) outlined the essential steps required for the elimination of patient abuse by implementing the following standards:

- opening communication and providing education
- establishing competency

- ending tolerance of unacceptable behavior
- creating a code of mutual respect that empowers health care professionals to contribute to safer quality care that benefits everyone from patients and family members to hospital personnel, the community, and health care nationwide [p. 77].

Understanding the complex array of serious issues related to patient abuse and identifying the different types of abuse that could materialize during patient-caregiver encounters place considerable emphasis on the need for administrators to offer on-going educational programs and in-service sessions that focus on empowering nurses to more readily identify and report abuse, thus enhancing interpersonal relationships and the communicative skills of nurses (Albina, 2016; Payne & Fletcher, 2005; Malmedal et al., 2014). Additionally, administrators, including nurse managers and supervisors, need to act as facilitators to engender open staff-member discussions and forums that focus on ethical issues encompassing patient care. Nurse leaders and administrators are responsible for laying the groundwork to create a culture of mutual respect and dignity, and for the ongoing dialogue highlighting the ethical issues that are encountered by staff nurses and other members of the health care team (Albina, 2016).

One essential component of the success of this strategy relies upon ensuring a comfortable, non-threatening atmosphere where the open exchange of ideas can take place (Albina, 2016). Facility-based prevention measures are discussed within the context of long-term care facilities (Payne & Fletcher, 2005). These measures refer to the policies and procedures that administrators and employees are expected to follow, thus ensuring the protection of patients residing in long-term care facilities and emphasizing the expectation that these measures are implemented within the organizational culture.

A number of these interventions can be readily applied in other institutional settings. Protections afforded to patients should include procedures and protocols to avert potential dangers (e.g., falls, medication errors, negligence in care) and imbue a heightened awareness to the serious consequences contributing to negative patient outcomes. Physical and emotional trauma leads to significant tolls on victims of abuse and can extend to families and loved ones in the suffering they experience. Maintaining adequate staffing is essential in providing a safe level of care and is dependent upon nurse managers, supervisors, and administrators who are dedicated in their efforts to maintain keen oversight of nurses and staff members, upholding the tenets of quality assurance (Payne & Fletcher, 2005).

Abuse of Patients and Reporting Abuse

Legal Definitions. Pennsylvania Regulations, 28 Pa Code §201.3 defines abuse within the context of nursing homes as:

> the infliction of injury, unreasonable confinement, intimidation or punishment with resulting physical harm or pain or mental anguish, or deprivation by an individual, including a caretaker, of goods or services that are necessary to attain or maintain physical, mental, and psychosocial well-being. This presumes that instances of abuse of all residents, even those in a coma, cause physical harm, or pain or mental anguish [para. 1].

Under 28 Pa Code §201.3, the term abuse is further qualified to delineate the specific types of abuse that are recognized under the statute. These include verbal abuse, sexual abuse, physical abuse, mental abuse, involuntary seclusion, and neglect. These terms are defined under Title 28 Pennsylvania Code in the following manner:

1. *Verbal abuse*—Any use of oral, written or gestured language that willfully includes disparaging and derogatory terms to residents or their families, or within their hearing distance, regardless of their age, ability to comprehend or disability.

2. *Sexual abuse*—Includes sexual harassment, sexual coercion or sexual assault.

3. *Physical abuse*—Includes hitting, slapping, pinching and kicking. The term also includes controlling behavior through corporal punishment.

4. *Mental abuse*—Includes humiliation, harassment, threats of punishment or deprivation.

5. *Involuntary seclusion*—Separation of a resident from other residents or from his room or confinement to his room (with/without roommates) against the resident's will, or the will of the resident's legal representative. Emergency or short-term monitored separation from other residents will not be considered involuntary seclusion and may be permitted if used for a limited time as a therapeutic intervention to reduce agitation until professional staff can develop a plan of care to meet the resident's needs.

6. *Neglect*—The deprivation by a caretaker of goods or services which are necessary to maintain physical or mental health [para. 1].

Abuse, as detailed in 28 Pa Code §201.3, underscores the serious ramifications that could jeopardize the safety and well-being of vulnerable patients under the control of caregivers in the clinical setting; such abuse would, no doubt, threaten positive patient outcomes. A refusal or failure of those responsible to provide food, shelter, health care, or protection for a vulnerable individual or group of individuals falls under the penumbra of abuse.

Identifying and reporting abuse is not an isolated issue impacting the U.S. health care system alone. Similar concerns are noted in the literature spanning the globe. Wijma et al. (2016) conducted a Swedish study to evaluate the silence, shame, and abuse that surface during patient care encounters. The researchers commented that health care is intended to alleviate the suffering of patients and should not be "inflicting unnecessary suffering on patients, and yet this happens" (p. 1). Abuse of patients by those entrusted to their care is a topic that is reluctantly "spoken" about, and when a discussion does come to the forefront, there are a wide range of terms that are used to denote abuse in health care (AHC). Examples include patient dissatisfaction, medical errors, and patient suffering that serve as indicators to describe negative patient outcomes resulting from the delivery of poor health care (Wijma et al., 2016).

A systematic review was conducted to integrate current evidence related to the disrespect and abuse of Nigerian women during childbirth in order to better understand its nature and extent, factors contributing to disrespect and abuse, and consequences that result from uncaring acts of caregivers (Ishola et al., 2017). The researchers articulated that promoting respectful care during childbirth is a critical component to the improvement of quality patient care and is considered to represent a key component in the attraction of pregnant women to the care facility and utilization of skilled delivery services (Ishola et al., 2017).

Results garnered from this research (Ishola et al., 2017) revealed the most frequently reported type of abuse was non-dignified negative care resulting from the poor and unfriendly attitudes of care providers. The least reported incidents of abuse were those involving physical abuse and detention in facilities. These undesirable behaviors were determined by researchers to be correlated to lower socioeconomic status, knowledge deficit or lack of education, low self-esteem of women, suboptimum provider supervision and training, weak health systems, failure to hold caretakers accountable for actions, and legal redress mechanisms to remediate cases where abuse directly led to the harm of patients. Ishola et al. (2017) stated that "overall, disrespectful and abusive behavior undermined the utilization of health facilities for delivery and created psychological distance between women and health providers" (p. 1).

The disrespectful and abusive factors contributing to these unfavorable caregiver behaviors call for educational programs to inform women of their patient rights, in addition to encouraging health care systems to take a proactive role in cases where abuse is identified. This includes improving caregivers' sensitivity to meet specific needs of pregnant women, improving educational opportunities for providers of care, and developing and enforcing institutional policies on maternity care. Furthermore, this research has clearly demonstrated that there is significant need for additional research in this important topical area (Ishola et al., 2017).

Hodges (2009) similarly discussed abuse of patients by physicians with medical authority in hospital-based birth settings, commenting that bullying and performing medical treatments under false pretenses are issues that are rarely recognized as abuse or violence against pregnant women giving birth in hospital settings; however, they represent a violation of basic human rights and denote patient abuse. Since physicians are viewed as experts in treating patients, women may be unable to determine if information is omitted or misrepresented by physicians.

Abuse also includes provider actions relative to the delivery of medical treatment without obtaining informed consent, superseding patient refusal of a treatment or procedure, omission of information, and misrepresenting the need for therapeutic interventions. Hodges (2009) discussed patient abuse in birth settings by physicians and the serious nature of abuse in this clinical setting, as she stated, "Some women have been treated with extreme hostility, including the withholding of appropriate pain relief and obvious sexual abuse" (p. 9). Physicians who did not normally appear to exhibit abusive tendencies may participate in these negative behaviors, with nurses feeling powerless to intervene through the reporting of abuse.

In situations where nurses are witnesses to the abuse of patients by physicians, prompt actions can be taken to intervene and protect vulnerable patients and improve health outcomes. Nurses should not hesitate to seek the input of psychologists who focus their practice on this specialty of human behavior, who could suggest effective techniques for nurses to implement in this challenging hospital setting.

Childbirth educators can also inform pregnant individuals of their basic rights, thus empowering patients. Women who are well-informed are more apt to ask questions regarding their care during delivery. Nurses can also encourage women who experience abuse during their pregnancy and birthing process to lodge a complaint against the abuser.

Hodges (2009) articulated:

> The power of medical authority, the lack of accountability in the hierarchical system, policies and protocols, and expectations of compliancy all make an environment ripe for abuse and present obstacles for both women and staff to recognize to stop abuse [p. 8].

Nurses need to develop a heightened awareness in the recognition of abuse and take appropriate action to halt the abuse of patients entrusted to their care. Ending abuse will, however, require a systematic change within the institution where care is given.

Reporting incidents within the health care system exposes negative events and contributes to positive patient outcomes by serving as a tool in the reduction of harmful patient outcomes. Despite the beneficial power of reporting incidents and its value in the prevention of repeat events, incidents are not always reported for the same reasons they are omitted in patient medical records: they are not identified or recognized. When incidents do surface, it is not unusual to find that these events were not efficiently or effectively handled by administrators (Evans et al., 2006).

For incident reporting to be more successful, physicians, nurses, and staff need to adopt measures to ensure a more robust system to account for errors that are identified in hospital environments. Evans et al. (2006) conducted a cross-sectional survey of physicians and nurses by individual profession, with study objectives that included: (1) awareness and use of the current incident reporting system; (2) types of incidents staff were more likely to report and believe should be reported; and (3) barriers to reporting.

Results gleaned from this study revealed that most physicians and nurses were aware that an incident reporting system was operational within their place of employment (Evans et al., 2006). Additionally, nurses were more familiar than physicians in the protocol requirements for submission of incident reports and had greater knowledge related to accessing incident reports, when compared to physicians surveyed. Furthermore, staff were more likely to report habitual incidents that they witnessed more often. These include incidents usually associated with immediate outcomes, such as patient falls and medication errors requiring corrective action. Near misses and incidents that are reported over time, including pressure injuries and deep vein thrombosis (DVT), resulting from sub-optimal prophylaxis, were representative of negative patient outcomes least likely to be reported. The absence or lack of feedback from administrators comprised the most frequently reported barriers related to the reporting of incidents. Evans et al. (2006) suggested, "Perhaps the most challenging task is ensuring that practice improvements resulting from reports are disseminated to clinicians, because only then will incident reporting be seen as worthwhile and relevant" (p. 42).

Kousgaard et al. (2012) conducted a qualitative study to explore reasons leading to the failure of reporting patient safety incidents in general practice clinics in a region of Denmark. The main outcome measures in this study included the reflections and experiences of 12 general practitioners and members of the project group. They were interviewed regarding a country-wide system to report safety incidents. Results unearthed several important concerns, which included the following:

- Although most respondents were initially receptive to the notion of reporting and learning from patient safety incidents, very few incidents were actually reported. Explanations included the lack of perceived usefulness, time constraints, and practitioner efforts involved in reporting incidents within busy clinical settings with competing priorities.
- Data also revealed that practitioners considered the reporting of sensitive issues in relation to other professionals (e.g., submitting incident reports on other health care professionals). This is an area where practitioners hesitated or

failed to report; respondents indicated that they viewed this measure to be "a formalistic and harsh step, especially if the incident had already been brought to the attention of the professionals involved" (p. 203).

The researchers concluded that formal, comprehensive, and systematic reporting of and learning from patient safety incidents are difficult in general practice. Although the study focused on general practitioners, the results can readily be applied to nurses who work in busy clinical settings who experience similar barriers in the reporting of incidents that threaten the safety and well-being of patients.

When uncaring and ineffective practices within the organizational context are tolerated or ignored, poor quality care or unsafe practices can result (Mannion & Davies, 2015). In these instances, it is critical that nurses and staff feel empowered to voice their concerns. It is crucial that organizations respond positively to safety threats when communicated, learn from errors of the past, and institute effective policies that prevent future incidents (Mannion & Davies, 2015).

Whistleblowers and Reporting Abuse

Whistleblowing, or the disclosure of information (usually by an employee) to management or a regulator that evidences waste, mismanagement, or violation of law, has become more palpable as the old mores of "being a rat" fade. The potential for abuse in the health care field, both patient and financial, is significant (29 U.S.C. §218c). Although nurses have acted when wrongdoing is detected in many instances, few whistleblower claims resulted in publicly reported legal cases (Mansbach et al., 2014).

When health care whistleblower cases resulted in litigation, many times it was the result of the termination of a claimant's employment or a dispute as to whether the reported actions met the legal definition under the designated whistleblower statute (29 U.S.C. §218c). Below are two such cases that demonstrate the perils of whistleblowing in health care.

In the matter of *United States ex rel. Vanessa Absher et al. v. Momence Meadows Nursing Center, Inc. and Jacob Graff*, 764 F.3d 699 (7th Cir. 2014), the claimants were two nurses who, at the time of the complaint, were employed by Momence Meadows Nursing Center. Momence was a 140-bed, long-term care facility. Most of its residents received Medicare or Medicaid. The nurses contended that, while employed at Momence, they found information that their employer was filing false reimbursement claims to the Medicare and Medicaid programs. The two nurses made their whistleblower allegations under the federal False Claims Act (FCA) 31 USC §3729–3733 (U.S. Department of Justice, n.d.) and the Illinois Whistleblower Reward and Protection Act (IWRPA) 740 ILCS175/1. (The federal Whistleblower Act is also accessible [U.S. House of Representatives, n.d.].) Following a jury trial, the jury concluded that Momence had, in fact, submitted numerous false claims, and further that, because of their whistleblower complaints, Momence had retaliated against the two nurses. Although this matter was ultimately concluded in favor of the violating facility on technical legal interpretations, it does exemplify the risks faced by a health care whistleblower.

Another matter that resulted in litigation was discussed in the Court of Appeals of Maryland case of *Lark v. Montgomery Hospice*, 994 A.2d 968 (2010), 414 Md. 215 (2010). The Claimant was employed as a registered nurse at Montgomery Hospice and brought this action for wrongful termination and violation of the Maryland Health Care Worker Whistleblower Protection Act, Md. Code Ann., Health Occ. § 1–501 to 1–506. The Claimant contends that she raised issues related to charting that was not consistent with the health and safety of Montgomery's clients. The Claimant's employer did nothing to correct these issues. Subsequently, the Claimant raised concerns with management regarding various practices that she believed to be contrary to generally accepted professional standards of registered nursing practice, which threatened the health and safety of patients. The Claimant's allegations included: narcotic provided to non-hospice patients, improper documentation of narcotic drugs, and unauthorized treatments delivered to patients. Shortly after the Claimant nurse's allegations were submitted to her supervisors, she was issued a memo during her review that she used practices "outside the acceptable and safe standards of nursing practice." Thereupon, the Claimant's employment with Montgomery was terminated. The Claimant's lawsuit followed her termination.

The trial court granted Montgomery's motion for summary judgment and dismissed the litigation (*Lark v. Montgomery Hospice*, 994 A.2d 968 [2010], 414 Md. 215 [2010]). However, on appeal, the Maryland Court of Appeals, in reinstating the case, recognized the important public duty to blow the whistle on certain behavior, even in the absence of a specific statutory obligation to do so. That is, exposing certain statutory or regulatory violations, including health and safety violations, is sufficiently important that "under certain conditions, an employee who does so is protected from being discharged for that conduct" (994 A.2d 982).

Whistleblowing applies to both current and former employees of the organization. The objective of whistleblowers is to halt the behavior causing harm to patients and to obviate this conduct in the future. Incident reports can be made to supervisors and administrators within the organization where the whistleblower is employed and can also be shared with agencies external to the organization that are positioned to lend assistance. These include regulatory agencies that assume the responsibility of oversight, journalists, and if applicable, law enforcement agencies (Mansbach et al., 2014).

Whistleblowing is itself a course of action. It is at best a thorny dilemma for individuals contemplating the option of reporting incidents that cause harm to patients, because the whistleblower has to decide whether protecting public interest trumps loyalty to coworkers, supervisors, and/or the employer (Mansbach et al., 2014). The dilemma of reporting abusive incidents causing injury or harm to individuals becomes more complex in health care settings when the recipient of abuse is a vulnerable patient. When physicians, nurses, and staff fail to report abuse, or do not take immediate action to curtail the detrimental conduct of administrators or colleagues, they may be violating ethical and professional standards of practice that are central to safeguarding the health and welfare of the patients they serve (Mansbach et al., 2014).

Various federal and state statutes, including those related to health care, contain whistleblower protections. For example, within the Patient Protection and Affordable Care Act, Pub. L. No. 111–148, 124 *Stat.* 119 (2010) ("ACA"), employees receive protections against retaliation by an employer when the employee is engaged in protected activity. The ACA, 29 U.S.C. §218c, sets forth specific protections for whistleblower employees by amendment to the Fair Labor Standards Act of 1938, adding the following:

Protections for Employees
  (a) PROHIBITION. No employer shall discharge or in any manner discriminate against
  any employee with respect to his or her compensation, terms, conditions, or other privileges

of employment because the employee (or an individual acting at the request of the employee) has:

> (1) received a credit under section 36B of the Internal Revenue Code of 1986 or a subsidy under section 1402 of this Act.
>
> (2) provided, caused to be provided, or is about to provide or cause to be provided to the employer, the Federal Government, or the attorney general of a State information relating to any violation of, or any act or omission the employee reasonably believes to be a violation of, any provision of this title (or an amendment made by this title).
>
> (3) testified or is about to testify in a proceeding concerning such violation.
>
> (4) assisted or participated, or is about to assist or participate, in such a proceeding; or
>
> (5) objected to, or refused to participate in, any activity, policy, practice, or assigned task that the employee (or other such person) reasonably believed to be in violation of any provision of this title (or amendment), or any order, rule, regulation, standard, or ban under this title (or amendment).

(b) COMPLAINT PROCEDURE.

> (1) IN GENERAL. An employee who believes that he or she has been discharged or otherwise discriminated against by any employer in violation of this section may seek relief in accordance with the procedures, notifications, burdens of proof, remedies, and statutes of limitation set forth in section 2087(b) of title 15, United States Code.
>
> (2) NO LIMITATION ON RIGHTS. Nothing in this section shall be deemed to diminish the rights, privileges, or remedies of any employee under any Federal or State law or under any collective bargaining agreement. The rights and remedies in this section may not be waived by any agreement, policy, form, or condition of employment.

The failure of nurses to report abuse in the institutional setting is a serious topic of concern as nurses struggle to report abusive acts that are morally charged, particularly when reporting these incidents creates angst for nurses when they report coworkers who abuse patients. Retaliation is a feared reality for those who report coworkers, offering them little protection. Legislation was passed to protect whistleblowers, with court decisions favoring the whistleblower in many instances; however, despite any compensatory damages awarded to the whistleblower, there remains a price to be paid. These include the loss of collegial friendships and blackballing, which threatens the future of the whistleblower (Curtin, 2013).

Many explanations are offered as to why the whistleblower is unfairly punished. These explanations are complex in depth and breadth of concern and give reason for nurses to pause when contemplating the reporting of abuse (Curtin, 2013). Coworkers who have not blown the whistle may feel uncomfortable and awkward with the situation at hand. Additionally, the protection of the team places considerable psychological pressure on individual team members, demanding protection of the team, rather than the patient. Team members learn early on in their employment the importance of getting along with others. Furthermore, the influence that figures of authority maintain over team members reinforces the notion that most people will engage in something that they know to be wrong if they are asked to do so by persons of authority. Individuals have the tendency to evaluate themselves by assessing their good intentions rather than their actions, even if the facts disagree with what they believe is right. If individuals place the abusive act within the context of survival, behaviors that are otherwise unacceptable are more easily tolerated, or even encouraged. Curtin articulated that:

> an overemphasis on expediency "justifies" conduct that would otherwise be condemned as unethical. Group pressure to conform, the pull of team affiliation, and the "all or nothing"

attitude of group think leads otherwise moral people into, at the very least, the complicity of silence [p. 2].

Nurses assume considerable risk when they speak out and report abuse. Nurse advocacy is a widely accepted role of the nurse, as it is valued by the profession as a means of protecting vulnerable patients. When nurses blow the whistle on coworkers and staff who abuse patients, they believe that they are acting in the best interest of the patient while maintaining integrity in their professional role, thus ensuring the safety of those under their care. Conversely, as nurses advocate for patients, they do not want to be recognized as a whistleblower, because this term is perceived with negativity and frequently carries with it an unpleasant stigma that follows those who bring abuse to the forefront. Nurses become whistleblowers when their attempts to intervene on patients' behalf prove to be futile efforts within health care systems and organizations where they are employed, ultimately imbuing a culture that condones silence (Curtin, 2013).

Workplace factors that impact patient advocacy and nurses' (RNs') inclinations to report unsafe practices have been studied (Cole et al., 2018). Constructing safe work environments for nursing practice in acute care settings must include quality improvement strategies, integrated into institutional culture to reduce unfavorable health outcomes, in patients presenting with complex health care requirements (Agency for Health Care Research & Quality [AHRQ], 2019). Establishing an institutional culture of safety includes the incorporation of the following essential elements:

- acknowledgment of the high-risk nature of an organization's activities and the determination to achieve consistently safe operations
- a blame-free environment where individuals are able to report errors or near misses without the fear of reprimand or punishment
- encouragement of collaboration across the ranks and disciplines to seek solutions to patient safety problems
- organizational commitment of resources to address safety concerns (AHRQ, 2019, p. 1).

These four key elements are important measures in the reduction and prevention of errors and in improving the overall quality of health care. AHRQ (2019) shared that "safety culture is fundamentally a local problem, in that wide variations in the perception of safety culture can exist within a single organization" (p. 1). Hence, "the perception of safety culture might be high in one unit within a hospital and low in another unit, or high among management and low among frontline workers" (p. 1). Additionally, extant research demonstrates that individual provider burnout negatively impacts the perception of safety culture. A combination of these two research findings are likely contributors of the mixed record of interventions intended to reduce errors and improve the safety climate (AHRQ, 2019).

Recognizing that nurses were more likely to report wrongdoing with a patient than physicians, a qualitative study by Jackson et al. (2010) examined reasons nurses decided to blow the whistle when confronting unethical situations. Semi-structured interviews with 11 nurse whistleblowers were conducted in Australia. Interviews also addressed experiences of being whistleblowers. Autobiographical stories were provided during the implementation of the narrative inquiry design. The ethical principle of justice framed analysis of participants' stories. The first main theme, *Reasons for whistleblowing: I just couldn't advocate*, incorporated the tension between patient advocacy and the stigma of being a whistleblower. Nurses were unable to gain support and had to protect patients from harm by whistleblowing. The second theme, *Feeling silenced: nobody speaks out*, described a conspiracy of silence in organizations. Fear of losing their job hindered whistleblowing. Their working lives became unbearable. The last theme, *Climate of fear: you are just not safe*, noted the fear that infuses organizational culture. Repercussions were feared, such as for personal welfare and that of children, financial loss, and litigation. They felt unsafe and vulnerable, and some coworkers refused to work with them. The researchers acknowledge a limitation of the study: perhaps a larger sample from different sources might reveal more positive experiences. The nurses interviewed carried out their duty to protect patients and to improve the quality of care. Nonetheless, a major concern in this study's findings is the pressure in health care organizations to maintain the status quo.

Fear of retaliation remains a significant barrier in the reporting of unsafe patient care practices, even though nurses may not have been personally involved in retaliatory actions by coworkers. Nurse leaders carry the burden of responsibility as facilitators to instill a culture of safety within the clinical setting where patient safety takes priority and where comprehensive measures are set in place, thus creating an optimum level of comfort for nurses as they advocate for patients and report harmful incidents. Prevailing protection laws, on-going in-service education, and professional nursing organizations (e.g., ANA) also serve as valuable mechanisms that support nurses in health care organizations (Cole et al., 2018).

Perron et al. (2020) explored nurses' whistleblowing and defined the process as the act of disclosing unethical and/or illegal practices to persons who may directly or indirectly bring about change (Perron et al., 2020, p. 115 citing Near & Miceli). The authors noted that as nurses identify serious shortcomings and wrongdoings in the workplace out of their concern for patient safety, they are at great personal risk for negative outcomes. As the process of whistleblowing unfolds, the nurse reports the serious problem to a leader in a health care institution. Both operate in different power situations.

The authors (Perron et al., 2020) argued that despite policies and laws that safeguard whistleblowers, they have often not been protected from reprimand, ostracism, institutional loyalty, depression, and even disciplinary actions. Internal reports of wrongdoing may not result in change based on an intra-institutional review of the whistleblowing complaint. Reporting a serious safety threat or event can disrupt an organization.

According to Perron et al. (2020), nurse whistleblowers are often caught in the complexity of the diverse aspects of their role, and this is increasingly complicated after reporting whistleblowing events. Power imbalance, knowledge, and the blind spots of organizations leave nurses in a precarious, hypervisible state as compared to their typical position of invisibility. As whistleblowers, they can be seen as "faulty care providers and problematic information brokers" (Perron et al., 2020, p. 116). Perron et al. (2020) proposed an alternate perspective to whistleblowing by applying the lens of the sociology of ignorance. In this context, ignorance includes "that which is not known, cannot be known, or refused to be known" (p. 116). Consequently, social and economic processes, such as whistleblowing, "rest more on what we do not know than on knowledge" (Perron et al., 2020, p. 116 citing Proctor & Schiebinger & McGoey).

Organizations' restricted definitions of safety, quality, risk, and other major concepts are compounded by failure to question other factors that affect health care. This restricts being able to benefit from other forms of knowledge. As nurses report wrongdoing, their knowledge of the details of whistleblowing events might be interpreted by their complicated position in organizations. They could be considered unreliable as judged by prevailing knowledge and ignorance; this complicates the distance between administrators and nurses and reduces the likelihood of corrective actions. Again, reporting may result in distrust of whistleblower nurses.

The reporting procedures of organizations, the extent of corporate responsibility, and the treatment of whistleblowers varies by institution. Access to nurse whistleblowers' information about the institutional response to a specific serious event is often limited. Administrators manage both the knowledge and the ignorance. Although legislation and policies can protect whistleblowers' position in organizations, they might suffer harassment or demotion. Finally, administrators can influence institutional attention to increasing the knowledge and dispelling the ignorance of different roles and policy and reporting constraints when employees act as whistleblowers.

Implications for Nursing

Organizations need to account for nurses' experiences and embrace workplace principles that encourage and support collaborative efforts through the leadership of nurse managers and administrators. Protocols for reporting abusive incidents should be operationalized and well-disseminated to nurses and staff to empower those witnessing abusive acts or situations where patient safety may be compromised. Furthermore, nurses providing direct care are well-positioned to identify unsafe conditions and intervene in near misses to mitigate more serious events from occurring. The responsibility to facilitate reporting systems, ones that do not penalize the individual who is reporting abuse or violations in safety, lies in the hands of nurse managers and administrators (Cole et al., 2018).

The impetus to become a High Reliability Organization (HRO) has motivated health care organizations to create a safety culture. Committing to the principles of HROs means that patient care is provided error-free and zero harm is achieved (Chassin & Loeb, 2013). Staff become expert in recognizing and preventing errors and conditions that otherwise might seem to be minor. In HROs, intimidating behaviors that restrict reporting are eliminated by organizational leaders. Nurses and other frontline staff help to create and to maintain an HRO (Smith, 2018).

Abuse of a patient is a harmful event and is not a small problem nor an error. In the case of abuse, the harm reached the patient. Patient abuse is the ultimate deviation from the expected performance of health care providers and contrasts dramatically with the principles of HROs.

Abuse shows staff's intent to harm patients. With such an event, any organization's achievement of patient safety is compromised. Frontline staff are obligated to provide descriptions to leaders of incidents they witness and judge to be abuse. The benefits of upstream reporting should help an institution to develop trust and to improve care processes and employee evaluation. Therefore, following the disturbing discovery of patient abuse, the organizational culture most likely recommits and continues the journey by following the HRO principles of zero harm (Chassin & Loeb, 2013).

In contrast, an option for nursing homes and long-term care settings is hiring or contracting for the services of advanced practice registered nurses (APRNs). These experts not only affect residents' readmissions to acute care institutions, but also improve the quality of patient care (Rantz et al., 2017). Combined with an interprofessional intervention team, nurse practitioners and other APRNs can intervene early and provide direct care to residents and mentor, role model, and educate nursing staff. With an established track record of increasing quality care, patient satisfaction, and health outcomes, they provide in-service education, round with physicians, examine and treat residents with acute problems, and participate in quality improvement efforts. As such, they can alert the health care team to potential and actual incidents of abuse, and once again report upstream to leaders in facilities.

Next, the dependence of patients and residents on staff could help nursing staff understand patients' need to receive basic nursing care. Insights into adult patients' perspectives of nursing care dependence was examined through a metasynthesis of 18 qualitative research studies using Johanna Briggs Institute approaches (Pirreda et al., 2015). Based on the view that high care dependence was linked to increased mortality risk in older institutionalized persons, the researchers critically appraised studies as patients were cared for in a variety of settings. Interviews were used for data collection for all studies; only those with patient participants were included.

The researchers found that when patients' bodies required care, such as needing help for intimate care and elimination support, patients experienced a decline in social position (Pirreda et al., 2015). Nurses' attention to bodily needs reduced their attention to patients' feelings. As care was shared by several staff members, patients suffered and felt shame by virtue of becoming common property. In contrast, dependency on competent caregivers resulted in feelings of being liberated for people with functional impairments. Adult patients also felt the love of altruistic caregivers and learned to rely on them for help. Elderly patients appreciated having some autonomy yet adjusted to some limitations in obtaining care. On the other hand, the contexts of some organizations that were inflexible enhanced patient dependency and failed to show nurses' responsiveness to patients' needs and for continuity of care.

Good personal contacts and relationships might assist nursing staff to see the inner being of patients when bodily care predominates (Pirreda et al., 2015). Perhaps patients' experiences of care dependence could be explored with nursing staff so that the humiliation and suffering associated with dependence on staff for bodily care might explain some persons' resistance and aggression in response to episodes of bodily care. However, nursing staff are at times victims of patient violence. In a situation with a resident who has dementia and is aggressive, a member of the nursing staff might be hurt, and they fear caring for them. To prevent a staff member impulsively harming a patient in return, nursing staff need to learn de-escalation and interventional techniques for patients whose behavior is difficult to manage.

Nurses need to review laws in their home states to become informed on regulations covering incidents of abuse. The promulgation of laws and regulations is a helpful mechanism that offers a level of protection to professionals in reporting abuse. One example includes the State of New Jersey Health Care Professional Responsibility and Reporting Act, also known as Chapter 83 or the Cullen Act. This law was enacted in July 1985 after Charles Cullen, a nurse, confessed to murdering anywhere between 29 and 40 patients assigned to his care while employed in a number of hospitals in New Jersey and Pennsylvania. Despite a questionable record of employment, Cullen succeeded in moving from hospital to hospital for 16 years. The purpose of the Cullen Act is to "facilitate the sharing of information about health care professionals who may present a risk of harm to patients" (p. 1). Essentially, the Act protects health care entities in New Jersey by allowing them to report the "impairment, incompetence, negligence, and professional misconduct of health care professionals to the New Jersey Division of Consumer Affairs or other health care entities without fear of reprisal by the health care professional at issue" (p. 1).

This and similar laws that mandate reporting of inappropriate conduct in the health care setting provide appropriate protections to health care professionals who witness and report abusive conduct. Eliminating the old school bunker mentality of hide/cover-up incompetence, negligence and abuse, not only assists in eradicating ill-treatment, but upgrades the quality of health care services. Kousgaard et al. (2012) commented that considerable emphasis needs to be placed on the integration of effective strategies and resources to establish organizational structures that manage the ongoing promotion, support, and feedback that are site specific to the institution.

Summary

This chapter considered abuse within the context of failure to report acts of abuse within the health care setting as nurses continue to grapple with the balance of professional standards of practice, moral obligations, and legal mandates that encompass reporting and the lack thereof. Nurses who witness abuse are often placed in uncomfortable positions in their attempts to uphold their responsibility in reporting unsafe practices and the ill treatment of vulnerable patients. Wijma et al. (2016) noted that abuse in health care is complex; additional research needs to be framed by theoretical perspectives. Additional research into this important area of nursing is warranted to safeguard and to protect nurses in their efforts to protect patients from harm and to expose nurses to the complexity of issues that arise from the failure to report abuse in clinical settings.

Retaliatory actions post-reporting abuse appear in the literature (Cole et al., 2018; Curtin, 2013), as a number of nurse managers, administrators, and coworkers chose to retaliate after abuse was reported. Mechanisms of dissuasion (e.g., psychological pressure) are a reality for professional nurses and serve as an unremitting reminder of the implicit risks associated with reporting and the courage required to transcend the status quo of silence to report abuse. When the voices of nurses reporting abuse are not supported by nurse managers and administrators, nurses have the option of stepping into the murky waters of the whistleblowing process. Whistleblowing carries with it a distinct stigma and instills a level of fear for whistleblowers, as the loss of collegiality and friendship, harsh sanctions, and employment security are threatened (Curtin, 2013).

Quality improvement initiatives need to be strengthened and integrated into the institutional setting, thus ensuring the safety and well-being of patients who are the recipients of care. Implementing safety measures and strategies that protect patients from near misses and unsafe practices promotes a culture of safety within the institution (AHRQ, 2019).

Table 16 identifies and summarizes the types of abuse that appear in the literature.

Table 16. Types of Abuse

Type	Definition	Example
Verbal abuse	Any use of oral, written, or gestured language that willfully includes disparaging and derogatory terms to residents or their families, or within their hearing distance, regardless of their age, ability to comprehend or disability (28 Pa Code §201.3)	Threats of harm Saying things to frighten a resident, such as telling a resident that the resident will never be able to see his family again (28 Pa Code §201.3)

Type	Definition	Example
Sexual abuse	Nonconsensual sexual contact or any unwanted sexual contact (ALTSA, 2019)	Includes sexual harassment, sexual coercion or sexual assault Any unwanted touching, rape, sodomy, coerced nudity, sexually explicit photographing (ALTSA, 2019)
Physical abuse	Intentional bodily injury (ALTSA, 2019)	Includes hitting, slapping, pinching, and kicking. The term also includes controlling behavior through corporal punishment (28 Pa Code §201.3)
Mental abuse	Deliberately causing mental or emotional pain (ALTSA, 2019)	Includes humiliation, harassment, threats of punishment or deprivation (28 Pa Code §201.3)
Involuntary seclusion	Separation of a resident from other residents or from his room or confinement to his room (with/without roommates) against the resident's will, or the will of the resident's legal representative; emergency or short-term monitored separation from other residents will not be considered involuntary seclusion and may be permitted if used for a limited period of time as a therapeutic intervention to reduce agitation until professional staff can develop a plan of care to meet the resident's needs (28 Pa Code §201.3)	Caretaker viewed as indifferent to patient
Neglect	The deprivation by a caretaker of goods or services which are necessary to maintain physical or mental health (28 Pa Code §201.3)	Not providing basic items such as food, water, clothing, a safe place to live, medicine, or health care (ALTSA, 2019)

Adapted from: 28 Pa Code §201.3 Pennsylvania Regulations, Title 28 Health and Safety, and Aging and Long-Term Support Administration (ALTSA), 2019.

Strategies

Table 17 presents strategies to effect change based on the reviewed literature.

Table 17. Strategies to Eliminate Abuse
in Health Care Settings

Strategies to Effect Change	Evidence-Based Citations
Avoid blaming members of the health care delivery team directly involved in the care of patients who were abused	Albina (2016)
Offer educational sessions to direct caregivers on how to identify and report abuse	Malmedal et al. (2014)
Administrators and managers consistently follow adopted policies and procedures aimed at protection of residents of long-term care settings and hold staff accountable for actions deemed abusive	Payne & Fletcher (2005)
Supervise detention facility staff closely when guarding pregnant women	Ishola et al. (2017)
Teach pregnant women about their rights as patients and ways to report abuse to administrators	Hodges (2009)
Administrators and managers consistently provide feedback to staff about practice improvements and strategies to correct or report abuse	Evans et al. (2006)
Incorporate content on complaint procedures in employee orientation programs consistent with state-based whistleblowing laws	Patient Protection and Affordable Care Act, Pub. L. No. 111–148, 124 *Stat.* 119 (2010)

Conclusion

Nurses working in health care institutions are expected to deliver patient care that aligns with personal accountability and ethical codes of conduct that define the profession (Fagerström, 2006). In daily practice, nurses satisfy their duties by maintaining a connection between being good (character) and doing good (action), notwithstanding time constraints and conflicting demands that are known to surface in the workplace (Wolf, 2012).

Emboldening nurses with the courage to report incidents of abuse that jeopardize the health status and safety of patients has been historically problematic and continues to raise significant concerns in current practice settings. A change in institutional climate, in addition to adopting a culture that supports nurses and assists them in identifying processes of reporting, is indicated to protect patients and improve care outcomes (Bolsin et al., 2011).

Whistleblowing as an option for reporting abuse carries with it a real stigma, despite the recognized contribution this reporting mechanism has made to protect the safety of patients. Additionally, whistleblowing and staff fearfulness of the negative consequences that can occur by nurses and staff going outside official boundaries to bring unsafe care to the forefront remains a reality, mandating health care institutions to initiate proposals on how to improve situations of this nature (Bolsin et al., 2011).

Future research on this topic area should focus on how to implement and organize the reporting of violations within the organizational structures of health care institutions, as they manage the promotion, support, and feedback required for reducing incidents in nurse practice (Kousgaard et al., 2012).

Discussion Questions

1. Define abuse and describe the different types of abuse that contribute to negative outcomes in hospital settings.

2. Discuss barriers that arise in clinical settings that could inhibit the reporting of patient abuse.

3. Evaluate workplace strategies that could be implemented in the health care arena that support nurses in the prevention of abusive acts and assist in the improvement of patient outcomes.

4. Analyze differing viewpoints of nurses and health care professionals related to whistleblowing in institutional settings.

5. Examine various laws and regulations enacted to protect patients from abuse in hospital settings.

AUTHOR SELECTION

Belle, J. (2013, April). *Touching poem by an older man* [Poem]. AgingCare. https://www.agingcare.com/discussions/touching-poem-by-an-older-man-157056.htm.

REFERENCES

Agency for Healthcare Research & Quality. (2019). *Patient safety primer: Culture of safety.* https://psnet.ahrq.gov/primers/primer/5/safety-culture.
Aging and Long-Term Support Administration. (2019). *Types and signs of Abuse.* Washington State Department of Social and Health Sciences. https://dshs.wa.gov.
Albina, J.K. (2016). Patient abuse in the healthcare setting: The nurse as patient advocate. *Association of Perioperative Registered Nurses, 103 (1),* 74–80. http://dx./doi.org.10.1016/j.acrn.2015.10.021.
American Nurses Association. (2015). *Code of ethics for nurses with interpretive statements.* https://www.nursingworld.org/practice-policy/nursing-excellence/ethics/code-of-ethics-for-nurses/.
Bolsin, S., Pal, R., Wilmshurst, P., & Pena, M. (2011). Whistleblowing and patient safety: The patient's or the profession's interests at stake? *Journal of the Royal Society of Medicine. 104,* 278–282. doi 10.1258/jrsm.2011.110034.
Burr Road Operating Company II, LLC v. New England Health Care Employees Union, District 1199. (Appellate Court of Connecticut, No. 33954. January 26, 2016).
Chassin, M.R., & Loeb, J.M. (2013). High-reliability health care: Getting there from here. *Milbank Quarterly, 91*(3), 459–490.
Cole, D.A., Bersick, E., Scarbek, A., Cummins, K., Dugan, K., & Grantoza, R. (2019). The courage to speak out: A study describing nurses' attitudes to report unsafe practices in patient care. *Journal of Nursing Management. 27,* 1176–1181. https://doi.org/10.1111/jonm.12789.
Curtin, L. (2013). When nurses speak up, they pay a price. *American Nurse Today, 8*(10), 1–5.
Evans, S.M., Berry, J.G., Smith, B.J., Esterman, A., Selim, P., O'Shaughnessy, J., & De Wit, M. (2006). Attitudes and barriers to incident reporting: A collaborative hospital study. *Journal of Quality and Safety in Health Care, 15,* 39–43. doi: 10.1136/qshc.2004.012559.
Fagerström, L. (2006). The dialectic tension between 'being' and 'not being' a good nurse. *Nursing Ethics, 13,* 622–632.
Hodges, S. (2009). Abuse in hospital-based birth settings. *Journal of Perinatal Education, 18*(4), 8–11.
HomeCare Council of New Jersey (2019). *Cullen Act: Requirements and Protections.* [PDF]. http://www.homecarecouncilnj.org/CullenAct.pdf.
Ishola, F., Owolabi, & Filippi, V. (2017). Disrespect and abuse of women during childbirth in Nigeria: A systematic review. *PLOS One 12*(3), 1–17. https://doi.org/10.1371/journal.pone.0174084.
Jackson, D., Peters, K., Andrew, A., Edenborough, M., Halcomb, E., Luck, L., Salamonson, Y., & Wilkes, L. (2010). Understanding whistleblowing: Qualitative insights from nurse whistleblowers. *Journal of Advanced Nursing, 66*(10), 2194–2201. doi: 10.1111/j.1365-2648.2010.05365.x.

Kim v. Lakeside Adult Family Home. (No. 91536–9, S. Ct. Wash., May 12, 2016).

Kousgaard, M.B., Joensen, A.S., & Thorsen, T. (2012). Reasons for not reporting patient safety incidents in general practice: A qualitative study. *Scandinavian Journal of Primary Health Care, 30*, 199–205. doi: 10.3109/02813432.2012.732469.

Lark v. Montgomery Hospice. 994 A.2d 968 (2010), 414 Md. 215.

Malmedal, W., Hammervold, R., & Saveman, B.I. (2014). The dark side of nursing homes: Factors influencing inadequate care. *Journal of Adult Protection, 16*(3), 133–151. doi: 10.1108/JAP-02-2013-0004.

Mannion, R., & Davies, H.T. (2015). Cultures of silence and cultures of voice: The role of whistleblowing in healthcare organisations. *International Journal of Health Policy and Management, 4*(8), 503–505. doi: 10.15171/ijhpm.2015.120.

National Council of State Boards of Nursing. (2011). TERCAP.

The Patient Protection and Affordable Care Act, Publ. L. 111–148, 124 Stat. 119 (2010). https://www.congress. gov/111/plaws/publ148/PLAW-111publ148.pdf.

Payne, B.K., & Fletcher, L.B. (2005). Elder abuse in nursing homes: Prevention and resolution strategies and barriers. *Journal of Clinical Justice, 33, 119–125.* doi: 10.1016/j.crimjus2004.12.003

Pennsylvania Code. Pennsylvania Long Term Care Facilities Regulations, Definitions 28 Pa Code §201.3. Definitions. http://www.pacodeandbulletin.gov/Display/pacode?file=/secure/pacode/data/028/ chapter201/s201.3.html&d=reduce.

Perron, A., Rudge, T., Gagnon, & M. (2020). Hypervisible nurses: Effects of circulating ignorance and knowledge on acts of whistleblowing in health. *Advances in Nursing Science, 43*(2), 114–131. doi: 10.1097/ ANS.0000000000000311.

Pirreda, M., Matarese, M., Mastroianni, C., D'Angelo, D., Hammer, M.J., & De Marinis, M.G. (2015). Adult patients' experiences of nursing care dependence. *Journal of Nursing Scholarship, 47*(5), 397–406. doi: 10.1111/jnu.12154.

Rantz, N.M., Birtley, N.M., Flesner, M., Crecelius, C., & Murray, C. (2017). Call to action: APRNs in U.S. nursing homes to improve care and reduce costs. *Nursing Outlook, 65,* 689–696.

Senate and General Assembly of the State of New Jersey. (2005, May 3). CHAPTER 83: Health Care Professional Responsibility and Reporting Enhancement Act. C.26:2H-12.2b.

Smith, C. (2018). Promoting high reliability on the front line. *American Nurse Today, 13*(3), 30–32.

United States Congress. 31 U.S. Code § 3729. *False claims.* https://www.law.cornell.edu/uscode/text/31/ 3729.

United States Department of Justice. (n.d.). *False Claims Act: A primer.* https://www.justice.gov/sites/ default/files/civil/legacy/2011/04/22/C-FRAUDS_FCA_Primer.pdf

United States House of Representatives. (n.d.). 50 USC CHAPTER 42, SUBCHAPTER VI, Part A: Personnel Management: §2702. Whistleblower protection program. https://uscode.house.gov/view. xhtml?req=granuleid%3AUSC-prelim-title50-chapter42-subchapter6-partA&edition=prelim.

Wijma, B., Zbikowski, A., & Brüggemann, A. (2016). Silence, shame, and abuse in health care: Theoretical development on basis of an intervention project among staff. *BMC Medical Education, 16*(75). doi: 10.1186/s12909-016-0595-3.

Wolf, Z.R. (2012). Nursing practice breakdowns: Good and bad nursing. *MEDSURG Nursing, 21*(1), 16–36.

Multiple-Choice Questions

1. Which of the following actions should nurses carry out when overhearing a nursing assistant share that she slapped a person with dementia "hard" to induce him to better behave?

    A. Call a lawyer for advice

    B. Report the incident to a colleague

    C. Make a note to remember to share her suspicions

    D. Describe the incident during a meeting with the nurse manager

2. Which of the following standards needs to be implemented by health care institutions to prevent patient abuse?

    A. Administer the Culture of Safety instrument to all employees

    B. Treat once-witnessed disrespectful behavior as behavior to tolerate

    C. Advertise the end to institutional tolerance of disrespectful behavior

    D. Share examples of disrespectful behavior on the institution's intranet

3. **Which of the following staff positions in nursing is obligated to report patient abuse? Select all that apply.**
   A. Registered nurse
   B. Nurse manager
   C. Chief nurse
   D. Licensed practical nurse

4. **Which of the following aspects of climates in health care organizations inhibits nurses from reporting incidents of abuse involving patients?**
   A. Litigation
   B. Financial losses
   C. Fear of personal harm
   D. Loss of status

Chapter 14

Homicide and Nursing Staff

Zane Robinson Wolf, PhD, RN,
CNE, ANEF, FCPP, FAAN

Objectives

1. Analyze personal and behavioral characteristics of serial murderers.
2. Examine outcome data suggesting the possibility of nefarious activity in clinical settings.
3. Contrast different checklists used by health care professionals to assess critical indicators of malfeasance against patients.
4. Explore the Collins and Mikos (2008) model of legal and professional regulation of nurses in the context of nurses convicted of murder.

Critical Incidents

Neils Hoegel was accused and convicted of killing many patients. Different drugs, including lidocaine and calcium chloride, were used to poison patients. During the first trial, the ex-nurse admitted that he caused cardiac events and enjoyed resuscitating patients. Fatality rates increased on his shift (Noack, 2018). Health care workers noticed an increased number of resuscitations at clinics where he worked (Moulson, 2017).

News stories on the ex-nurse's clinical crimes revealed initial convictions and incarceration for two murders in 2015, followed by additional charges of deaths in the German cities of Delmenhourt and Oldenburg (Moulson, 2017, 2018). Toxicological examinations of patients who died led to another trial. The second trial charged Hoegel in the deaths of 62 patients in Delmenhorst and 35 patients in Oldenburg. Former staff at the two health care settings were also implicated in criminal cases (Associated Press, 2017).

Hoegel may have murdered more patients than Charles Cullen, a former American nurse who will spend the rest of his life in prison (Graeben, 2013). A more recent example of a nurse who murdered patients is Canadian Elizabeth Wettlaufer (Canadian Broadcasting Corporation, 2017). She administered insulin and killed eight elderly patients in Ontario nursing homes. In addition to murder charges, attempted murder and aggravated assault charges were filed. Her crimes were committed between 2007 and 2016. She was never fired from positions for murder, but for making medication errors.

Wettlaufer (Casey, 2017) confessed murdering patients to attendees of Alcoholics Anonymous meetings, a pastor, and fellow health care providers. Some thought she was lying. Few took Wettlaufer seriously, until a nursing student and staff in a psychiatric hospital reported claims to authorities. Patients killed were vulnerable, either because of having dementia, of being difficult to manage, or of just being old. Wettlaufer said she received a message from God to act.

Another example of nurses who allegedly killed patients, described by Curtin (2019), occurred in Novus hospice settings. Jessica Love, a nursing supervisor of the largest hospice in North Texas, pled guilty to committing health care fraud. Patients were fatally overdosed for profit and died earlier than expected. Patients were killed by the nurses turning off oxygen, "increasing Ativan and morphine, and rolling the patient onto the left side" (Curtin, 2019, p. 48). Novus billed Medicare and Medicaid for services.

The alleged creator of the fraud and murder scheme was Bradley Harris, CEO, a certified public accountant; however, a total of 16 individuals have been charged with fraud (Wigglesworth, 2018a). Documents were falsified and may have been shredded. Murder and conspiracy to commit murder charges against employees were pending (Wigglesworth, 2018b).

These three examples point to the crime of homicide. "Criminal homicide occurs when a person purposely, knowingly, recklessly, or negligently causes the death of another" (Cady, 2009, p. 11). Murder and manslaughter, examples of criminal homicide, are serious crimes or felonies, and prison terms and death sentences often follow. Murder, or unlawfully taking human life, is often contextualized by power, personal gain, and brutality. The terms murder and homicide are used interchangeably (Douglas et al., 1992).

Serial murder is defined as "the unlawful killing of two or more victims by the same offender(s), in separate events" (Morton & Hilts, 2013, p. 9). Killers among health care professionals have been distinguished by the phrase carer associated serial killers (CASK) (Forrest, 1995). Another label for providers that murder a number of patients is health care serial killers (HSK) (Yardley & Wilson, 2016). Additionally, nurses accused of murder are often termed angels of death (Yardley & Wilson, 2016). Some may fit the classifications of mercy/hero or hero homicide (Douglas et al., 1992).

Background

Nursing staff who harm or kill patients commit interpersonal violence (Sumner et al., 2015). They intentionally use their power and access against patients. Interpersonal violence is considered a public health problem; however, few nurses and other health care providers commit murder, compared to other occupations.

Many risk factors are associated with interpersonal violence. These include child maltreatment, youth violence, and partner violence. Individual (poor impulse control), family (familial economic stress/socioeconomic status), community (exposure to neighborhood violence), and societal (high prevalence of poverty) factors also have been implicated. Multiple adverse experiences can be linked to acts of violence; risk factors can also be reduced by nurturing families and community support. Examples of violence prevention initiatives are early childhood visitation (Nurse-Family Partnership), parenting training (Oregon Model, Parent Management Training), and school-based, social-emotional learning approaches (Life Skills Training) (Sumner et al., 2015).

Nurses may not recognize that it is possible that a coworker could be murdering patients. Lacking awareness of the possibility may help them to ignore higher than normal death rates on a shift or an unusually high number of cardiopulmonary arrests in an ICU (Park & Khan, 2002). Higher incidences of death on a nurse's shift have been carefully evaluated (Yardley & Wilson, 2014) and have stimulated local investigations. Additionally, awareness of stories describing nurses accused and convicted of murder and strategic institutional policies and procedures could help nurses respond more quickly to suspicious activities and occurrences and report them to clinical leaders (McNamara, 2012; Tilley et al., 2019).

Objective measures that can suggest murder by health care providers are reviewed routinely by morbidity and mortality committees in acute care institutions. Deaths and serious adverse events are also evaluated by quality improvement and risk management departments of hospitals (Sullivan, 2009) and patient safety committees. Statistically based reports that address incidence, showing clusters of these outcomes, can trigger investigations by health care leaders, yet have to be carefully interpreted (Standing Bear, 1996). However, time may elapse before committee members analyze possible indicators of intentional patient harm (Graeber, 2013).

In the Cullen case (Graeber, 2013), certain medications were being ordered at the unit level in increased number. Therefore, patterns in dispensing triggered by medication orders may also need to be monitored closely by pharmacists. For example, a centralized comprehensive refill authorization program was created in an electronic medical record system, Epic, so the pharmacy team could refill prescriber requests in a clinic. Similar programs may be used in acute care institutions (Rim et al., 2018).

Studies confirm that registered nurses are more frequently involved in patient murders compared to other nursing staff. Injected medications (poisoning by drugs) are the most frequent method (Wolf et al., 2019; Yorker et al., 2006). Regrettably, nurses have been accused, tried, and convicted of murdering one or more patients.

The sites of homicides performed by employees in health care settings differ from those of other murderers due to accessibility. The opportunity for health care providers to commit harm is present at work because of regular contact with vulnerable persons: older, very young, and very ill (Yardley & Wilson, 2016). Therefore, nurses and other caregivers are classified as contact killers (Cotter, 2010). Anchor points or comfort zones for HSKs are the places where they work (Morton & Hilts, 2013).

The reputations of an accused person, employing institutions and their staff, and administrators are threatened by allegations of murder. When unexplained deaths are being investigated, disharmony can result among health care providers (Forrest, 1995; Graeber, 2013). News accounts of these egregious crimes keep the public engaged in the progress of charges and subsequent judicial processes (Shellen, 2006).

Standards and Nursing Theory

Many professional organizations have promulgated patient safety and helped to set standards for quality health care for constituents. For example, the National Quality Forum (2011) shared a consensus report in which 29 serious reportable events (SRE) were examined. The agenda was to facilitate the education of health care organizations and systems so that patient safety was promoted and harm prevented. The NQF obtained consensus through a systematic process and emphasized outcome measurement.

Potential criminal events were among the selected categories. The categories functioned as a classification scheme.

The National Quality Forum (2011), when referring to SREs, acknowledged the difficulty with attributing the intent of health care providers' actions when harming patients. They included the word *potential* because on discovery, intent might not be identified. Their report acknowledged the rarity of SREs. Of potential criminal events, impersonating a licensed health care provider, abduction of a patient/resident of any age, sexual abuse/assault of a patient or staff in a health care setting or on its grounds, and death or serious injury of a patient or staff member resulting from a physical assault (i.e., battery) that occurs within or on the grounds of a health care setting include examples. Also noted in the report's care management event category were patient deaths in a health care setting associated with medication errors, blood product administration, maternal death or serious injury associated with labor or delivery in a low-risk pregnancy, a neonate death or serious injury associated with labor or delivery in a low-risk pregnancy, a fall, and unstageable pressure injuries after admission/presentation. Others included artificial insemination with wrong donor sperm or wrong egg, irretrievable loss of an irreplaceable biological specimen, and failure to follow up or communicate laboratory, pathology, or radiology test results. Settings identified included hospitals, outpatient/office-based surgery centers, ambulatory practice settings/office-based practices, and long-term/skilled nursing facilities. Murder is definitely a serious reportable event.

The principles of beneficence and nonmaleficence orient health care providers to their responsibilities. The American Nurses Association (ANA, 2010), like other nursing organizations, publishes positions that emphasize nursing's commitment to the common good and described in the ANA's Code of Ethics (2015). Murder of patients violates the basic commitment of all health care providers not to harm persons in their care. Murder is the worst breach of professional ethics and personal moral codes.

It is not surprising that the negative side of nursing is not often represented in nursing theory. However, Halldorsdottir (1991) depicted caring and uncaring behaviors on a continuum, the five basic modes of being with another. Two of the types or modes of being with another frame the harmful behavior of nurses. These include: (1) the life-restraining or biostatic mode is uncaring; the patient perceives the nurse as indifferent, insensitive, and detached; the patient is discouraged and his or her life is negatively impacted; and (2) the life-destroying or biocidic mode represents the most negative, destructive, uncaring mode; the patient is depersonalized; the joy of life is destroyed, and the vulnerability of the patient is increased (Halldorsdottir, 1991). Nurses who murder patients provide a definitive example of the biocidic mode. Nurse-patient relationships and professional action are destroyed. This typology provides a standard by which to classify harmful actions of nurses.

Literature

According to Field (2008), nurses kill patients out of compassion, to end suffering, accidentally, and intentionally out of malice. Nurses who murder patients may be labeled either insane and/or profane, argued Field. He suggested that serial killers might be both. Profane behaviors show callousness, premeditation, and absence of empathy and remorse about persons murdered. Serial killers might be insane, according to Field, but insanity is a legal concept.

Field (2008) pointed out that serial killers who are nurses demonstrate similar characteristics of other serial killers. However, they do not typically violate victims sexually or take trophies. More often they are women, compared to men. Nonetheless, it is difficult to profile the characteristics of nurses who kill, in the hope of identifying them before they kill more victims. He proposed that power was the chief motivation.

Field and Pearson (2010) asserted that nursing had been almost silent about nurse murderers. Field and Pearson's study focused on the following clusters: killing and consequences, constructions of nurses who murder, and reactions to the murder of patients. A consistent demographic pattern was not identified in the nurse examples evaluated. Patients were often murdered in ICUs, CCUs, emergency, residential aged care, and community settings. They were very young, very old, very ill, and physically or mentally disabled.

Nurses who murdered patients worked alone for short time periods and changed jobs when alerted by suspicions of their wrongdoing (Field & Pearson, 2010). They killed patients by physical abuse, lethal doses of medications, and suffocation. Evidentiary patterns showed the relationship between shifts worked and death counts. Motives varied, including thrill killing, attention seeking, sexual gratification, power, and pleasure in killing. Some coworkers denied being suspicious.

The researchers noted silence about nurse murderers by employing organizations, governmental regulatory agencies, and consumers of health care (Field & Pearson, 2010). They cautioned that nurses need to recognize that coworkers could be murderers; reporting suspicious behavior was essential. One indicator for administrators to evaluate on job applications is the number of jobs held in various health care agencies; administrators need to consider not hiring these applicants. Monitoring deaths and resuscitation counts were also recommended. However, these statistics provide circumstantial evidence only (Graeber, 2013).

Morton and Hilts (2013) reported results of a symposium hosted by the Federal Bureau of Investigation in San Antonio, Texas, in 2005. Mental health professionals, academics, officers of the court, and members of the media from the U.S. and other countries attended as a multidisciplinary group of experts; they shared perspectives on serial murder. They worked to identify common knowledge on serial murder. The monograph produced distilled information on major issues related to serial murder. For example, a distinction was made between forensic or behavioral evidence. In the case of Cullen (Graeber, 2013) and other accounts of nurse murderers (Wolf et al., 2019), behavioral evidence exceeded forensic evidence.

Miller (2014) described serial killers by presenting various typologies and motives. A type that fits nurse serial killers was custodial killer. They murder patients by medication overdose or asphyxiation and were most often female, motivated by a need to put patients out of their misery. Another type that can represent nurse murderers is spatial mobile killers: patients were murdered in a geographically same or nearby area. Some nurse killers shared that they killed because of a religious imperative. They were also power/control serial killers. Very few identified in one study were couple serial killers (Wolf et al., 2019).

Yardley and Wilson (2016) studied serial nurse killers that committed the crimes in hospitals. They described factors that might alert health care leaders to behaviors that indicate serious harm to patients. They used Ramsland's (2007) Red Flag checklist and other studies' findings to identify the sample. Most health care serial killers ($N = 16$) were from North America and Europe, with the U.S. having most (38 percent). They were split equally by gender, and the mean age when convicted was 38.1.

Most were convicted based on five to nine murders committed in one hospital. They frequently killed adults and old persons and used a single method, poisoning, most often with medications. The highest prevalence of items on Ramsland's checklist was higher incidence of death on his/her shift, history of mental instability/depression, and makes colleagues anxious/suspicious. They recommended greater scrutiny and warned that hospital administrators and others should be cautious about basing accusations of murder on available evidence. Prevention and detection demand further efforts.

Personality characteristics of four female serial killers (killer of two or more victims by same offender[s] in separated events) were explored (Hildebrand & Culhane, 2015). The researchers emphasized the reliance on media accounts and studies of male murderers. Of the U.S. pool of 49 females meeting study criteria as convicted serial killers, four incarcerated women were sampled. Researchers administered the Minnesota Multiphasic Personality inventory-2, Million Clinical Multiaxial Inventory-III, Levenson Psychopathology Scale, Psychopathy Personality Inventory-Revised, and Self-Report Psychopathy Scale-III, and elicited demographic characteristics. A former nurse's aide and registered nurse were part of the sample. The former nurse's aide killed frail people only and fit the usual angel of death label. The registered nurse killed terminally ill patients. Both could be classified as occupational serial killers. A common finding about the four women was depressive symptoms. Motivations and behaviors varied. A prototypical female serial killer was not identified.

The National Violent Death Reporting System (NVDRS) is a state-based active surveillance system that records data on victims, perpetrators, caregiver roles, and circumstances that precipitated homicides by a caregiver (Karch & Nunn, 2011). Karch and Nunn used the NVDRS to examine demographics, mechanism of injury, location of injury, and location of death for adults killed by caregivers for the years 2003 to 2007. For 68 killed by caregivers, four persons were injured in a hospital/medical facility or supervised residential facility. Places of death for 68 persons were hospital inpatient ($N = 20$), emergency department ($N = 3$), nursing home/long-term care facility ($N = 2$), and victim's home ($N = 43$). Health care providers comprised 14.3 percent of perpetrators. Three health care providers intentionally poisoned patients with digoxin, dilantin, and hydrogen peroxide.

Nurses have an opportunity to respond to the impact of homicide on secondary victims, such as family members and friends of homicide victims and health care providers who witness and care for victims of homicide. In addition to the state and the wider society affected by homicides, the impact is often at the local community level and felt as communal sadness (Morrall et al., 2011). Of note is the restorative justice movement that created programs offered in different countries in support of secondary victims. Forensic nurses, nurse lawyers, and mental health nurses, including psychiatric/mental health nurse practitioners, are involved in supporting secondary victims of homicide at crime scenes, emergency units, and primary care offices. Secondary victims of homicide suffer from traumatic bereavement and may evidence post-traumatic stress disorder. Secondary victims require ongoing support due to the devastating murders of persons close to them or for whom they cared.

Regulatory Initiatives

Administrators and managers who have employed nursing staff whose unprofessional conduct has spurred these leaders to action, such as termination or suspension, have often questioned whether they should report this activity to administrators of nearby institutions. In the case of Charles Cullen, administrators shared unofficial warnings (Graeber, 2013); however, he was employed at various institutions despite warnings. His case raised the issue of what to report. Most references for former employees like Cullen typically cited only the dates a job applicant was employed.

The State of New Jersey, as a response to the crimes of Charles Cullen, enacted the Health Care Professional Responsibility and Reporting Enhancement Act (HCPRREA) (Bennett, 2016). The Act led to the creation of the Health Care Professional Information Clearinghouse Coordinator in the Division of Consumer Affairs (DCA) of the Systems Branch of the Department of Health. The law emphasizes the conduct of professionals when performing patient care, treatment, or diagnosis. It asserts that professionals' clinical practice conduct aims to promote patient safety by not physically or emotionally harming a person in their care. Practices by health care professionals, described as adversely affecting patient safety and dangerous, place patients in imminent danger, demonstrate decreased levels of competence, or lack capacity to practice (alcohol or chemical use, psychiatric or emotional disorder, senility or disabling physical disorder) (New Jersey Administrative Code, Title 13 Law and Public Safety Chapter 45E, 2011).

New Jersey health care entities and health care professionals are protected when they report impairment, incompetence, negligence, or professional misconduct (Home Care Council of New Jersey, n.d.). Written reports are mandated for both and are filed with the DCA (New Jersey Administrative Code, Title 13 Law and Public Safety Chapter 45E, 2011). A clearing house is available for submitting reports and is under DCA. Health care entities must also demonstrate action. For example, health care professionals' privileges to practice may be revoked, suspended, permanently reduced, removed from a list of a health services firm or staffing agency, discharged, terminated, or rescinded. Conditions or limitations on the exercise of clinical privileges or practices may also be imposed. The specific actions implemented by employing agencies must be reported.

Event reporting instructions are available for the HCPRREA (Rutgers, n.d.). A specific person is designated as a reporter in each entity or organization (Herbert & Lopez, 2014). An example of a university policy that illustrates compliance with HCPRREA is provided in University of Medicine & Dentistry of New Jersey (2010).

Many states and universities have required that applicants to state professional licensing boards or health care educational programs complete criminal background checks (Collins & Mikos, 2008) and provide biometric fingerprints. Administrators have questioned the worth of adding federal criminal record clearances to state and university requirements and as ongoing evidence of criminal clearance when students are enrolled in prelicensure programs. Health care organizations have also required that clearances are completed and guaranteed, supported by requirements in affiliation agreements, prior to allowing students' access to clinical practice agencies. Another consequence of Charles Cullen's criminal history was the New Jersey Board of Nursing's decision to add criminal history background checks on license renewals along with the requirement for new license applicants (Herbert & Lopez, 2014).

Some consider background checks the first defense (AHC Media, 2005) to avoid hiring dangerous staff. Advice on background checks includes knowing both the state's and the adjacent states' requirements for background checks, verifying applicants' identity using fingerprinting, obtaining Form DD-214 for persons discharged from the military, and acquiring applicants' last performance reviews. Risk managers might also conduct toxicology screens immediately following cardiac arrests in all patients, without suspecting foul play; review and compare monthly code and death statistics by unit, shift, and hospital; require pharmacies to account for unit-based doses of medications; and incorporate data from associated policies into root-cause analyses following suspicious or unexpected deaths.

In contrast, the Integrated Automated Fingerprint Identification System (IAFIS) is a national, computerized system for storing, comparing, and exchanging fingerprint data in a digital format. The FBI's Division of Criminal Justice Information Services (CJIS) manages the system (FBI, CJIS, n.d.). Criminal history information, fingerprints, criminal subject photographs, and information on military and civilian federal employees are included. Individuals can be identified through IAFIS, and other data can also be shared. The rapidity of the automated system could assist members of the law enforcement community to link criminals to fingerprints left at crime scenes. Also, in Pennsylvania, fingerprints obtained from employees in regular contact with children and hired by licensed entities (employing agencies), as contracted by the Department of Health, Pennsylvania with Cogent Systems, are sent to IAFIS by Pennsylvania employing agencies. Pennsylvania Criminal History Record Checks are managed by the Pennsylvania State Police (Commonwealth of Pennsylvania, Department of Health, n.d.).

The National Council of State Boards of Nursing (NCSBN, 2014) consulted with forensic experts and published guidelines for criminal background checks. The Board noted that the criminal background checks represent a legitimate regulatory purpose; the Board document also acknowledged the laws of states. Furthermore, the NCSBN's Uniform Licensure requirements have mandated that nurse license applications should include a question about past criminal history. Misdemeanors, felonies, and plea agreements are to be identified in addition to biometric data. Statements of applicants with a positive history are required to expand on the nature of all offenses.

Applications are screened in the case of a positive criminal history (NCSBN, 2014). The applicant's explanation is either accepted or proceeds to advanced screening. Reasons requiring advanced screening are minor offenses with lack of honest disclosure, serious offenses suggesting a pattern of behavior, crimes of a sexual nature, and history of substance abuse. Serious or minor offenses are reviewed; a state's board of nursing or related group then determines the applicant's possible threat to public safety if licensed as a nurse. Resources and forensic psychological consultation and testing (16 Personality Factors, California Psychological Inventory, Personality Assessment Inventory, Minnesota Multiphasic Personality Inventory-2, and PsychEval Personality Questionnaire) may be recommended. Risk assessment is gauged as high, medium, or low. A decision to license or not to license is made (NCSBN, 2014).

Allegations of unprofessional conduct are reported to nurse regulatory authorities, including state boards of nursing. State boards of nursing respond to complaints and usually do not revoke licenses when allegations of unprofessional conduct are made. These professional boards revoke licenses when nurses are convicted of serious crimes. Nurses disciplined for substance use may join board-supported programs. For example, the Pennsylvania Nurse Peer Assistance Program (n.d.) is an option for nurses struggling with substance use. The Pennsylvania Code (n.d.) regulates the professional conduct of nurses and disciplines nurses for unprofessional conduct.

In contrast, the contributions of nursing practice to population health are important to evaluate as related to patient outcomes. A study by Choi et al. (2020) examined if scope of practice and ease of practice laws from 50 states for registered nurses and nurse practitioners were associated with U.S. suicide and homicide rates. The study's framework applied the Centers for Disease Control and Prevention (CDC) Social-Ecological Framework for Violence Prevention concepts—sociodemographic variables, health care system factors, and firearms and firearm policy—on the outcomes of suicide and homicide rates. The state-level, five-year analysis (2012–2016) included post–Affordable Care Act data obtained from the CDC's Web-based Injury Statistics Query and Reporting System. Predictor variables were nurse practitioner scope of practice laws (limited, partial, full) and RN ease of practice (nursing licensure compact member or non-member). Covariates were state sociodemographic characteristics (urban/rural, poverty rate, Medicaid generosity, worker index, population density), health care system factors (primary care physician rate, NP rate, distance to trauma center), and firearm factors (hunting license rate, firearm prohibition laws). Fixed linear regression statistical results showed that full NP scope of practice was related to fewer suicides and homicides. RN licensure compact membership was related to lower suicide and homicide rates. The study makes a case for nurses' contributions to population health through injury outcomes, such as suicide and homicide. Laws favorable to full nursing practice protect the population from negative outcomes like injuries. Although this is one study, the findings make a case for nursing practice on homicide outcomes. Additional research on this topic is needed.

Algorithms, Checklists, and Databases

Several strategies have been created to analyze patterns in data that might identify serial killers. For example, Hargrove (Wilkinson, 2017) created a serial-killer detector, the basis of the Murder Accountability Project (MAP, 2019), and applied the algorithm to murder reports. At first, Hargrove became a crime reporter and eventually obtained FBI data on reported murders and began to develop a computer program to identify serial killer victims. Factors were grouped, such as geography of victims and their killers. Another professional, Witzig, a retired homicide detective and former FBI intelligence analyst, contributed to the FBIs Violent Criminal Apprehension Program (VICAP). The MAP continues to present material on murders in the U.S. on a webpage. Hargrove and Witzig are members of MAP's Board of Directors. An IBM SPSS program has been created and copyrighted (MAP, 2019) to encourage data entry and analysis of serial murderers' characteristics.

Ramsland (2007) studied serial killers who were health care professionals. She was concerned that murders of patients might not be identified, as explained by the public's trust in health care providers. Ramsland (2007) compared single murderers to serial killers and reported the pathologies and methods of physicians, nurses, and other health care providers known as serial killers. She created a 29-item Red Flag list of serial killer characteristics, including difficult personal relationships, mental instability, predictions of death, craving attention, enthusiasm about his or her skills, and disciplinary problems at work. The list includes murder patterns such as statistically higher death rates, code blue rates, and clusters of unexpected deaths when a suspect was on duty.

Wolf et al. (2019) described the attributes of nurses who killed patients in acute care institutions or residents of long-term care agencies and characteristics of murder events. They generated a checklist based on literature obtained from news reports, popular press publications, court records, and theoretical and empirical citations and compared it to Ramsland's (2007) Red Flag list. Personality and behavioral indicators manifested by nurses who murdered or were accused of murdering patients and characteristics of murder events were compared to checklist items. See Table 18 for an example of a checklist (Wolf et al., 2019).

Table 18. Red Flags for Nursing Staff Convicted of or Accused of Killing Patients*

Increased Number of Patient Deaths and Emergency Situations	
Suspicious deaths	
Deaths unrelated to reason for hospital admission	
High number of deaths for intensive care units	
High number of deaths for nursing home or long-term care units	
Code blues, cardiac arrests, arrhythmias, respiratory crises, emergency situations on suspect's shifts	
Unexpected Changes in Patient Conditions	
Conditions changed dramatically	
Unexplained seizures and complications	
Increased illness episodes	
Excellent condition prior to deaths	
Suspicious circumstances surrounding unexpected deaths	
Unexpected and/or "unnatural" deaths among "difficult" patients	
Changes in Medication Patterns	
Marked increase in supply of medications suspected in deaths during employment	
Decreased supply of specific medications suspected in deaths during employment	
Medications ordered did not match ICU patients' medication profile	
Drug Tampering or Missing Drugs	
Syringes and needles with residual amounts medications involved in deaths	
Vial tampering: multiple punctures unexplained	
Drug packages show evidence of tampering	
Missing medication doses or vials	
Staff Member Personal Patterns: Suspicious	
Called multiple codes	
Suspected of creating emergencies	
Emergency situations increased during staff member's shifts	
Patients more likely to die on staff member's shifts	

Staff Member Personal Patterns: Suspicious	
Staff member present during many deaths	
Staff member present at sudden, unexpected deaths	
Patient became ill whenever nurse cared for patient	
Demonstrates expert cardiopulmonary resuscitation technique	
Elected to perform cardiopulmonary resuscitation during code blues	
Resuscitated patients close to dying "peacefully"	
Relatives suspicious of staff member	
Complaints reported about staff member's abuse of patients	
Unexpected injuries in patient: bruises, fractured ribs, punctured lungs	
Seen resetting equipment	
Statements by Suspected Staff Member	
Wanted patients to finish dying	
Spoke about patients' "time to go"	
Predicted deaths of patients	
Elderly patients should be "gassed"; elderly patients "a waste"	
Talked about killing patients	
Bragged about murders	
Phoned reports of killing residents to TV station	
Shared stories about murders: dismissed as sick jokes	
Stated wish that patient would hurry up and die to give staff member something to do	
Complained about difficult patients and family members; quoted saying: annoying, ornery, pushy, whiny, heavy workload, demanding	
Provided contradictory explanations about suspicious incidents when interviewed	
Fascinated with Suffering and Death	
Morbid fascination with blood, symptoms before dying, such as red and blue skin changes	
Curious about manner of patients' deaths	
Observed patients as they were dying	
Excited by Crises	
Needed excitement and attention	
Enjoyed resuscitating patients	
Evidence of Wrongdoing Points to Staff Member	
Sharps box stuffed with drugs used to poison patients	
Broken containers of suspicious drugs found in disposal bucket	

Evidence Directly Implicating Staff Member	
Empty ampules found in staff member's possession	
Syringe with trace of missing drug found in staff member's home garbage	
Morphine possession at home	
Vials of pavulon or anectine (skeletal muscle relaxant) found at staff member's home	
Empty syringes in staff member's possession	
Performance Problems of Staff Member	
Made medication errors	
Administered improper doses of medications	
Demonstrated poor charting patterns	
Opened charts of patients not assigned to him/her	
Falsified records	
Exceeded Scope of Practice for License or Certificate	
Gave IV medications to patient: not within scope of practice	
Overstepped authority when giving care	
Considered skills superior to others: disparaged physicians	
Employment Patterns of Staff Member	
Changed jobs frequently	
Hired by health care agencies in two states	
Employed by more than one health care agency	
Spent long hours on ward	
Worked two shifts	
Preferred working night shift: fewer staff present	
Disciplinary Problems	
Coworkers suspicious: reported suspicious behavior	
Investigated by administrators	
Dismissed from one or multiple jobs	
Fired from job once or more than once	
Asked to resign; forced to resign twice	
Suspended with pay; suspended without pay	
Lied about license	
Failed to present license; was employed without license	
Psychiatric Diagnoses and Other Mental Health Indicators	
Dissociative identity disorder; bipolar; multiple-personality disorder; Münchausen syndrome; Münchausen by proxy; substance abuser	
Mentally unstable	
Medical discharge from armed services	
Suicide attempts	

Criminal History: Convicted or Accused	
Drug dealer; forger; embezzler; domestic violence; assault; substance abuse	
Evidence	
Tissue specimens tested positive for drug	
Medications identified in syringes and needles used as poisons	
Syringes in sharps container tested positive for bleach; dialysis lines tested positive for bleach; blood tested positive for biomarker 3-chlorotrosine; bleach substituted for Zemplar; LDH blood values increased	
Funeral director reported evidence of assault	
Coworker Descriptors of Positive and Negative Characteristics of Staff Member	
Staff nicknames for suspect: angel of death, compassionate angel of death	
Shy; religious	
Lied; stole; exploited others; secretive; lazy; physically abusive; difficulty with personal relationships	
Model nurse; efficient; competent leadership award; reliable; capable employee; jolly; compulsive helper	

*Reprinted with permission granted by Dr. Shirley Gordon, 1/3/2020 email.

Checklists must be used cautiously by administrators and members of morbidity and mortality, risk management, quality improvement, and patient safety committees to make decisions about staff behavior or patterns in data that demonstrate unusual spikes in deaths, cardiopulmonary resuscitations, increased orders of certain medications, etc. Health care leaders are charged with making decisions to investigate nursing staff's suspicious behavior. However, since much of the evidence in murder cases is circumstantial, leaders are cautious about alleging murderous intent and about referring their suspicions to law enforcement personnel (Graeber, 2013).

Additionally, Aamodt developed the Radford Serial Killer Data Base (Florida Gulf Coast University, 2019). The comprehensive source is updated and supported by sources, such as websites, books, court documents, and government agencies. Case study data on serial killers can be obtained. It is a non-governmental database and extensive, with details on 3,304 subjects, including serial killers, mass murderers, spree killers, and others.

Summary

Single murders and serial murders of hospitalized patients or long-term care residents are carried out by perpetrators, who at times are health care providers, and include nursing staff. Their occurrence is undeniable. Historical and recent cases illustrate the persistence of the problem, along with challenging all health care providers and administrators to prevent the worst of crimes against persons in their care (NQF, 2011).

of nurses, and (2) categories of sanctions. Murder as framed by the first model is situated in the criminal domain, with criminal law as the regulatory structure. Criminal charges are made (interaction) and criminal sanctions (outcome) are instituted with the aim of public protection. Violator types of sanctions for such crimes include suspension/termination/revocation and incarceration; these types fit categories of sanctions: retribution, deterrence, and incapacitation. The models presented by Collins and Mikos (2008) help to categorize and compare different types of unprofessional conduct performed by nursing staff.

Discussion Questions

1. What reporting obligations, as required by the Cullen Law, do health care entities or organizations and health care professionals have when suspicions of potentially harmful activity against patients are identified?

2. What behaviors and personal factors distinguish nurses who murder patients?

3. How might checklists function to validate the need for frontline staff and managers to pursue validated behavioral indicators of unprofessional conduct and to initiate investigations?

4. How might pharmacists monitor very frequent orders of dangerous drugs for hospital units?

5. How do institutional committees, such as quality improvement, risk management, mortality and morbidity, and patient safety, monitor harmful patient outcomes and raise the alarm for patterns needing the involvement of law enforcement and regulatory agencies?

AUTHOR SELECTIONS

Hebert, G., & Lopez, B.J. (2014, June). Response to Case of Charles Cullen [Video]. National Council of State Boards of Nursing. 2014 Discipline Case Management Conference. Park City, UT. https://www.ncsbn.org/1238.htm.

Netflix. (2016). *Nurses Who Kill*. [Film]. https://www.netflix.com/title/80185622.

REFERENCES

AHC Media. (2005, December 1). Want to detect dangerous staff? Use background checks, monitoring. *Healthcare Risk Management*, 1–4.

American Nurses Association. (2010). *Nursing's social policy statement: The essence of the profession.* https://cmjantha.files.wordpress.com/2017/06/ana-social-policy-statement.pdf.

American Nurses Association. (2015). *Code of ethics for nurses with interpretive statements.* https://www.nursingworld.org/practice-policy/nursing-excellence/ethics/code-of-ethics-for-nurses/.

AMN Healthcare Education Services. (2014). *Forensic evidence collection for nurses.* https://lms.rn.com/getpdf.php/2071.pdf.

Associated Press. (2017, August 28). *Convicted killer nurse suspected of 41 more murders.* https://www..cbsnews.com/news/germany-killer-nurse-neils-hoegel-suspected-84-murder-delmenhorst-oldenburg/.

Bennett, C.D. (2016, April 18). *Department of Health Proposes New Rules at N.J.A.C. 8:30 Implementing the Health Care Professional Responsibility and Reporting Enhancement Act.* https://www.state.nj.us/health/news/2016/approved/20160418a.shtml.

Berge, K.H., Dillon, K.R., Sikkink, K.M., Taylor, T.K., & Lanier, W.L. (2012). Diversion of drugs within health care facilities, a multiple-victim crime: Patterns of diversion, scope, consequences, detection, and prevention. *Mayo Clinic Proceedings, 87*(7), 674–682.

Cady, R.F. (2009). Criminal prosecution for nursing errors. *JONA's Healthcare Law, Ethics and Regulation, 11*(1), 10–16.

Canadian Broadcasting Corporation. (2017, June 26). *Canada nurse Elizabeth Wettlaufer jailed for life for murders*. http://www.bbc.com/news/world-us-canada-40412080.

Casey, L. (2017, June 2). Former nurse Wettlaufer felt 'urge to kill.' *Edmonton Journal*, NP2.

Choi, K.R., Takada, S., Saadi, A., Esterlin, M.C., Buchbinder, L.S., Natsui, S., & Zimmerman, F.J. (2020). The relationship of nursing practice laws to suicide and homicide rates: A longitudinal analysis of US states from 2012 to 2016. *BMC Health Services Research, 20*, 176. https://doi.org/10.1186/s12913-020-5025-x.

Collins, S.E., & Mikos, C.A. (2008). Evolving taxonomy of nurse practice violators. *Journal of Nursing Law, 12*(2), 85–91.

Combs, L. (2017). Certified forensic nurse and consultant. *Journal of Legal Nurse Consulting, 28*(1), 20–21.

Cotter, P. (2010). The path to extreme violence: Nazism and serial killers. *Frontiers in Behavioral Neuroscience, 3*(Article 6), 1–5. doi: 10.3389/neuro.08.061.2009.

Curtin, L. (2019). Killing for profit: Reinforcing hospice's valuable services after disturbing court case. *American Nurse Today, 14*(6), 48.

Douglas, J.E., Burgess, A.W., Burgess, A.G., & Ressler, R.K. (1992). *Crime classification manual: A standard system for investigating and classifying violent crimes*. Lexington Books.

Federal Bureau of Investigation, Criminal Justice Information Services Division. (n.d.). Privacy Impact Assessment Integrated Automated Fingerprint Identification System National Security Enhancements. https://www.fbi.gov/services/information-management/foipa/privacy-impact-assessments/iafis.

Field, J. (2008). Why nurses kill. *Nursing Standard, 23*(9), 24–25.

Florida Gulf Coast University. (2019). *Radford FGCU Serial Killer Database Research Project*. http://skdb.fgcu.edu/info.asp.

Forrest, A.R. (1995). Nurses who systematically harm their patients. *Medical Law International, 1*, 411–421.

Graeber, C. (2013). *The good nurse*. Hatchette Book Group.

Halldorsdottir, S. (1991). Five basic modes of being with another. In D. Gaut, & M.M. Leininger (Eds.), *Caring: The compassionate healer* (pp. 37–49). National League for Nursing Press.

Hebert, G., & Lopez, B.J. (2014, June). Response to Case of Charles Cullen [Video]. National Council of State Boards of Nursing. 2014 Discipline Case Management Conference. Park City, UT. https://www.ncsbn.org/1238.htm.

Hildebrand, M.M., & Culhane, S.E. (2015). Personality characteristics of the female serial murderer. *Journal of Criminal Psychology, 5*(1), 34–50. doi: 10.1108/JCP-04-2014-0007.

Holz, C.L. (2014). Nursing the dead: Medicolegal death scene investigation. *American Nurse Today, 9*(7), 37–38.

HomeCare Council of New Jersey (2019). *Cullen Act: Requirements and Protections*. [PDF]. http://www.homecarecouncilnj.org/CullenAct.pdf Hoyt, C.A. (2006). Integrating forensic science into nursing processes in the ICU. *Critical Care Nursing Quarterly, 29*(5), 259–270.

International Association of Forensic Nursing, American Nurses Association. (2015). *Forensic Nursing Scope and Standards 2015*. https://cdn.ymaws.com/www.forensicnurses.org/resource/resmgr/Docs/SS_Public_Comment_Draft_1505.pdf.

McNamara, S.A. (2012). Incivility in nursing: Unsafe nurse, unsafe patients. *AORN Journal, 95*(4), 535–540.

Miller, L. (2014). Serial killers: I. Subtypes, patterns, and motives. *Aggression and Violent Behavior, 19*, 1–11.

Morrall, P., Hazelton, M., & Shackleton, W. (2011). Homicide and its effect on secondary victims. *Mental Health Practice, 15*(3), 14–19.

Morton, R.J., & Hilts, M.A. (Eds.). (2013, July 17). *Serial murder: Multi-disciplinary perspectives for investigators*. Behavioral Analysis Unit, National Center for the Analysis of Violent Crime. Federal Bureau of Investigation, U.S. Department of Justice. https://www.fbi.gov/stats-services/publications/serial-murder.

Moulson, G. (2017, August 29). German nurse now believed to have killed 86 people or more. *The Philadelphia Inquirer*, A3.

Moulson, G. (2018, January 22). A nurse already serving a life sentence was charged with killing 97 more patients. *Time*. https://news.yahoo.com/nurse-already-serving-life-sentence-140315536.html.

Murder Accountability Project. (2019). *SPSS Algorithm*. https://www.dropbox.com/s/49i2mw0caswn8y0/Algorithm.pdf?dl=0.

Murder Accountability Project. (2019). *Tracking America's unsolved homicides*. http://www.murderdata.org/.

National Council of State Boards of Nursing. (2014). *Criminal Background Check (CBC) Guidelines*. https://www.ncsbn.org/final_14_cbc_guidelines_052914.pdf.

National Quality Forum. (2011). Serious reportable events in healthcare.

New Jersey Administrative Code, Title 13 Law and Public Safety Chapter 45E. (2011, June 20). Health Care

Professional Reporting Responsibility. https://www.njconsumeraffairs.gov/regulations/Chapter-45E-Health-Care-Professional-Reporting-Responsibility.pdf.

New Jersey Division of Consumer Affairs, Office of the Attorney General. (n.d.). *Top Tips for License Applicants.* https://www.njconsumeraffairs.gov/Documents/Top-Tips-for-License-Applicants.pdf.

Noack, R. (2018, October 31). Ex-nurse in Germany admits to killing 100 patients. *The Philadelphia Inquirer.* A3.

Park, G.R., & Khan, S.N. (2002). Murder and the ICU. *European Journal of Anaesthesiology, 19,* 621–623.

Pennsylvania Code. (n.d.). Chapter 21. State Board of Nursing. Subchapter A. Registered Nurses. https://www.pacode.com/secure/data/049/chapter21/chap21toc.html.

Pennsylvania Department of Health. (n.d.). *Frequently Asked Questions: Records and fingerprints.* https://www.health.pa.gov/topics/Documents/Facilities%20and%20Licensing/faq7379emprecordchecks0109.pdf.

Pennsylvania Nurse Peer Assistance Program. (n.d.). *FAQ.* http://pnap.org/faq/.

Pugh, D. (2011). A fine line: The role of personal and professional vulnerability in allegations of unprofessional conduct. *Journal of Nursing Law, 14*(1), 23–31.

Ramsland, K. (2007). *Inside the minds of healthcare serial killers: Why they kill.* Praeger Publishers.

Rim, M.H., Thomas, K.C., Hatch, B., Kelly, M., & Tyler, L.S. (2018). Development and implementation of a centralized comprehensive refill authorization program in an academic health system. *American Journal of Health-System Pharmacy, 75,* 132–138.

Rutgers, The State University of New Jersey (n.d.). Health Care Professional Responsibility and Reporting Enhancement Act (HCPRREA) Event Reporting Instructions. https://uhr.rutgers.edu/sites/default/files/form_applications/HCPRREAReportingForm_0.pdf.

Shellem, P. (2006). The killer next door: An analysis of investigative journalism. *Journal of Forensic Nursing, 2*(3), 134–141.

Standing Bear, Z.G. (1996). Using crime statistics in nursing. *Journal of Psychosocial Nursing & Mental Health Services, 34*(1), 16–23.

Sullivan, M.K. (2009). Serial murder in health care. *Nursing Management, 40*(6), 32–36.

Sumner, A.A., Mercy, J.A., Dahberg, L.L., Hillis, S.D., Klevens, J., & Houry, D. (2015). Violence in the United States: Status, challenges, and opportunities. *JAMA, 314*(5), 478–488.

Szulecki, D. (2017). Ann Burgess: Studying victims of trauma–and perpetrators, too. *American Journal of Nursing, 117*(2), 70–71.

Tilley, E., Devion, C., Coghlan, A.L., & McCarthy, K. (2019). A regulatory response to healthcare serial killing. *Journal of Nursing Regulation, 10*(1), 4–14.

University of Medicine & Dentistry of New Jersey. (2010, January 20). University Policy: Compliance with Health Care Professional Responsibility & Reporting Enhancement Act (HCPRREA). https://rbhs.rutgers.edu/oppmweb/university_policies/human_resources/PDF/00-01-30-15_05.pdf.

Wigglesworth, V. (2018, June 15). Nursing supervisor pleads guilty in health care scheme that led to early deaths of hospice patients. *The Dallas News.* https://www.dallasnews.com/news/crime/2018/06/15/nursing-supervisor-pleads-guilty-in-health-care-scheme-that-led-to-early-deaths-of-hospice-patients/.

Wigglesworth, V. (2018, June 21). Nurse overmedicated patients under orders from hospice CEO to hasten deaths, plea documents say. *The Dallas News.* https://www.dallasnews.com/news/2018/06/21/nurse-overmedicated-patients-under-orders-from-hospice-ceo-to-hasten-deaths-plea-documents-say/.

Wilkinson, A. (2017, November 20). The serial-killer detector. *The New Yorker.* https://www.newyorker.com/magazine/2017/11/27/the-serial-killer-detector.

Winfrey, M.E., & Smith, A.R. (1999). The suspiciousness factor. *Critical Care Nursing Quarterly, 22*(1), 1–7.

Wolf, Z.R., Donohue-Smith, M., & Wolf, K.C. (2019). Nurses who murder or who are accused of murdering patients. *International Journal for Human Caring, 23*(1), 51–70.

Yardley, E., & Wilson, D. (2016). In search of the 'angels of death': Conceptualizing the contemporary nurse healthcare serial killer. *Journal of Investigative Psychology and Offender Profiling, 13,* 39–55.

Yorker, B.C., Kizer, K.W., Lampe, P., Forrest, A.R., Lannan, J.M., & Russell, D.A. (2006). Serial murder by healthcare professionals. *Journal of Forensic Sciences, 51*(6), 1362–1371.

Multiple-Choice Questions

1. Which of the following work patterns provides a stimulus for health care institutions to pursue the possibility of patient murders? Select all that apply.

    A. Missing intravenous medications

    B. Resuscitation patterns

    C. Breaches of professional ethics

    D. Shift correlates with death counts

2. **What change to license renewal did the New Jersey Board of Nursing impose on license holders?**
   A. Add criminal history background checks
   B. Mandate health care clearances
   C. Require fingerprinting
   D. Document biometric data

3. **Which of the following ICU red flags might alert critical care units to potential indicators of criminal wrongdoing?**
   A. Persistent intuitions
   B. Stable mortality trends
   C. Drug toxicities/overdoses
   D. Suspicious behavior

4. **Which of the following types of evidence is characteristic of patient murders?**
   A. Circumstantial
   B. Anecdotal
   C. Documentary
   D. Digita

CHAPTER 15

Mistakes Versus Crimes

Zane Robinson Wolf, PHD,
RN, CNE, FCPP, ANEF, FAAN

Objectives

1. Compare the chief differences between mistakes and crimes made by health care providers.

2. Contrast counseling or disciplinary approaches health care leaders use to address errors and crimes in health care settings.

3. Examine clinical situations in which nurses are in jeopardy for making health care errors and for being charged with crimes.

4. Define health care error, negligent conduct, reckless conduct, and intentional rule violation.

Critical Incidents

Error

Kimberly Hiatt, RN, committed a medication error, having realized that she overdosed an eight-month-old infant, Kaia Zautner, with 10 times the safe dose of calcium chloride. She reported the error and had cared for the infant prior to the mistake. Kaia died five days later; Ms. Hiatt was fired. The first victims were the infant and her family; the second, the nurse who made the mistake and lived through subsequent events. Kimberly committed suicide. The error may or may not have led to the infant's death.

Crime

Charles Cullen is incarcerated for life. He held professional nursing licenses in New Jersey and Pennsylvania, practiced nursing in several health care organizations, and received positive performance evaluations. He was convicted of murdering adult, critically ill and older patients, estimated at over 40 individuals admitted to hospitals or nursing homes. Cullen's preferred shift was nights. He had no remorse and had a compulsion to kill. His history included mental instability, depression, suicide attempts, stalking a nurse, domestic violence, and debt. He was fired five times and forced to resign twice. He poisoned patients with digoxin and lidocaine, and his suspicious behavior was reported by coworkers (Wolf et al., 2019).

Background

These examples, a health care error or mistake and murders, differ significantly. They remind health care providers of conversations held whenever a health care provider is charged with a crime that is a mistake made at work (Mongeau, 1998). In addition, news stories show that, following errors, nurses have been charged with crimes by the law enforcement community. When reporters publish stories of patients' deaths and attributions to health care providers are made, accounts are sensationalized (Kalisch & Kalisch, 1982; Knowles, 2019). Such health care incidents are unintentional, and therefore miss the important factor of criminal intent (Tilley et al., 2019).

The Institute for Safe Medication Practices (ISMP, 2019) presented a news release in which health care leaders were exhorted to examine systems causes of errors rather than blaming nurses or other providers that made mistakes resulting in a patient's death. ISMP (2007) has consistently pointed out the public's need to examine systems' flaws in health care agencies. The organization's continued position that blame and prosecution of a clinician who made a health care error challenges the Just Culture approach (model used as prerequisite to safety and reliability in health care; promotes nonpunitive, transparent approach in situations arising from unintended medical injury; supports prompt investigation to determine whether recklessness or risk taking [actions that would require discipline, coaching, or remediation], Halpern, 2016) espoused by Marx (2001) and supported by Reason's (1990) human error theory.

The American Association of Nurse Attorneys (TAANA) and the American Association of Legal Nurse Consultants (AALNC, 2011) encouraged reporting and analysis of health care errors with a focus on contributing factors and system flaws. Their statement revealed the organization's opposition to punitive approaches to error; fear results in decreased error reports and endangers patient safety. The joint statement proclaimed that criminal prosecution of unintentional mistakes undermines safety, supports the culture of blame, and continues the perfect practice expectation of clinicians, thus contributing to health care provider shortages. Moreover, the joint statement emphasized and referred to the responsibility of state boards of professional practice to investigate complaints as compared to the judicial system. The American Operating Room Nurses (AORN, 2018) also published a position statement on the organization's opposition to criminalizing errors in perioperative settings. They advocated a systematic investigation by quality and risk management staff and recommended that further concerns be followed in accordance with current state and federal regulatory requirements and as related to licensure.

Allegations of criminal behavior and prosecution of clinicians who have made fatal errors can result in decreased reporting and limit the possibility of correcting errors associated with systems flaws. In the face of fatal errors, health systems are challenged to provide corrective action plans to sustain reimbursements (Kelman, 2019) and improve patient safety outcomes. Health care errors threaten the confidence of health care professionals (Scott et al., 2010). They live in fear of harming patients. Criminal prosecution of fatal errors adds to that fear (Sofer, 2019) and may inhibit reporting of near miss or actual errors.

Definitions

Criminal charges must be proven in court after individuals are charged and tried (Philipsen, 2011). *Mens rea* (criminal intent), *actus reus* (deliberate engagement in criminal act), concurrence of *mens rea* and *actus reus* (intent and act: intent triggered act), and causation must be present. Causation means that harm must have occurred resulting from criminal action.

A crime is broadly defined as a diverse range of behaviors criminalized by the modern state (Farmer, 2019). A definition of crime may reflect the following moral category: public wrongs have been performed and rights and duties to the entire community have been violated. The community is owed respect of the law by its citizens. Alternatively, a procedural definition of crimes represents them as acts that "might be prosecuted or punished under criminal procedure" (Farmer, 2019, para. 3).

In contrast, health care errors are defined in different ways. For example, the National Coordinating Council for Medication Error Reporting and Prevention's (NCCMERP's, 2019) definition of medication error follows:

> A medication error is any preventable event that may cause or lead to inappropriate medication use or patient harm while the medication is in the control of the health care professional, patient, or consumer. Such events may be related to professional practice, health care products, procedures, and systems, including prescribing, order communication, product labeling, packaging, and nomenclature, compounding, dispensing, distribution, administration, education, monitoring, and use [para. 1].

This definition does not specify a clinician's intention; the presumed intent of medication administration is to do no harm and improve the welfare of patients. In the case of the error, the health care provider did not intend to make a mistake (Philipsen, 2011). There was no intent to harm. However, nurses may be accused of malpractice in situations in which patients are harmed; their defense attorneys need to describe how a standard of care was violated (Philipsen, 2011).

The phrase, adverse event, is commonly used in health care to describe a negative occurrence in the delivery of services. Adverse events are defined below and can be categorized as preventable and unpreventable (Bates et al., 1995).

> Adverse events were defined as: unintended injuries resulting in prolongation or hospitalization of disability at the time of discharge. "Severe adverse events" were adverse events resulting in death … preventable adverse events were adverse events judged by a reviewer as probably or definitely preventable using current technology [p. 453].

Another definition is: "An adverse event is an injury secondary to medical care and not a result of a patient's underlying condition" (Weissman et al., 2007, p. 449). Later, the National Patient Safety Foundation (2019) defined adverse event as an untoward incident, therapeutic misadventure, iatrogenic injury, or other occurrence of harm or potential harm directly associated with care or services provided. A common definition of adverse event might foster interprofessional communication and consistent research definitions.

Bates et al. (1995) noted in a classic study that preventable and unpreventable adverse events need to be identified to determine defect rates. The researchers sampled admissions to a hospital's medical service for five months using medical record, chart analysis. They used a six-point scale to judge the presence of adverse events and preventability. Billing screens (re-admissions, death, etc.) and record-review screens (hospital-incurred trauma, cardiopulmonary arrest, etc.) were used. The screens were used to correlate with and classify the types of adverse events. A total of 3,137 comprised the sample. Adverse events ($N = 365$) were identified; severe adverse events were seen in

9 percent of admissions; 5 percent were preventable; and 3 percent were preventable and severe. Overall categories of adverse events identified in another study (Stockwell et al., 2018) were hospital-acquired infection, body system (respiratory, gastrointestinal, renal or endocrine, neurologic, cardiovascular, hematologic), surgical or obstetrical, allergic reaction, non-allergic rash, pressure ulcer, fall, death, pyrexia, hypothermia, and tube complication in pediatric patients. It is difficult to know whether adverse events are the result of intentional or unintentional acts, as the first definition suggests. Adverse events might be a result of errors, reckless behavior, or even crimes. The underlying cause may be difficult to detect.

Marx (2001) provided definitions of behavioral concepts related to health care errors when explaining the relationship between discipline and patient safety. He identified four categories—human error, negligent conduct, reckless conduct, and intentional rule violation—and applied them to mishaps or accidents in health care. He suggested that, depending on the behavioral category, disciplinary sanctions might be appropriate. The definitions follow:

- Human error is characterized as a social label when "there is general agreement that the individual should have done other than what they did, and in the course of that conduct inadvertently causes or could cause an undesirable outcome, the individual is labeled as having committed an error" (p. 6). The error is unintentional, the outcome is undesirable and may be life threatening.
- Negligent conduct, more serious than human error, is a legal term used when an individual has been harmed by the health care system. In common law, the negligent person must pay for damages. It is described as "failure to exercise expected care. Should have been aware of substantial and unjustifiable risk" (p. 8).
- Reckless conduct, or gross negligence, is more blameworthy than negligence. Civil and criminal liability are implicated. There is "conscious disregard of substantial and unjustifiable risk" (p. 8).
- Intentional rule violations occur when a person makes a choice. An individual "knowingly violates a rule or procedure" (p. 8) when performing a task [Marx, 2001].

Although the category of human error does not suggest a crime, past and recent cases show that health care providers are charged with negligence and felonies for their accidents or errors. Negligent conduct, reckless conduct, and intentional rule violations may also result in criminal complaints lodged in the justice system. In a Just Culture environment, employees invoke a philosophy of caring and look out for one another (Pastorius, 2007).

Health care leaders might recommend that supervisors deal with safety threats, such as errors, negligent conduct, reckless conduct, and intentional rule violations, within the institution and require counseling or disciplinary sanctions. It seems prudent to track these occurrences in error reports to patient safety and mortality and morbidity committees. Reckless behaviors are not necessarily excluded from the concept of intentionality. Clinicians take chances and violate procedures. However, patient harm may result, and law enforcement may charge them with wrongdoing (Yorker, 1998). In the nursing context, an unsafe action resulting in such harm is similarly classified as human error (an inadvertent slip), at-risk behavior (a drift toward unsafe habits;

potential negligence of a justifiable reason), or reckless behavior (intentional disregard for safety to taking an unjustifiable risk) (Harris et al., 2013).

The Just Culture model most likely has influenced creation of National Patient Safety Foundation tools (NPSF, 2016) to evaluate clinical behavior. Instruments have been adopted to assist patient safety officers, quality improvement, patient safety committee staff, and others to evaluate adverse events, determine if a standard of care was met, evaluate intent, and intervene with consoling, coaching, training, or disciplining involved clinicians. Use of such tools to assist supervisors to counsel staff could provide clarity in relation to discussions with staff involved in errors. In a Just Culture environment, perhaps the best work environment, employees may look out for one another. Consequently, errors and other safety threats could be reduced.

Literature

Ethical Perspectives and Clinical Jeopardy

Ethical principles guide nurses and other health care providers; they are expected to provide care consistent with rules and rights based on ethical principles of autonomy, beneficence, justice, and nonmaleficence (Devettere, 2016). In an example of a study in which complaints against nursing staff were reported, verbal or written complaints were filed against nurses with a regional board of nursing in Brazil (da Silva et al., 2016). Complaints were analyzed retrospectively, based on breaches of legal or bioethical principles. For example, the principles of autonomy, justice, beneficence, and nonmaleficence were used to classify case examples. Once a complaint was made, disciplinary proceedings began. Complaints were often made against young professionals by health care providers and community members, such as patients and family members. The autonomy of coworkers and patients (users) was violated most frequently. Most complaints were made against registered nurses. Allegations of the unlicensed practice of nursing were brought most often against registered nurses. Many involved issues with unprofessional, interprofessional relationships, such as abuse of power and harassment. Specific infractions were not described.

From this (da Silva et al., 2016) and other accounts, it is evident that health care teams work in situations framed by ethical principles and witness or participate in unexpected clinical events and errors they or their colleagues make (Scott et al., 2010). Complications associated with medical treatments, surgical procedures, diagnostic tests, and patients' acute or chronic health status are commonly seen by providers. Whether events signify tragic circumstances for patients or result in less serious outcomes, health care professionals experience pain as witnesses and participants in difficult and unfortunate situations in which patients suffer and die.

Clinicians care for patients and families in many settings. Examples include community and university hospitals, long-term care agencies and nursing homes, primary care offices, and patients' homes. Care is delivered with the implicit but lived intent of improving the welfare of those served. However, the work of health care providers positions them in situations in which outcomes for patients and families can be negative.

Situations in clinical settings have presented nurses with remarkable challenges, such as illustrated in accounts of a well-publicized disaster. In a dramatic series of difficult events, nurses' actions attracted national attention following Hurricane Katrina (Mason, 2006). The ethical principles of autonomy, beneficence, justice, and nonmaleficence may have been violated.

Two nurses and a physician were accused of intentionally killing critically ill and well patients who received two medications. They and their colleagues were involved in a sustained crisis situation during and following the hurricane. The physician and the two nurses implicated in deaths during Katrina had cared for patients just before and after generators failed, hospital temperatures were 90° to 100°, staff were extremely fatigued and carried patients downstairs for evacuation, evacuations were slow, and gunshots were heard in the vicinity of the hospital (Fink, 2009).

Physicians and nurses conferred during and after the full force of the hurricane made landfall in New Orleans. Decisions were made and three triage levels were set for evacuation (Fink, 2009). Healthier patients were evacuated first, more critical patients last. However, all patients were not evacuated. Some died, and the number of deaths exceeded that of comparable hospitals in the area.

Questions on how long staff should stay with patients, who should be assigned to triage levels, who should not be evacuated, and which patients should be eased into death took place during chaotic situations. Ultimately, the medication order for the patients on one unit was based on prior discussions with a few health care colleagues. The physician and the nurses administered morphine alone or with midazolam intravenously. They may have hastened the deaths of 45 patients, some of whom were extremely ill and others who were not seriously ill (Fink, 2009).

The coroner conducted autopsies on many bodies during the immediate aftermath of the hurricane; forensic experts were also consulted on evidence (Fink, 2009). The bodies of nine patients had toxic levels of morphine or morphine and midazolam. Four deaths were labeled homicides, not euthanasia. Patient autonomy was violated, because able patients, for example, were not asked about whether they would agree to receiving the medications. One physician was charged with second-degree murder and conspiracy to commit second-degree murder; the two nurses who testified at the grand jury hearing supported the physician's order. The physician was not indicted as a result of the grand jury decision. She and others have subsequently explored reasons for shielding health care workers from civil and criminal liability in disasters.

Nurse and physician fatigue could have complicated a most difficult and extreme set of circumstances during the Katrina disaster. For example, nurse fatigue has been linked to patient safety threats, especially for those providing direct care of patients; they are on their feet throughout 12-hour shifts in hospitals (Wisconsin Nursing Coalition, 2007), much longer in disasters. News accounts of the acute care problems associated with the COVID-19 pandemic demonstrate the extreme situations in which many health care providers are working. Accrediting bodies have considered prohibiting the number of work hours performed per week by employees. Health care provider fatigue is but one example of safety threats. Provider fatigue and unusual stress, associated with numerous problems, including resources and staffing, operated during the Katrina disaster and have occurred in other crisis situations.

The situation of health care providers caring for patients at Memorial Hospital in New Orleans is very different from the nurses and physicians who killed patients during Nazi Germany in compliance with Hitler's orders (Benedict et al., 2007). Propaganda films of the time promoted euthanasia. Persons with disabilities and psychiatric conditions were murdered because they were thought as not contributing to the economy and a drain of resources. Psychiatric patients were gassed, and their bodies were cremated. The gassing stopped due to public outcry; nonetheless, psychiatric patients were given high doses of barbiturates dissolved in water and administered orally. Morphine, scopolamine, or an air embolus was also used. Two mass graves were located with 1,000 bodies in each. A total of 18,232 patients were killed during a three-year period. Nurses were told that they had no choice to refuse physician orders and were not to be held responsible for their actions. Some physicians and nurses were charged in the deaths, convicted, and executed; others were not.

Major disasters, such as Katrina, and the atrocities of Nazi Germany have resulted in charges against health care providers and been investigated in criminal justice systems. They contrast greatly with the daily challenges of health care providers who carry out their goals of improving the welfare of patients and of maintaining their safety.

Many health care decisions and interventions are carried out in institutional, community, and home-based settings. As natural environments, they provide the space for positive and negative outcomes. Because of this reality, many opportunities for providing safe care are also within reach.

Discipline, Malpractice, and Education

News stories report that crimes are committed by nurses; most of the data on the crimes are available in professional boards of nursing's reports of disciplinary decisions. Data available about nurses who have committed crimes are published in ongoing state board of nursing accounts of disciplinary sanctions when, for example, nurses have diverted medications or have been convicted of felonies, such as murder. Licenses may be revoked. Therefore, complaints to state boards of nursing require that nurses be vigilant in facing charges (Brown, 2002).

A classic study was conducted in one state in the Upper Midwest for 1998 and 1999 (Powers et al., 2002). A total of 413 cases for disciplinary action were reviewed; 339 complete records were analyzed. RN cases were 58.11 percent of the cases and LPN, 41.88 percent. Of the disciplined nurses, 82.5 percent were female and 17.4 percent were male; 17.9 percent had more than one violation reported. Substance abuse complaints were at 26 percent. Types of violations included competency violations ($N = 148$), drugs/alcohol ($N = 90$), no license or license not current ($N = 36$), medication error ($N = 22$), sexual misconduct ($N = 13$), felony (conviction reported by law enforcement, courts, licenses) ($N = 15$), and other ($N = 48$) (overdue taxes, psychological conditions, violation of a vulnerable adult act requirement, refused or denied license in another state, practicing outside scope of practice). Reporters to the board were often employers, licensees, colleagues, patients, department of health, law enforcement, and courts.

Four types of basic nursing education were compared by non-disciplined and disciplined nurses (Powers et al., 2002). Female practical nurses were disciplined more often than male and other type-educated (BSN, ADN, diploma) nurses. Male ADN-educated nurses were disciplined more than other type-educated nurses, except female practical nurses. Female disciplined nurses exceeded males on the following type of violations: competence, drugs/alcohol, no license, medication error, sexual misconduct, and felony. The researchers emphasized the importance of evaluating nursing staff competency in preventing health care errors.

Perhaps nurses and other health care providers may not have a clear understanding of professional liability related to health care errors. They may learn malpractice and criminal law concepts when they or their colleagues are notified of complaints against them. It is doubtful that undergraduate and graduate nursing programs include detailed instructional content on nurse crimes, liability, and malpractice claims.

Nurses, physicians, and other health care providers have often dealt with malpractice claims. To examine patterns in the claims, Miller (2011) presented a retrospective comparison of four years, divided into two periods, of litigations seen in National Practitioner Data Bank (NPDB) data. States with the highest malpractice claims were stable compared to previous years: Florida, New York, California, and Massachusetts. Reasons for high claims, in addition to population size, were attorneys that named all parties involved, the influence of multiple chronic health problems on increased patient vulnerability to injury, and when patients were diagnosed. Most cases focused on diagnosis (failure to diagnose, delay in diagnosis, improper performance), treatment, and medications. Obstetrical incidents were among the top five claims and associated with neurological injury to infants.

Forty-three percent of malpractice claims resulted in serious injury, including death, permanent injuries, and temporary injuries; frequency of death was the highest for both time periods (Miller, 2011). Most cases were settled outside of the judicial system for both periods; only four out of 501 (2007–2008) versus four out of 550 (2009–2010) were judicial judgments. Mean payments ranged from $206,375 (2010) to $232,549 (2007). Determination of root causes of incidents and identification of causes were recommended. Education of staff on types of malpractice claims might be beneficial in deepening their understanding of personal and institutional liability.

Sweeney et al. (2017) identified the need to add malpractice content to nurse practitioner (NP) education programs. They analyzed NPDB data to identify common types of medical errors involving nurse practitioners, to inform nursing education curricula of error-prone clinical processes and situations, and to share results with regulatory and accrediting agencies that develop NP educational standards. The retrospective data analysis addressed reports for 1990 to 2014 on NP events leading to malpractice payments ($N = 1715$, main outcome). Diagnosis-related claims predominated; most were failure to diagnose and delay in diagnosis. The most frequent treatment-related error was delay in treatment. Medication-related allegations represented 12.77 percent of claims. Most claims (82 percent) originated in outpatient settings. The most frequent patient outcomes were death ($N = 545$), major permanent injury ($N = 190$), and significant permanent injury ($N = 158$). Most claims (76.81 percent) involved one provider.

The researchers (Sweeney et al., 2017) recommended that NP malpractice data inform curricular revisions and include citations targeting specific NP safety threats. They advocated an emphasis on patient-provider communication to improve patient-centered care. Evaluation of diagnostic test findings at point-of-care and referrals to physicians were also stressed. The number of liability claims could decrease based on patient-centered care and more active engagement of patients and family members in care planning and decision making.

Crimes and Clinical Situations

Nurses may not have studied concepts related to criminal charges for practice errors or crimes. Cady (2009) provided a review of criminal law concepts as a resource.

She described characteristics of criminal neglect (failure to provide adequate medical care leading to danger), negligent homicide (killing of a person by act of omission), and criminal homicide (murder and manslaughter). Grand jury involvement, criminal complaints, bail, plea bargains, preliminary hearings, indictments, the need to hire defense attorneys, and the work of prosecuting attorneys were examined. Cady (2009) also contrasted differences between civil and criminal systems. Nurses could benefit from education that helps them to understand legal concepts (Coomber et al., 2015).

Acknowledging that few nurses have murdered patients, the most extreme example of intent to harm a person under their care, Jones (1998) questioned the hazardous situation of nurses who work in intensive care units (ICUs). He suggested that ICU nurses might be accused and convicted of murder when they made errors. Nurses have access to medications that could be administered as poisons. He compared cases where nurses were convicted of murder to those released from charges in which evidence was insufficient, yet negative reporting of them as angels of death led to long-lasting stigmatization. Jones (1998) also warned that when caring for patients near death, nurses should avoid comments interpreted as dark humor (e.g., bleak, callous). Statements could be offered later as evidence of wrongdoing, despite the possibility that it could be a coping mechanism for witnessing the deaths of many patients. The fact that nurses who murder patients do it where they work, presents an occupational hazard (Jones, 1984, citing Charbonneau).

Jones (1998) suggested that nurses' proximity to patients provides an opportunity to implicate them in crimes, and publicity then tempers public opinion. Acknowledging Yorker (1988), he identified indicators that raise suspicion, for example, increased cardiopulmonary arrests or deaths in patient groups, and deaths or cardiopulmonary arrests inconsistent with patients' conditions or localized to a specific shift. When foul play is suspected, he advised nurses to retain evidence, record incidents in detail, and monitor potentially harmful drugs.

Yorker (1988) has asserted that, by virtue of nurses' presence in hospitals around the clock, they are targets of suspicion when death rates increase. For example, statistical evidence of deaths or codes alerts fellow clinicians, managers, and performance improvement committee members to the need to consider data on health care providers' hours worked. They also consider staffing patterns that could implicate employees in patients' deaths during specific or other patient safety threats.

According to Sackman (2015), ICUs can be described as crime scenes. Because the context is one in which near-death events occur followed by codes, patterns can suggest that a crime was committed. Health care providers consequently could be subjected to formal investigations when counts of deaths increase. To avoid the publicity and lawsuits that follow accusations of employee wrongdoing, administrators have preferred that such an employee leave the institution. However, detecting murders or murderers does not necessarily follow identification of suspicious deaths and codes, as found in accounts of serial killers convicted of murder.

Sackman (2015) acknowledged that ICU deaths can be a result of infections, errors, and complex patient conditions. However, he called for a *suspicious* death policy, so that cases are reviewed and documented. Data include staff being present just before suspicious events, medications audited in automated dispensing systems and crash carts, and other evidentiary items, including waste receptables and sharps containers, IV fluid containers, specimens, etc. Securing evidence was recommended as was a new hospital policy. Most clinicians do not have forensic skill. However, investigators, as members of the law enforcement community, have the skills to examine evidence in relation to accused health care providers when suspicions of wrongdoing are referred to criminal justice systems.

Nurses and other health care professionals in Turkey (Büken et al., 2006) may also be charged with a crime if, when working in clinical settings, they fail to inform or delay to report a situation in which a crime might be committed. As a result of an Article in the Turkish Penal Code and contextualized by concerns about terrorism, patients' secrets that might suggest they were involved in a crime, and discovered during the provision of health care services, must be reported. This is considered a special circumstance. The situation overrides the right to health care treatment and confidentiality. However, the authors saw the law as a violation of their ethical responsibility to treat patients prior to reporting criminal indicators discovered during care episodes and the importance of protecting patients' information confidentially. They argued that patients' lives come first, before suspicion of crime is reported. In addition, providers are responsible to give care and to protect patient rights.

The authors (Büken et al., 2006) were concerned that a reaction to the law could be that patients hesitate to provide sufficient detail about their condition to physicians, and that trust in health care providers could erode. The authors questioned that health care workers might not know what constitutes a crime or are able to decide that a crime has been committed. Their dilemma is the nursing obligation to patients and to society. Consequently, consultation with experts was recommended when conflicts arise. This legal code is another example of nurses' and other providers' risk of criminal charges just based on being present at work and caring for patients.

Boothman (2016) addressed the problem of caregivers that routinely engage in dangerous behavior. He asserted that experienced health care providers know colleagues whose risky behavior constitutes a safety threat. Coworkers remain silent; they fail to report dangerous behavior over time and may want to avoid subsequent institutional processes resulting in disciplinary proceedings for colleagues (Boothman, 2016). Boothman (2016) advocated that organizations seek information from their staff about dangerous behavior.

Vanderbilt University Medical Center (VUMC) (Webb et al., 2016) developed a process to promote coworker accountability by sharing coworker concerns about safety. They have had success with a patient system. They adopted a program in which the Co-Worker Observation Reporting System (CORS) process was used to identify safety threats. They launched different phases of the program so that employees would accept the process.

The CORS process (Webb et al., 2016) began when a coworker submitted a report on a professional's unsafe or disrespectful conduct. Reports were entered using their online occurrence reporting system or by telephone. A risk manager retrieved and reviewed reports to identify egregious behavior or potential liability. The Center for Patient and Professional Advocacy performed coding and analysis. Three levels of approach were used in the process: single-report sharing (private review with a messenger with an opportunity for self-regulation); sharing multiple reports–awareness interventions (patterns identified in accumulated reports; report created on concerns; messenger has session with coworker using nonpunitive approach); and advanced interventions (guided intervention by authority policy; referrals for illness, cognitive impairment, or psychiatric illness; possible corrective/disciplinary institutional action).

Key actions were recommended to identify potential murderers in health care settings (Tilley et al., 2019). Raising awareness was advised, that is when employees need to consider the possibility that an institution could employ a nurse who was murdering patients. Information sharing was also offered in the creation of a clearing house on work histories, so that regulators and supervisors could be alerted. Expanded reference checks were also emphasized. However, some state regulations might restrict sharing employee information. Next, early intervention was suggested for providers needing support; problems with mental health or addiction could trigger the provision of support. Monitoring the drug supply was also advocated, specifically drugs known to be used in murders. Adding such actions to the ongoing development of a culture of safety augments reporting of safety threats and supports whistleblowers, so that seeing something is followed by saying something (Tilley et al., 2019). Tracking mortality data with follow-up by regulators has also been recommended by many researchers.

Support of Health Care Providers

Clinicians are committed to earning and maintaining the trust the public places in them and in health care systems. Consequently, when errors and adverse events occur, providers are often devastated; they are saddened that patients are harmed, suffer, and may experience permanent injury or die. Their personal and professional anguish and suffering takes a toll; they have been termed second victims or wounded healers (Scott, 2011; Wu, 2000).

Second victims are health care providers who are involved in an unanticipated adverse patient event, in a medical error and/or a patient-related injury and become victimized in the sense that the provider is traumatized by the event. Frequently, they feel personally responsible for patients' outcomes. Many think they have failed patients, second-guessing their clinical skills and knowledge base (Scott et al., 2011). They may be the working wounded (Wright, 2011).

Often the guilt and regret that follow errors are shared across professional boundaries when health care providers make mistakes. They may openly admit their guilt, blame themselves and each other, and expect punishment. The Just Culture strategy (Marx, 2007) supports discipline for reckless behavior, consolation for human error, coaching at-risk behavior, and training as an opportunity for improvement (National Patient Safety Foundation, 2016). Self-confidence is shaken, whether student or seasoned provider. Therefore, the distress associated with errors is not only limited to patients and families, but also is experienced by health care providers who are also harmed (Jones & Tieiber, 2012). The distress may be so overwhelming that seasoned nurses might end their career (Philipsen, 2011) or commit suicide (Smetzer, 2012).

Implementation of the Just Culture framework has resulted in improved health care environments in which safety efforts are supported because a distinction has been made between error and intentional unsafe acts, such as clinicians' reckless behavior (American College of Healthcare Executives, 2017). Clinicians work in settings in which moral and ethical principles shape health care practices. In advocating a balance between systems improvements and provider accountability for errors, the Just Culture promotes the reporting of safety threats and errors.

Second victims are supported now more than previously. For example, principles of critical incident stress management (CISM), an intervention developed for military combatants and first responders, have been more widely applied in support of individuals who have experienced traumatic events (Wolf, 2005). CISM encourages those individuals by encouraging sharing experiences, learning about stress reactions and symptoms, and providing referrals.

Additionally, Medically Induced Trauma Support Services (MITSS, 2017) is an organization whose mission is aimed at creating a more compassionate health care system aimed at the well-being of patients, families, and health care providers. The vision of MITSS is for individuals involved in a medically induced trauma to access healing support services. In addition to an organizational assessment for clinician support, they offer a clinical support tool kit for health care.

The Crime of Murder

Crimes against patients are distinguished from errors in that they are intentionally, deliberately committed by nurses and other health care providers (Tilley et al., 2019). Registered nurses, licensed practical nurses, and nursing assistants have been accused of and convicted of murder (Brous, 2008; Field, 2007; Field & Pearson, 2010; Wolf et al., 2019; Yorker, 1988; Yorker et al., 2006) as have other health care providers. Compared to the number of nursing staff who commit murder, those who murder patients are the exception and very few.

Key actions were recommended by Tilley et al. (2019) to identify potential murderers in health care settings. Raising awareness is essential, so the possibility that health care personnel could murder patients is supported by fact. While unusual, nursing staff could be murdering patients (Eddy, 2019). Information sharing about nurses' work histories in a clearing house might alert supervisors and regulators to the possibility. Reference checks need to be expanded. (Tilley et al., 2019). However, state laws dictate what may be disclosed in reference checks. Early intervention of providers needing support, for example, those with mental health or addiction problems, was proposed as an intervention that might prevent criminal acts. Tracking mortality data and coroner reports and monitoring drug supplies of medications used to poison patients were emphasized. Lastly, the need to support whistleblowers who report seeing something and saying something was recommended.

Of note are the different approaches to reviewing errors and adverse events that local health care leaders carry out. For example, chief nurse executives and chief nursing officers often issue complaint reports about nursing staff to state boards of nursing (Martin et al., 2018). Delays in reporting unprofessional conduct could result, for example, when noting diversion of medications from patient prescriptions, substance abuse indicators in nurses, and allegations that might include assault and murder. Having policies in place and being satisfied with policies were associated with increased likeliness to report violations of nurse practice acts to state boards of nursing. Barriers included not knowing what is reportable, lacking skill in filling out a report, being concerned with legal ramifications, and facility culture, for example not requiring reporting.

Tilley et al. (2019) analyzed literature for factors and then proposed recommendations to detect serial killers in health care settings. According to Tilley et al. (2019), characteristics of serial killers include mental health problems, a history of mental instability, and a hero complex. They may make colleagues anxious and suspicious, have nursing practice issues, such as falsifying records or not documenting administered medications, and have difficult interpersonal relationships. They might have unauthorized medications in their home or locker at work and change places of employment frequently. Victims of serial murders are very vulnerable; for example, sedated or disoriented patients, adults in intensive care units, etc., have been killed (Wolf et al., 2019).

Serial killers work during evening and night shifts, are less supervised, and often work in hospitals and long-term care settings (Tilley et al., 2019; Wolf et al., 2019). Easily accessed medications, for example, insulin, muscle relaxants, opioids, and potassium, are administered intravenously and poison patients. Tilley et al. (2019) offered clues to detect serial killers among health care providers. They include increased death and cardiac events, direct witness reports, and employee reports. However, some employees do not report their concerns or suspicions.

Adverse events could be caused by both intentional actions and unintentional errors by nursing staff and other health care providers. Consequently, vigilance is called for among nursing staff, managers, directors, and all members of the health care team. In the case of serious outcomes for patients shown in increased frequencies of death and codes and calculated rates based on census, quality improvement, risk management, and patient safety committee staff need to investigate specific time periods. They also might conduct a root cause analysis (RCA) and a failure mode and effects analysis (FMEA) (Brous, 2008).

Nurses might benefit from education on state board of nursing regulations and disciplinary actions published when professional misconduct charges are confirmed following complaints and investigations. However, nurses charged with malpractice and other serious charges need to obtain legal counsel.

Summary

The literature on errors and criminalization of errors reiterates that punitive approaches to health care errors and adverse events result in decreased reports of at-risk factors. Therefore, opportunities are lost for systems improvement of care processes and for review of employees' performance. Errors provide opportunities for improvement of processes.

Many safety processes are implemented to eliminate health care errors. Health care providers continue to monitor safety threats when faced with errors with and without harmful effects for patients. Support of providers has increasingly been used in health care institutions to assist second victims. However, the intentional reckless and persistent behaviors of some employees need to be dealt with directly, fairly, and with sufficient evidence of intent and disregard for patients and other employees.

Strategies

See Table 20 for several strategies that might assist health care providers to reduce errors. Many more strategies are also relevant. The strategies represent actions that focus on different aspects in health care institutions and highlight the complexity of health care errors and crimes.

Table 20. Strategies to Reduce Health Care Errors

Strategies to Effect Change	Evidence-Based Citations
Administer NPSF Just Culture tool when reviewing provider errors; carry out interventions: consoling, coaching, training, disciplinary actions	National Patient Safety Foundation (2016)
Recommend psychological counseling for providers with persistent pattern of reckless behaviors and who display angry, hostile, behavior	Tilley et al. (2019)
Conduct workshop for patient safety committee members and leaders on health care monitoring of data sources as indicators of intentional patient harm	Scott et al. (2010)
Abandon silence when seeing reckless behavior in colleagues and other professionals	Boothman (2016) Maxfield et al. (2005)
Map committees and functions of health care institutions that are responsible for monitoring patient safety and data reviewed by those committees	Sackman (2015)

Conclusion

This chapter reviews some issues associated with errors and crimes in health care settings. Literature cited provides selected aspects of differentiating human error from crimes. At the same time, the gray zone of health care errors is revealed and shows the challenges that direct care providers and health care leaders confront when faced with how to differentiate human error from crime and the responsibility to involve the criminal justice system and state boards of nursing.

Discussion Questions

1. What specific content on malpractice, liability, and negligence are included in undergraduate and graduate nursing program curricula and in education sessions for employees of health care institutions?

2. What are the distinctions among health care error, negligent conduct, and intentional rule violation?

3. What behavioral indicators, associated with patient safety patterns in nursing staff, require a review by nurse leaders?

4. What is the demarcation between reckless behavior and criminal behavior?

5. What current practices are used in health care agencies to demonstrate implementation of Just Culture model initiatives?

AUTHOR SELECTIONS

Fink, S. (2013). *Five days at Memorial*. Broadway Books.
Seys, D., Wu, A.W., Van Gerven, E., Vleugels, A., Euwema, M., Panella, M., Scott, S.S., Conway, J., Semeus,

W., & Vanhaecht, K. (2012). Health care professionals as second victims after adverse events: A systematic review. *Evaluation & the Health Professions, 36*(2), 135–162. doi: 10.1177/0163278712458918.

REFERENCES

American Association of Nurse Attorneys & American Association of Legal Nurse Consultants. (2011, August 12). *TAANA/AALNC Joint Position Statement Criminal Prosecution of Health Care Providers for Unintentional Human Error.*

American College of Healthcare Executives. (2017). *Zero Harm blueprint: The high reliability framework to help your organization build a Zero Harm culture.* https://www.scha.org/files/documents/zeroharmblueprint_fullbook_18.pdf.

American Operating Room Nurses, Inc. (2018). AORN Position Statement on Criminalization of Human Errors in the Perioperative Setting. *AORN Journal, 108*(1), 64–65. http://doi.org/10.1002/aorn.12292.

Bates, D.W., O'Neil, A.C., Petersen, L.A., Lee, T.H., & Brennan, T.A. (1995). Evaluation of screening criteria for adverse events in medical patients. *Medical Care, 33*(5), 452–462.

Benedict, S., Caplan, A., & Page, T.L. (2007). Duty and 'euthanasia: The nurses of Meseritz-Obrawalde. *Nursing Ethics, 14*(6), 781–794.

Boothman, R.C. (2016). Breaking through dangerous silence to tap an organization's richest source of information: Its own staff. *Joint Commission Journal on Quality and Patient Safety, 42*(4), 147–148.

Brous, E. (2008). The criminalization of unintended error: Implications for TAANA. *Journal of Nursing Law, 12*(1), 5–12.

Brown, L.A. (2002). Your state board of nursing. Friend or foe? *Nursing 2002, 32*(12), 48–50.

Büken, E., Sahinoğlu, S., & Büken, N.O. (2006). Statutory disclosure in Article 280 of the Turkish Penal Code. *Nursing Ethics, 13*(6), 573–591. doi: 10.1177/096733006069692.

Cady, R.F. (2009). Criminal prosecution for nursing errors. *JONA's Healthcare Law, Ethics and Regulation, 11*(1), 10–16.

Charbonneau, I. (1984). Paech speaks out on Grange. *Canadian Nurse, 80*(11), 14.

Coomber, R., Donnermeyer, J.F., McElrath, K., & Scott, J. (2015). *Key concepts in crime and Society.* SAGE Books. http://dx.doi.org/10.4135/9781473919693.

Da Silva, L.A., Candido, M.C., & Duarte, S.J. (2016). Complaints against nursing professionals: Mapping a Brazilian reality. *Nursing Ethics, 24*(8), 889–901.

Devettere, R.J. (2016). Medical and behavioral research. In R.J. Devettere, *Practical decision making in health care ethics* (pp. 463–528). Georgetown University Press.

Farmer, L. (2019). Crime, definitions of. In P. Crane, & J. Cunningham, *New Oxford Companion to Law.* www.oxfordreference.com/view/10.1093/acref/9780199290543.001.0001/acref-9780199290543-e-527.

Field, J. (2007). *Caring to death: A discursive analysis of nurses who murder patients.* University of Adelaide.

Field, J., & Pearson, A. (2010). Caring to death: The murder of patients by nurses. *International Journal of Nursing Practice, 16*, 301–310.

Fink, S. (2009, August 20). The deadly choices at Memorial. *The New York Times Magazine.* https://www.nytimes.com/2009/08/30/magazine/30doctors.html.

Halpern, K.J. (2016). A medication error and legislation designed to punish: The American Association of Nurse Attorneys defends Just Culture in nursing. *Journal for Nurse Practitioners, 12*(2), 109–112.

Institute for Healthcare Improvement. (2019). *Patient Safety Dictionary A-E.* https://www.npsf.org/page/dictionaryae.

Institute for Safe Medication Practices. (2007, March 8). *Criminal prosecution of human error will likely have dangerous long-term consequences.* https://www.ismp.org/resoures/criminal-prosectution-human-error-will-likely-have-dangerous-long-term-consequences.

Institute for Safe Medication Practices. (2019, February 13*). ISMP calls for a system-based response to errors, not criminal prosecution.* https://www.ismp.org/news/ismp-calls-system-based-response-errors-not-criminal-prosecution.

Jones, J.H., & Treiber, L.A. (2012). When nurses become the "second" victim. *Nursing Forum, 47*(4), 286–291.

Kalisch, B.J., & Kalisch, P.A. (1982). When nurses are accused of murder: The melodramatic effects of media coverage. *Nursing Life, 2*(5), 44–47.

Kelman, B. (2019, February 4). Vanderbilt ex-nurse indicted on reckless homicide charge after deadly medication swap. *Nashville Tennessean.* https://www.tennessean.com/story/news/health/2019/02/04/Vanderbilt-nurse-reckless-homicide-charge-vercuronium-versed-drug-error/2772648002/.

Knowles, M. (2019, February 20). Former Vanderbilt nurse pleads not guilty to reckless homicide in fatal medication error. Becker's Hospital Review. https://www.beckershospitalreview.com/quality/former-vanderbilt-nurse-pleads-not-guilty-to-reckless-homicide-in-fatal-medication-error.html.

Martin, B., Reneau, K., & Jarosz, L. (2018). Patient safety culture and barriers to adverse event reporting: A national survey of nurse executives. *Journal of Nursing Regulations, 9*(2), 9–17.

Marx, D. (2001). *Patient safety and the "Just Culture": A primer for health care executives*. Columbia University.

Mason, D.J. (2006). In their shoes. *American Journal of Nursing, 106*(10), 11.

Maxfield, D., Grenny, J., McMillan, R., Patterson, K., & Switzier, A. (2005). *Silence kills: The seven crucial conversations for healthcare*. VitalSmarts.

Medically Induced Trauma Support Services. (2017). *Our Purpose*. http://mitss.org/about-us/our-purpose/.

Miller, K.P. (2011). Malpractice: Nurse practitioners and claims reported to the National Practitioner Data Bank. *Journal for Nurse Practitioners, 7*(9), 761–763, 773.

Mongeau, C. (1998). Voices from Colorado. *Nursing98, 28*(6), 48–49.

National Coordinating Council for Medication Error Reporting and Prevention. (2019). *About medication errors*. https://www.nccmerp.org/about-medication-errors.

National Patient Safety Foundation. (2016, September 22). *A Just Culture Tool. Version No. 1*. www.psf.org/just culturetool.

Pastorius, D. (2007). Crime in the workplace. Part 1. *Nursing Management, 38*(10), 18, 20, 22, 24, 26–27.

Philipsen, N.C. (2011). The criminalization of mistakes in nursing. *Journal for Nurse Practitioner, 7*(9), 719–726.

Powers, P., Maurer, R., & Wey, H. (2002). Characteristics of disciplined nurses. *Journal of Nursing Law, 8*(2), 7–19.

Scott, S.D. (2011). The second victim phenomenon: A harsh reality of health care professions. *AHRQ M & M Morbidity & Mortality Round on the Web*. http://www.webmm.ahrq.gov/perspective.aspx?perspectiveID=102.

Scott, S.D., Hirschinger, L.E., Cox, K.R., McCoig, M., Hahn-Cover, K., Epperly, K.M.,…Hall, L.W. (2010). Caring for our own team: Deploying a systemwide second victim rapid response team. *Joint Commission Journal on Quality and Patient Safety, 36*(5), 233–240.

Smetzer, J. (2012). Don't abandon the "second victims" of medical error. *Nursing 2012, 42*(2), 54–58.

Sofer, D. (2019). Is a medical mistake an error or crime? The case of a Tennessee nurse has rekindled an old debate. *American Journal of Nursing, 119*(5), 12.

Stockwell, D.C., Landrigan, C.P., Toomey, S.L., Loren, S.S., Jang, J., Quinn, J.A., Ashrafzadeh, S., Wang, M.J., Wu, M., Sharek, P.J., Classen, D.C., Srivastava, R., Parry, G., Schuster, M.A., & GAPPS Study Group. (2018). Adverse events in hospitalized pediatric patients. *Pediatrics, 142*(2). https://doi.org/10.1542/peds.2017-3360.

Sweeney, C.F., LeMathieu, A., & Fryer, G.E. (2017). Nurse practitioner malpractice data: Informing nursing education. Journal of Professional Nursing, 33(4), 271–275. doi: 10.1016/j.profnurs.2017.01.002.

Tilley, E., Devion, C., Coghlan, A.L., & McCarthy, K. (2019). A regulatory response to healthcare serial killing. *Journal of Nursing Regulation, 10*(1), 4–14.

Webb, L.E., Dmochowski, R.R., Moore, I.N., Pichert, J.W., Catron, T.F., Troyer, M., Martinez, W., Cooper, W.O., & Hickson, G.B. (2016). Using coworker observations to promote accountability for disrespectful and unsafe behaviors by physicians and advanced practice professionals. *Joint Commission Journal on Quality and Patient Safety, 42*(4), 149–161, AP1-AP3.

Weissman, J.S., Rothschild, J.M., Bendavid, E., Sprivulis, P., Cook, F., Evans, R.S.,…Bates, D.W. (2017). Hospital workload and adverse events. *Medical Care, 45*(5), 448–455.

Wisconsin Nursing Coalition. (2007). WNA and Wisconsin Nursing Coalition issue working draft in nurse fatigue and patient safety research and recommendations. *STAT Bulletin, July*, 3–4.

Wolf, Z.R. (2005). Stress management in response to practice errors: Critical events in professional practice. *Patient Safety Advisory, 2*(4), 7–10.

Wright, S. (2011). The working wounded. *Nursing Standard, 25*(31), 14.

Wu, A.W. (2000). Medical error: The second victim. The doctor who makes the mistake needs help too. *BMJ, 320*(7237), 726–727.

Yorker, B.C. (1988). The legal side: Nurses accused of murder. *American Journal of Nursing, 88*(1), 1327–1328.

Yorker, B.C., Kizer, K.W., Lampe, P., Forrest, A.R., Lannon, J.M., & Russell, D.A. (2006). Serial murder by healthcare professionals. *Journal of Forensic Sciences, 51*, 1362–1371.

Multiple-Choice Questions

1. In addition to contributing to health care provider shortages, which of the following outcomes has been attributed to the culture of blame in health care institutions?

    A. Decreased error reports

    B. Identified system flaws

    C. Increased perfection in clinical practice

    D. Decreased risk taking

2. **Which of the following is difficult to determine about adverse events?**
   A. They are unintentional acts.
   B. They are intentional acts.
   C. They can be a result of intentional or unintentional acts.

3. **Among several institutional committees, which of the following established committees in health care organizations track safety threats?**
   A. Ethics
   B. Interprofessional Education
   C. Human Resources
   D. Morbidity Mortality

4. **Which type of statements might later suggest wrongdoing when spoken about patients near death?**
   A. Hospital jargon
   B. Thoughtless
   C. Callous
   D. Critical

Answers to Multiple-Choice Questions

Chapter	Answers
Chapter 1. The Dark Side of Nursing	1. A 2. A 3. C 4. B
Chapter 2. Justifying Coercion in Patient Care	1. C 2. A 3. C 4. A
Chapter 3. Lying to Patients for Therapeutic Ends	1. C 2. D 3. B 4. D
Chapter 4. Blurred Lines: Professional Boundary Violations	1. A 2. B 3. A 4. C
Chapter 5. "Difficult" Patients	1. A, D, E 2. A 3. B 4. D
Chapter 6. Neglect and Negligence of Patients	1. D 2. B 3. A 4. D
Chapter 7. Physical Abuse of Patients	1. B 2. A 3. B 4. D
Chapter 8. Bullying by Nurses	1. D 2. A 3. A 4. B
Chapter 9. Relational Incompetence: The Witnessing Nurse	1. C 2. B 3. A 4. B

Chapter	Answers
Chapter 10. Reckless Nursing Care	1. B 2. A 3. C 4. D
Chapter 11. Missed Nursing Care: A Covert Error of Omission	1. B 2. D 3. A, B, C 4. A
Chapter 12. Shielding from Bad News	1. D 2. B 3. A 4. B
Chapter 13. Failure to Report Abuse and Whistleblowing	1. D 2. C 3. A, B, C, D 4. C
Chapter 14. Homicide and Nursing Staff	1. B, D 2. A 3. C 4. A
Chapter 15. Mistakes Versus Crimes	1. A 2. C 3. D 4. C

About the Contributors

Denise Nagle **Bailey**, EdD, RN, MEd, MSN, CSN, FCPP, has been an associate professor and director, La Salle Neighborhood Nursing Center at La Salle University. As appointed Independence Foundation Chair of Nursing Education at La Salle, she fostered public health programs and secured grant funding. She has authored numerous publications and reviews articles for nursing journals. She has BSN, MEd, and EdD degrees and CSN certification from Widener University, and an MSN degree, Public Health Nursing, La Salle.

Deborah **Byrne**, PhD, RN, CNE, is an assistant professor at La Salle University, School of Nursing and Health Sciences. Her BSN and MSN in nursing education were earned at Holy Family University, and PhD at Villanova University. She teaches courses on professional nursing, fundamentals of nursing, and adult health. Her professional practice includes adult acute care settings and home health nursing. Her research focus is on cultural competence, caring, end-of-life, undergraduate nursing education, simulation, and health disparities.

Maureen **Donohue-Smith**, PhD, PMHNP, is an associate professor of psychiatric nursing and director of the Psychiatric Mental Health Nurse Practitioner Program at La Salle University. She holds a PhD in human development, an MS in psychiatric nursing, and bachelor's degrees in nursing and English literature. She is a board-certified Psychiatric Mental Health Nurse Practitioner. Her research interests include the incorporation of the humanities into professional education and the representation of mental illness in film and literature.

Joanne R. **Duffy**, PhD, RN, FAAN, is an adjunct professor at Indiana University. She holds a BSN from Salve Regina University and earned her MSN and PhD from the Catholic University of America. She teaches graduate level nursing research and nursing theory, and she has conducted federally funded research on nurse caring and patient outcomes. She is the executive vice president and senior consultant at QualiCare, consults internationally on nursing leadership and evidence-based practice, and is a fellow of the American Academy of Nursing.

Beth Marie **King**, PhD, APRN, PMHNP-BC, is an associate professor at Florida Atlantic University. Her PhD was earned at Iowa State University; MS, University of Maryland; BSN, Grand View College; and RN diploma, Iowa Methodist Hospital. She coordinates the Post Graduate PMHNP Certificate program and teaches mental health and caring science concepts. She is an associate editor of the *Journal of Art and Aesthetics in Nursing and Health Sciences* and a board member of Anne Boykin Institute for Advancement of Caring in Nursing.

Colleen **Maykut**, DNP, RN, FCAN, is a professor at MacEwan University. Her BScN and MN were earned at the University of Alberta, and her DNP at Case Western University-Frances Payne Bolton School of Nursing. Her scholarship and teaching, grounded in the Science of Caring, focuses on curriculum development for student success, mentorship and collegiality for clinicians, and advancing nursing theories. She is an associate editor of the *International Journal of Caring Sciences* and is the treasurer for the International Association for Human Caring.

Jeannine **Uribe**, PhD, RN, is an assistant professor at La Salle University. She earned her PhD at the University of Pennsylvania, her MSN at La Salle University, and her BSN at Purdue

University. She teaches public health nursing in the undergraduate program and international public health nursing. In the doctoral program, she teaches foundations of the DNP and epidemiology. Her historical research topics include global public health nursing and nursing education. She is a board member of the Museum of Nursing History, Inc.

Doris C. **Vallone**, PhD, RN, PMHCNS-BC, is a clinical nurse specialist at the Corporal Michael Crescenz Veterans Administration Medical Center in Philadelphia, Pennsylvania, where she provides evidence-based psychotherapy for veterans with posttraumatic disorder. She earned her PhD at the University of Pennsylvania, her MSN at La Salle University, and her BSN at Gwynedd-Mercy University. Prior to joining the VA, she coordinated graduate and undergraduate Psychiatric-Mental Health Nursing courses at Widener University.

Mary L. **Wilby**, PhD, MSN, MPH, RN, CRNP, ANP-BC, is an associate professor at La Salle University School of Nursing and Health Sciences. She earned her BSN, MSN, and MPH at La Salle University and her PhD at Union Institute and University. She is the coordinator for the nurse practitioner tracks and teaches courses on primary care of adults, advanced pharmacology, advanced health assessment, and end-of-life care. Her clinical practice focuses on the care of adults with cancer and palliative and end-of-life care.

Zane Robinson **Wolf**, PhD, RN, CNE, FCPP, ANEF, FAAN, is a Dean Emerita and an adjunct professor at La Salle University. Her BSN and PhD were earned at University of Pennsylvania, and her MSN at Boston College. She teaches courses on patient safety and evidence-based practice and conducts research on medication errors, nurse caring, and nursing education. She is the editor-in-chief of the *International Journal for Human Caring*, and a Board member of the Pennsylvania Patient Safety Advisory.

Index

Index